AQUATIC EXERCISE THERAPY

AQUATIC EXERCISE THERAPY

Andrea Bates, BSc, PE
Norm Hanson, BSc, PT
A.E.T. Consulting
Kelowna, British Columbia
Canada

W.B. SAUNDERS COMPANY
A Harcourt Health Sciences Company

Philadelphia London New York St. Louis Sydney Toronto

W.B. SAUNDERS COMPANY
A *Harcourt Health Sciences Company*

The Curtis Center
Independence Square West
Philadelphia, Pennsylvania 19106

Library of Congress Cataloging-in-Publication Data

Bates, Andrea.

Aquatic exercise therapy / Andrea Bates and Norm Hanson.—1st ed.

p. cm.

ISBN 0-7216-5681-1

1. Aquatic exercises—Therapeutic use. I. Hanson, Norm.
II. Title. [DNLM: 1. Hydrotherapy—methods. WB 520 B329a 1996]

RM727.H8B38 1996 615.8′53—dc20

DNLM/DLC 95-19485

AQUATIC EXERCISE THERAPY ISBN 0-7216-5681-1

Printed in the United States of America.

Last digit is the print number: 9 8 7 6 5 4

AUTHORS' DEDICATION

So he went down and dipped himself in the Jordan seven times,
as the man of God had told him,
and his flesh was restored and became clean like that of a young boy.

II Kings 5:14

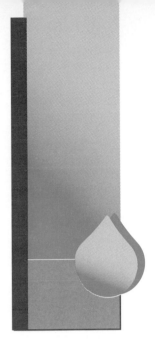

FOREWORD

Water has been used since time immemorial as a therapeutic medium. From ice packs to hot packs to whirlpools to Hubbard tanks, aquatic therapy has evolved over the past 50 years.

Passive use of water is widely available in the home in the form of sitz baths and hot tubs and is normally considered to be recreational. Aquatic therapy is also available in various communities in the form of bath houses, spas, and hot springs, in which the mineral content and temperature of the water are important. Aquatic exercise therapy in these situations is done on the initiative of the individual, rather than being supervised.

The ideal is to provide aquatic exercise therapy under the supervision of a physical therapist or kinesiologist. In recent years, aquatic exercise therapy in North America has become more pool-based, a setting in which group programs are easily instituted and supervised. These can be based in community pools, but in Kelowna we have a therapeutic pool in the hospital and have found it to be an integral part of therapy for most musculoskeletal and neurologic conditions.

This book is particularly oriented toward the use of water as a medium for exercise therapy. Water has certain attributes that make it superior to air as a medium for exercising.

1. The buoyancy of water partially suspends the body. Hence, balance is more easily maintained, and the risk of falling is less. Also, if one does fall, the results are less damaging. Buoyancy also allows more effective partial weight bearing in orthopedic rehabilitation. It compensates for weak musculature by giving extra support. This support allows for the painful limb to be moved both passively and actively. Lastly, buoyancy allows the body or limb to be supported in a stretched position if so desired. Buoyancy can be enhanced by the use of flotation devices for the trunk or limbs.

2. Water, being denser than air, gives increased resistance to movement, which allows for effective feedback from isotonic strengthening exercises and decreases the speed of movement. As the patient becomes stronger, the movements of the limb being rehabilitated can be integrated in the effort of keeping the patient afloat.

3. The higher temperature of the water relaxes the patient and facilitates pain management during exercise.

Sensory feedback from the water makes it ideal for retraining the proprioception-deficient individual.

Fear of water is also a quality that should be addressed. In the majority of people, such fear is a result of a previous bad experience, either from near-drowning or from having been forcefully submerged. In some cases the individual has never overcome the fear of drowning and never learned to float as a child. It is possible to get such patients involved in aquatic exercise therapy. It is important initially to make them feel comfortable in water and to teach them to float using the minimum amount of effort to maintain the floating position.

An important goal of aquatic exercise therapy is to bring the patient to the level at which he or she can do a complete program in a community-based swimming area, be it pool, lake, river, or sea.

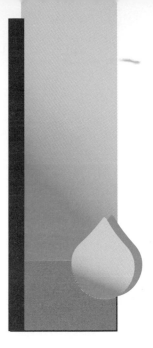

This book provides easy-to-understand protocols that can be followed by any exercise instructor. I think it will be a good addition to the literature on aquatic exercise therapy.

John Coghlan, MD
Physiatrist
Private Practice,
Kelowna, British Columbia

PREFACE

This project began when we started to search for a printed set of simple therapeutic exercise protocols for use in our facility. When our director, Chris Reuter, originally made dozens of inquiries to rehab facilities with pools across North America, it became apparent that no such set of protocols existed. He kept getting the response, "We don't have any, but if you develop some we would appreciate it if you would share them with us." Consequently, we started writing our own. Shortly thereafter, the energy and charisma of Darlene Swystun and Andrea Bates were added, and before we knew it we were on our way to self-publishing our first version of the book. Based on the response that we and our first handbook received, it was apparent that people from many different professions were looking for information on aquatic exercise therapy.

Our intent is that this book will facilitate communication between the doctor, physical therapist, aquatic therapist, and patient. Doctors and physical therapists can use it to quickly communicate to aquatic therapists which exercises they want their patients to perform. The aquatic therapist can also relate to the physical therapist how a patient is progressing through the different phases of a given protocol. If the patient is then discharged from the rehabilitation facility and wishes to continue the program at a community facility, an exercise instructor at that facility can easily find out which exercises have been done to that point. We have seen much successful communication even when the referring therapist and pool facility are not in the same building.

We do not envision this as a "cookbook" full of exercise "recipes" that can be applied without considering individual patients' needs. Neither should this book be used by untrained people to diagnose injuries or prescribe specific exercises. It is simply a reference source on which comprehensive aquatic exercise programs can be based. Ideally it will help provide some continuity of thought among the members of the rehabilitation team.

It was also not our intent to write another orthopedic assessment and treatment manual, since many great ones already exist. Our emphasis is on aquatic therapy. We try to point out specifically how aquatic exercises can be used to treat the common orthopedic conditions that we have outlined. We do, however, discuss the need to include land-based exercises at an appropriate time during the rehabilitative process.

Our logically progressive system of exercise routines is particularly beneficial to students. One of the most difficult concepts for a physical therapy student is to know when to advance a patient to more difficult exercises. Our approach breaks an exercise program into sequential levels. We don't present any new or radical treatment techniques, but we try to outline comprehensive exercise protocols in a clear, concise fashion.

Writing a book for such a broad market was not an easy task. It was, however, in the best interests of our patients to take this multidisciplinary approach. And it is for our patients, after all, that this book is really written.

Norm Hanson

ACKNOWLEDGMENTS

Mom, Dad, Ingrid, and Liz—
thanks for your encouragement. Love you.

Tim, Courtney, Quinn, and Mary—
thanks for everything; I couldn't have done it without you.

Dr. Mike Shaughnessy—
thanks for all the articles.

——— *AB*

Nancy Harms, KGH Physio—
thanks for the read on the FMS section.

Dr. Coghlan—
thanks for your support, books, and articles.

Margaret Biblis—
thank you for the vision and for seeing it through.

Deb, Amy, Lori, and Ted—
at WB Saunders.

The Father, Son, and Holy Spirit.

——— *NH and AB*

Pam—
for your patience, love, and countless hours of typing.
You are very special to me.

Hayden, Reid, and Spike—
for helping me keep things in perspective.

Chris Reuter and Hans Van Leehing—
for providing me with a great environment in which to develop.

Andrea—
for providing the spunk and energy necessary to get this project going.

——— *NH*

CONTENTS

Chapter 12

Chapter 13

Chapter 14

Chapter 15

Chapter 16

STRETCHES AND EXERCISES

AQUATIC EXERCISE THERAPY

WHAT IS AQUATIC EXERCISE THERAPY?

CHAPTER 1

AN INTRODUCTION TO AQUATIC REHABILITATION

What is Aquatic Exercise Therapy?

Aquatic exercise therapy (AET) is the union of aquatic exercise and physical therapy. It is a comprehensive therapeutic approach that uses aquatic exercises designed to aid in the rehabilitation of various conditions. Each exercise program is organized into specific components: the warm-up, stretching, muscular strength and endurance, and relaxation.[1] Each component requires a specific percentage of class time (Fig. 1–1).

AET is an innovative approach to aquatic therapy that promotes independence among patients, requires less staff time, and maximizes pool usage, compared with traditional pool programs. AET is more cost-effective than traditional programs and therefore more easily justified to administrators.

The Components of an Aquatic Exercise Therapy Class

The Warm-up

The warm-up is the prelude to the physical workout and should always be performed first. Physiologically, it allows the body to adjust to the onset of activity and to meet the necessary physical demands.

The warm-up should be gradual. It prepares the involved muscle groups to be stretched or strengthened by increasing the temperature and circulation of the muscles without causing fatigue or reducing energy stores. This, in turn, makes the muscles more pliable, decreasing the chance of injury.[1]

The warm water of a therapeutic pool allows the body's muscles and core temperature to increase very quickly. Therefore, the length of the warm-up depends on the temperature of the water and the profile of the patient group.

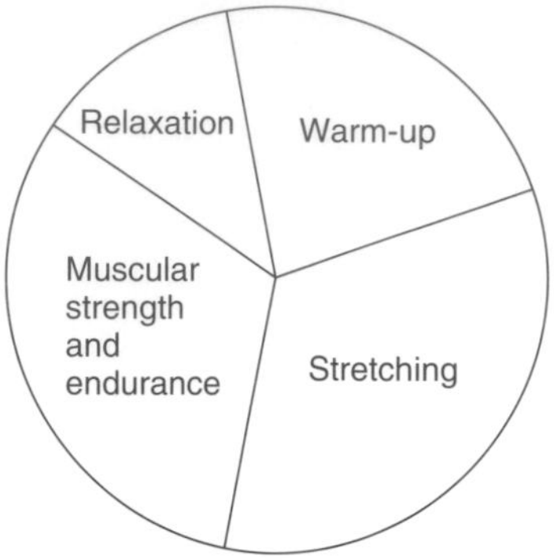

FIGURE 1–1. The components of an aquatic exercise therapy class and the relative amounts of time they occupy during a 1-hr session.

Indications

1. When stretching and strengthening exercises are to be performed.
2. When warming or loosening of a part or specific area of the body will help prevent injury.
3. When the water temperature is below the range for therapeutic waters: *92° to 98°F (33°–37°C).*

Goals

1. To increase the temperature of the body and the muscles.
2. To reduce the possibility of muscle tears and ligamentous sprains by warming specific muscles that will later be subject to stress.
3. To perform general active range of motion exercises with the areas of primary involvement, in preparation for more strenuous activity.
4. To identify painful or limited ranges of motion and areas of secondary involvement that may increase pain levels or interfere with recovery.
5. To help prevent muscle soreness.

Guidelines for the Therapist

1. The patient should always perform a warm-up before performing any stretching or strengthening exercises.
2. The cooler the water, the longer the warm-up should be.
3. The warm-up exercises performed should be relevant to the involved area and surrounding structures.

Stretching

Flexibility exercises are stretching exercises designed to increase the range of motion at a joint or a series of joints. A joint that has greater freedom of motion can improve the patient's ability to function and make movement more efficient. Increasing flexibility often makes the muscles and tendons more pliable and the supportive ligaments more supple.[2]

Passive stretching occurs while the patient is relaxed and requires the application of an external force. The force is applied either manually or mechanically in order to lengthen any tissues that have shortened. *Active stretching* requires the patient's participation to lessen the tightness in the muscle.[1, 2]

Flexibility is limited by the condition of the ligaments and layers of connective tissue surrounding the joint. Joint structure and muscle extensibility also limit the range of motion about a joint, as do disease and injury.

If a joint and its surrounding soft tissues are stretched beyond their normal range of motion, the joint is said to be overstretched. Overstretching often results in hypermobility. A contracture, on the other hand, is a shortening or tightening of the muscles or soft tissues that cross a joint. This tightness results in a reduction in the range of motion of the involved joint.[2]

When performing a flexibility exercise, the patient should avoid ballistic stretching (bouncing). Each stretching exercise should be performed with the joint slightly flexed. Any movement should be moderate in speed. Static stretches are best because they allow the muscle to lengthen without producing the microscopic tears in the muscle tissues that bouncing stretches produce. For maximum benefit, a stretch should be held from 10 to 60 seconds.[1]

Stretching exercises should involve the same muscles that will be involved in strengthening movements later. Many methods of elongating soft tissue, including manual passive stretching, stretch and hold, and self-stretching techniques, are described in this book.

Indications

1. When a joint's range of motion is restricted by contracture or other soft tissue abnormality that leads to the shortening of muscles, connective tissues, or epidermal tissues.[2]

2. When limited joint motion causes preventable skeletal deformities that can influence body symmetry and posture.[2]

3. When tight or shortened muscles interfere with active daily living or nursing care.[2]

4. When a muscle imbalance exists, or when one muscle is weak and the opposing tissue is tight. These muscles must be elongated enough to obtain a significant range of motion before strengthening exercises can be effective.

5. When muscular relaxation is necessary to reduce muscle soreness, tension, or stress in order to achieve a sufficient range of motion.

Goals

1. To restore normal range of motion to the involved joint and mobility to the soft tissues that surround the joint.

2. To prevent irreversible muscle tightness or shortening.

3. To facilitate muscular relaxation.

4. To increase the range of motion of one particular part of the body or of the body in general before the initiation of strengthening exercises.

5. To reduce the risk of musculotendinous injuries.[2]

Guidelines for the Therapist

1. The referring therapist must evaluate the patient to determine whether the range of motion is limited by the soft tissue or by the joint itself and whether stretching in warm water would benefit the patient.

2. Select each flexibility exercise according to the referring therapist's recommendations, and set realistic goals. Patients with hypermobility in a particular segment or area of the body should perform specific stretching exercises rather than engage in a generalized stretching program.[2, 3] These patients should refrain from using buoyant devices when stretching.

3. The patient should use whatever devices are necessary to ensure a comfortable and stable position; this will ensure the correct biomechanics during the execution of each exercise.

4. Stretches occur in direct opposition to tightness. The patient must remain relaxed throughout the execution of each exercise, and correct breathing patterns must be stressed.

5. Maintain a balance between the agonists and the antagonist muscle groups.

6. Static stretches rather than bouncing or ballistic stretches should be performed. The patient should maintain each position for a minimum of 10 seconds. An effective stretch should produce a "pulling" sensation in a tight muscle, not pain.[1]

7. Stretch the muscles that will be strengthened. Before starting an aggressive strengthening program, ensure that the joint has an adequate range of motion.

8. Do not stress joints and ligaments at the end of the range or lock hinge joints. The patient should always protect vulnerable joints by performing slow, controlled movements through the water.[1]

9. Use buoyancy to assist the patient if necessary, especially in the initial phase of rehabilitation after an injury.

10. Use the supportive properties of the water to provide stability for vulnerable joints.

Muscular Strength and Endurance

Muscular strength is the maximum tension that a muscle can exert in a single contraction. A contraction may be dynamically or statically produced and is specific for the muscle involved. The size and strength of a muscle increase with use and decrease if it is not used; hence the saying "Use it or lose it."

Restoration of muscle function is critical after an injury, surgery, or any period of restricted movement. The water provides a remarkable environment to produce very fine exercise progressions at an early stage, because it provides more resistance than air while supporting unstable or healing structures.

Muscular endurance is the ability of a muscle group to perform repeated contractions over a period of time. If muscular strength is considered in terms of how much a patient can lift or the greatest amount of resistance the patient can move through the water in a single effort, then muscular endurance refers to how many times the patient can lift or move a specified submaximal amount. Muscular endurance is specific to a muscle group and is important in the rehabilitation of an injury.

Indications

1. When there is muscle weakness after an injury, a surgical procedure, or a period of restricted movement.

2. When the support of buoyancy can reduce or eliminate pain that may be causing tension or spasticity in a muscle or group of muscles and thereby limit movement.

3. When a patient cannot walk on land because of disease or injury or cannot perform necessary daily living skills.

4. In cases of extreme deconditioning—water exercise is suitable for any level of muscular weakness.

5. To progress or advance the patient toward strengthening exercises on land.

Guidelines for the Therapist

1. All movements and exercises should be carefully controlled and initially should be guided by pain, unless otherwise stated.

2. Swollen limbs should be exercised in deep water, if possible. The hydrostatic pressure will help with edema. After the pain and swelling of an injury begin to decrease, isotonic or isokinetic exercise is best. This type of exercise helps to increase muscle function of a particular body part through a complete range of motion.

3. Always ensure that the patient is comfortably supported before initiating an exercise. The portion of the body that is not moving should be secured and stabilized by use of an external force, such as the pool wall or chair, or an internal force, such as musculature.

4. Use the resistance of water to achieve progressive strength adaptations by

- increasing the length of the lever arm
- moving a float from a proximal to a distal position or toward the bottom of the pool
- increasing the size or number of floats
- increasing the surface area of resistance
- moving through the water in a less streamlined position
- increasing the speed of movement
- moving weights toward the surface of the water

5. Maximize the weight-bearing effects of the water by exercising the lower limbs and spine in variable depths.

Relaxation

Relaxation is most commonly defined as *a conscious effort to eliminate tension in the muscles.*[3] Muscular tension can be produced physiologically, as a result of acute pain or injury, or psychogenically, as a result of anxiety or stress. Factors such as fatigue and overuse also contribute to the tension experienced by the muscle.[3]

Patients can be taught to recognize prolonged muscular tension and to control or inhibit it through therapeutic exercise.[4] During exercise, the active contraction of skeletal muscle is followed by a reflex relaxation response. The stronger the contraction, the greater the subsequent relaxation of the muscle; this is known as *Sherrington's law of reciprocal innervation.*[2, 5] If left untreated, prolonged muscular tension often becomes the primary factor in joint dysfunction. The affected joint enters a sustained cycle of pain, muscle guarding, stored metabolites, and impaired movement.[6]

The warmth of a therapeutic pool promotes muscular relaxation, increases circulation, reduces spasm, and effectively reduces pain levels.[7] These effects produce a significant disruption in the pain cycle (Fig. 1–2).

Many relaxation techniques can be used by the therapist, including combinations of local and general relaxation methods.

Local Relaxation Techniques

Local relaxation techniques include heat, massage, and joint traction.

HEAT. The application of superficial or deep heat to the soft tissues before the pool session helps to increase the extensibility of the shortened tissues. The application of heat after the pool session helps to maintain muscular relaxation.

MASSAGE. For patients who experience extreme pain or are awkward to work with on land, the water becomes an excellent medium in which to apply various massage techniques. Warm water immersion and massage have similar effects on tense or tight muscles. Massage increases circulation, decreases pain sensitivity, and promotes relaxation, as does submersion in warm water.[8] Because of the hydrostatic pressure of water, the therapist does not need to apply a lot of pressure to the involved area in order to decrease muscle spasm and stiffness. The therapist simply feels for abnormal tissue (hard and tender) and attempts to restore it to a normal soft, elongated, nontender state.

JOINT TRACTION. Traction occurs when the articulating surfaces of a joint are pulled apart or separated.[2] The use of joint mobilization or stretch-

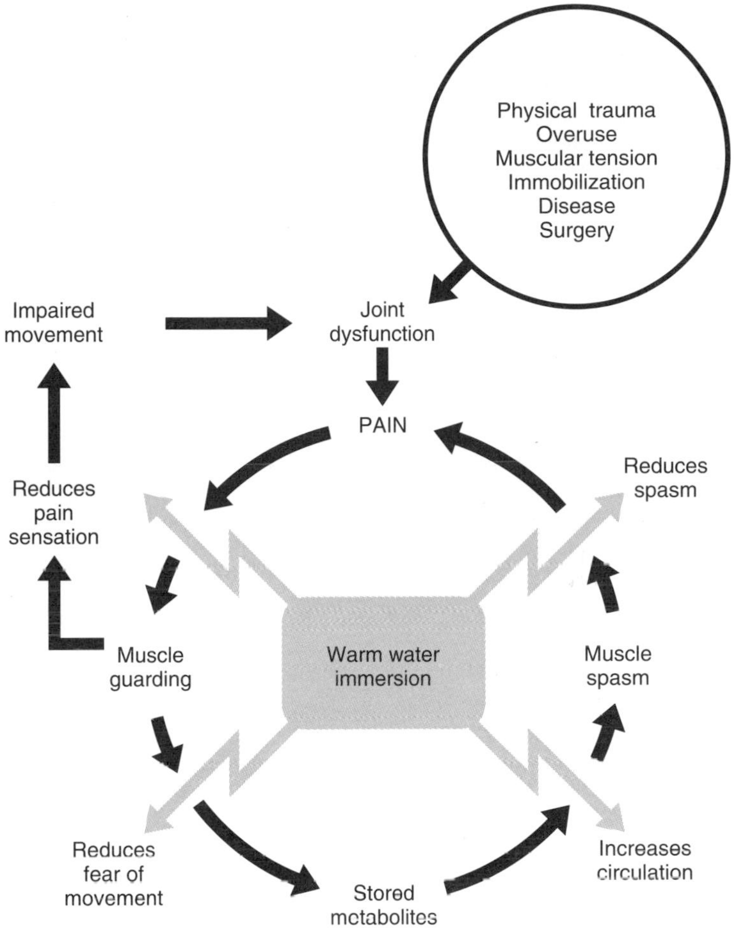

FIGURE 1–2. Warm water immersion disrupts the pain cycle and reduces joint dysfunction caused by impaired movement.

ing techniques before or in conjunction with joint traction can decrease pain and spasm of the muscles around a joint. Forms of joint traction used in the water include the following.

Weights. Weight works in opposition through the center of buoyancy. Holding a weight or placing a weight around a particular area can cause joint separation. Vertical floating traction is effective for some back conditions.

Manipulation. Joint manipulation involves bracing the body or the proximal aspect of the joint with one hand and pulling distally or outward with the other hand.

Pulling or Towing. This technique involves pulling or towing the body or limb in a long, continuous motion. It is performed very slowly and in one direction only.

Pendular Movements. Performed in the water, pendular movements provide an effective warm-up. These exercises involve the use of a weight on the limb to distract the joint surfaces and thereby relax and increase the mobility of the limb.

General Relaxation Techniques

Of the many general relaxation techniques available to the therapist, some require extensive training and practice until they are mastered. The patient may use one specific technique or a combination of techniques.

FLOATING. The patient may or may not be assisted by the use of flotation devices. The simple benefit of the "weightlessness" felt when submerged in warm water is often enough to provide relief to painful joints and facilitate relaxation.

AUTOGENIC RELAXATION. This technique involves decreasing muscular tension through conscious effort and thought. A complete autogenic training program may be divided into three exercise categories: autosuggestion about relaxation, single-focus meditation (as in yoga), and meditation on abstract qualities.[6]

BREATHING EXERCISE. Three- or four-part breathing involves taking progressively deeper breaths while consciously relaxing tense muscles.

PROGRESSIVE RELAXATION. This technique requires the patient to alternately tense and relax the involved muscles. The patient should be encouraged to develop a recognition for the tension signals when muscles are contracted.[2, 6]

Indications

1. When there is acute or chronic neuromuscular hypertension.
2. When poor sleeping patterns are present.
3. When tense muscles restrict joint motion or function.
4. When stress or anxiety produces physiologic ailments such as peptic ulcers.
5. After bouts causing overuse, fatigue, or exhaustion.
6. With various preoperative and postoperative conditions.[10]

Goals

1. To decrease muscular tension and facilitate relaxation.
2. To reduce stress and anxiety.
3. To recognize prolonged muscular tension and control or inhibit it through therapeutic exercise.
4. To maximize the therapeutic effects of warm water by increasing circulation, reducing pain sensitivity, and increasing muscular relaxation.
5. To break the pain cycle.

Guidelines for the Therapist

1. Be certain the patient is not afraid of the water, because muscular tension can inhibit rehabilitation.
2. Choose the technique or combination of techniques that is best suited for the patient's condition.
3. Explain the procedures to the patient so he or she can understand the rationale underlying the chosen relaxation techniques.
4. The patient should always be placed in a comfortable position, with all body parts well supported.
5. Stress the need for regular practice after the techniques have been learned.
6. Explain and set up long-term and short-term goals for relaxation training.

The Aerobic Component

There is no aerobic component in the initial phases of AET. Because of the high temperatures of therapeutic waters, high-intensity, long-duration activities are not advised. An injured patient can rarely exercise vigorously enough in the water to receive any aerobic benefit from increased heart rate.

After the patient has successfully restored an active range of motion to the involved joints and achieved adequate functional strength and endurance levels, aerobic exercise can be added to the patient's total program. Each program must be specifically designed for the individual patient, bearing in mind his or her condition, strengths, and weaknesses (see Chapter 17).

THE BENEFITS OF EXERCISING IN WARM WATER

The Physiologic Effects

Exercise in warm water is an effective treatment modality for a variety of conditions. Studies conducted on head-out-of-water immersion consider a water temperature of 95°F (35°C) to be *thermoneutral*—that is, it has no effect on core temperature.[11] Any minor deviations in water temperature can produce significant changes in the circulatory system. Instead of pooling in the limbs, blood is redistributed. This redistribution causes an increase in venous return and is considered the basis for all the physiologic changes associated with immersion.[11] The greatest physiologic changes are observed in an upright posture rather than in a supine or seated position.

The physiologic effects experienced by a patient immersed in warm water depend on the patient's posture and any elements that may alter the body's thermoneutral state. Elements that influence this state include the temperature of the water, the duration of the class, the type and intensity of the exercise, and the patient's pathologic condition.[7, 12]

Water temperature alone can increase the body's temperature if it is higher than the temperature of the skin. The magnitude of the temperature increase depends on what percentage of the body is immersed. During head-out-of-water immersion, heat is gained by the areas of the body that are under the water and is lost through the sweat glands of the areas exposed to the air. Temperature changes vary from patient to patient.[7, 11, 12]

The physiologic responses experienced by the body during warm water immersion are very similar to those of localized heat application but less concentrated.[7] The physical properties of water in conjunction with the heat are responsible for many general physiologic responses that affect a variety of body systems (Table 1–1).

TABLE 1–1. Physiologic Changes During Warm Water Exercise

Increased respiratory rate
Decreased blood pressure
Increased blood supply to the muscles[11, 14]
Increased muscle metabolism[11, 14]
Increased superficial circulation
Increased heart rate
Increased amount of blood returned to the heart[11]
Increased metabolic rate
Decreased edema of submerged body parts (owing to the hydrostatic pressure at the water surface, 14.7 psi, plus an increase of 0.43 psi for every foot increase in depth)[9, 11]
Reduced sensitivity of sensory nerve endings
General muscular relaxation

The Therapeutic Effects

In addition to the various physiologic changes that occur during warm water immersion, the physical properties of water offer many advantages in a rehabilitative setting. Although there are many conditions that benefit from aquatic therapy, this book focuses primarily on orthopedic and rheumatologic conditions, postsurgical rehabilitation, chronic pain, and athletic reconditioning. Some of the advantages of warm water AET should be considered in order to effectively treat the recovering patient (Table 1–2). These advantages are described more fully in the following paragraphs.

Promotion of Muscular Relaxation

The relaxation response depends on how comfortable the patient is in the water. The warmth of the therapeutic pool reduces muscular tension and helps prevent restricted joint movement. The warmer the water, the better.

Reduces Pain Sensitivity

Warm water helps patients with pain relax and feel more comfortable. Buoyancy counteracts gravity and alleviates body weight by reducing the compression forces on the joints. The water provides support for injured limbs, which allows for comfortable positioning without increased pain. The pain cycle is disrupted. The stimulatory effects of warm water promote the relaxation of "tight" spastic muscles, which reduces muscle guarding. Warm water "distracts" the pain by bombarding the nervous system. The bombardment of sensory input travels on fibers that are larger and faster and have a greater conductivity than the pain fibers.[6] During warm water immersion, the sensory inputs are competing with the pain input; as a result, the patient's pain perception is "gated" or blocked out. This reduction in pain is perhaps the most significant advantage of aquatic therapy.

Decrease in Muscle Spasm

Body parts immersed in water warmer than 95°F (35°C) begin to rise in temperature toward the temperature of the core.[11] The warmth reduces abnormal muscular tone and spasticity.

Increase in Ease of Joint Movement

The physical properties and the warmth of the water play an important role in improving or maintaining joint range of motion. The buoyancy of the

TABLE 1–2. Therapeutic Benefits of Warm Water Exercise

Promotes muscular relaxation
Reduces pain sensitivity
Decreases muscle spasm
Increases ease of joint movement
Increases muscular strength and endurance in cases of excessive weakness
Reduces gravitational forces (early ambulation)
Increases peripheral circulation (skin condition)
Improves respiratory muscles
Improves body awareness, balance, and proximal trunk stability
Improves patient morale and confidence (psychological)

water decreases the compression forces on painful joints and assists movement. The water also provides support and thus decreases the need for splinting or guarding. Movement is easier and occurs with less pain. The warmth of the water reduces spasticity, promotes relaxation, and helps prepare the connective tissue for stretching. Elongated tissue has a lower risk of injury and of muscle soreness after exercise.

Exercises to increase joint mobility should be taken to end range slowly and held for 30 seconds or more. The patient should be encouraged to go beyond the point of limitation, if possible, and then to relax.[8] Movements toward the surface of the water are assisted by buoyancy; the effect is greater if a flotation device is used.

Increase in Muscular Strength and Endurance in Cases of Excessive Weakness

The water provides a greater resistance to movement than air yet allows the joint to move more freely. The submerged body parts encounter resistance in all directions of movement, which requires a greater energy expenditure.[11] In the water, movements are more consistent and more easily graded using the principles of buoyancy without the pain of active movement. Equipment is not always necessary to produce strength gains in weak muscles. Performing exercises in the water can be very cost-effective.

Warm water promotes the relaxation of the spastic antagonists of a weak, exercising muscle. Strength training can begin in the water before it is possible on land. This helps prevent atrophy of skeletal muscles. The stimulatory effect of the water helps the patient to become more aware of the body parts that are moving and the mechanics involved in the movement.

Reduction of Gravitational Forces

The effects of gravity are reduced in the water. The more submerged the body, the smaller the compression forces acting on the body. After injury, a patient can stand and begin gait training and strengthening exercises earlier than on land, without being concerned about causing further damage to the healing structures.[8, 12] Walking earlier helps improve balance and increase muscle tone. A gradual reduction in the water level helps retrain the weight-bearing aspect of gait.

Increase in Peripheral Circulation

Circulation increases in water temperatures greater than 93°F (34°C). The redistribution of blood during immersion causes an increase in blood flow to the periphery.[11] Warm water immersion causes an increase in skin temperature toward that of the body core. This, in turn, produces cutaneous vasodilatation and an improved appearance of the skin.[11] Exercising causes an increase in the blood supply to the muscles and helps increase venous return. Tissue fluids move more freely through the injured structures, removing retained metabolites, which improves nutrition and helps speed up the healing process.[8] Exercising injured limbs in deep water increases circulation. As water depth increases, so does the hydrostatic pressure exerted on the submerged body part. Because of this, there is an increase in circulation.[11, 12]

Improvement of Respiratory Muscles

In chest-deep water, there is an increase in the hydrostatic pressure exerted on the walls of the chest and abdominals during breathing. The water resists inspiration. This is most evident in patients with low vital capacities (below 1500 mL), in frail older adults, and in cardiac patients.[13] Spastic respiratory muscles are relaxed by the neutral warmth provided by the water. Aquatic activities that require an increase in respiration (eg, swimming, aerobic exercise) or train the breathing component (eg, blowing bubbles) are beneficial to patients who have respiratory problems.[14]

Improvement of Body Awareness, Balance, and Trunk Stability

Warm water stimulates awareness of the moving body parts and provides an ideal medium for muscle re-education. The supportive properties of the water give patients with poor balance time to react when falling by slowing the movement. Vestibular stimulation helps to improve the equilibrium response by stimulating the antigravity muscles in the extremities and trunk.[14] Stabilization during exercise can also be obtained through the use of railings, parallel bars, underwater benches, submerged chairs, tubes, and other devices.

Improvement of Patient Morale and Confidence

For patients with pain and those who cannot yet exercise on land, the water provides a positive medium in which to move and relax. The ease of movement allows the patient to achieve much more than on land and provides the patient with confidence to aid rehabilitation. There is less fear of falling or of hurting the injured or painful sites. Group exercise encourages social interaction and provides support and motivation for patients with similar injuries at various phases of their recovery.

Although there are many other advantages of aquatic therapy, it can be seen that this type of treatment in orthopedic rehabilitation is both effective and enjoyable.

REFERENCES

1. Krejci V, Koch P. Muscle and Tendon Injuries in Athletes. Chicago, Year Book Medical Publishers, 1976.
2. Kisner C, Colby L. Therapeutic Exercise: Foundations and Techniques. 2nd ed. Philadelphia, F.A. Davis, 1990.
3. Arnheim D. Modern Principles of Athletic Training. 6th ed. St. Louis, Time Mirror/Mosby College Publishing, 1993.
4. Alter J. Stretch and Strengthen. Boston, Houghton Mifflin, 1986.
5. Jacobsen E. You Must Relax. New York, McGraw-Hill, 1970.
6. Kessler RM, Hertling D. Management of Common Musculoskeletal Disorders: Physical Therapy Principles and Methods. Philadelphia, Harper & Row, 1983.
7. Skinner AT, Thomson AM. Duffield's Exercise in Water. 3rd ed. East Sussex, Bailliere Tindall, 1983.
8. Thomson A, Skinner A, Piercy J. Tidy's Physiotherapy. 12th ed. Toronto, Butterworth-Heinemann, 1991.
9. Golland A. Basic hydrotherapy. Physiotherapy 67:258–260, 1981.
10. Jacobson E. Progressive Relaxation. 4th ed. Chicago, University of Chicago Press, 1962.
11. Hall J, Bisson D, O'Hare P. The physiology of immersion. Physiotherapy 76:517–521, 1990.
12. Dulcy F. Benefits of aquatic therapy, Part I. American Exercise Association, AKWA Newsletter, November 1988.
13. Haralson KM. Therapeutic pool programs. Clin Manage 5:510–513, 1988.
14. Charness A. Physiological and Psychological Values of Pool Therapy. Aquatics for the Physically Disabled, February 1983.

CHAPTER 2

DESIGNING AN EFFECTIVE AQUATIC EXERCISE THERAPY PROGRAM

ESTABLISHING THE FOUNDATIONS OF THE PROGRAM

Therapeutic Purpose

Before designing an aquatic facility, it is important to identify the various patient populations that will be using it and how it will be used.[1] Patients who have pain, pain with movement, limited joint motion, weakness, edema, and poor coordination or balance all benefit from aquatic programs.

A program can focus on just one or on all of these problems. Programs may be developed with one particular objective in mind, such as sports rehabilitation and work hardening programs. The individual sessions may focus on relaxation, aerobic conditioning, or a combination of objectives. Whatever the focus of the program, the design of the facility must meet the needs of the staff and patients who use it.

The Aquatic Facility

Before consulting with an architect, it is important to determine all the options that will be needed to implement the desired therapeutic programs. Considerations or restrictions relating to the site, dimensions, or position of the pool should also be addressed. The following factors must be considered.

Water Depth

The depth of the water must be acceptable for the type of program or for the conditions being treated. For example, therapists who use Bad Ragaz techniques need the water to remain at one depth, preferably no higher than chest level. If only adults are to be treated in the pool, then shallow water is not necessary. On the other hand, programs that focus on sports rehabilitation or aerobic conditioning use a variety of deep water exercises. These exercises may need deeper, cooler water.

Variation in water depth can be achieved by the use of a movable floor or a stepping or sloping pool floor. A movable pool floor works by a hydraulic lift system. The water acts as the lubricating fluid that allows the floor to move up and down. The floor can be adjusted to any depth during each session. The entire pool floor is at the set depth, which can be a problem if people of different heights are being treated. Movable floors are expensive and rare. A stepping pool floor allows for versatility, as does a sloping pool floor. The fall of the slope should be 1 in 16.[1]

Water Temperature

The temperature of a therapeutic pool is 92° to 98°F (33°–37°C). This temperature is not suitable for aerobic conditioning. The temperature of a swimming pool is usually between 80° and 85°F (27°–30°C).[2] If aerobic conditioning is an important focus of the program, a separate, warmer pool may be necessary for stretching, strengthening, and relaxation routines. The number and needs of the patients using the pool help justify the cost of adding a cooler or warmer second pool.

Design

Pool Surroundings

The pool area is a controlled environment within the facility. Direct access to the pool site from outside is not advised, because it is important to minimize heat loss and prevent drafts.

The pool areas and surrounding corridors should be wide enough for wheelchairs and stretchers. Handrails mounted to the walls of the approach corridors are beneficial for patients with poor balance or coordination and for those using crutches or walkers. The doors should open easily and remain open to allow patients on crutches, in wheelchairs, or on stretchers to enter the pool area safely.[1–3]

The outer doors should be equipped with locks, and if no staff are present in the pool area, the door should remain closed and secured. If there is a movable floor, it should be left all the way up and the key should be removed from the power box when the pool is not in use.

Reception and waiting areas should be large enough to allow patients in wheelchairs to maneuver safely and to park to one side of the hallway without blocking entrance ways.[3] Drinking water and other refreshments should be available to patients, as should access to a telephone.[4]

Patient change rooms should also be large enough to allow for manipulation of one or two wheelchairs. Benches or chairs, mirrors, sinks, and grounded outlets for hair dryers should be provided. A suitable change area and office are also necessary for pool staff.

The surrounding floor surfaces should be absolutely nonslip and should slope down slightly toward the drain. The fall of the slope should be 1 in 24.[1] Adequate drainage channels should be located by the showers and at any other place where water may accumulate.

A comfortable average air temperature is between 68° and 78°F (20°–25°C).[3, 5] Maintenance of an acceptable air temperature in the pool and surrounding areas is important for the comfort of patients and staff. In the pool area, an air temperature of 78°F (25°C) and a relative humidity of 55% is most comfortable.[1] The constant evaporation of the water from the pool requires an efficient ventilation system, one that is able to complete 10 to 12 air exchanges per hour.

Every therapeutic pool should have an alarm system and a telephone. The alarm must be unique to the pool area and be loud enough to be heard by other staff members in different areas of the building. An alarm that sounds different tells staff members exactly where the emergency is. The response time should be no longer than 10 seconds. Each staff member should be trained and regularly tested in one- and two-person cardiopulmonary resuscitation. Emergency procedures should be posted and reviewed on a regular basis with all staff members.

An effective alarm system may involve alarm cords that hang over the pool or buttons that are by the pool within reaching distance, or both. The therapist may also wear a small, remote emergency system activator on a neck chain. This type of system is best because the therapist can stay with the patient in distress and still activate the alarm system.

The utility room should be near the pool. It provides a secure area for the storage of pool chemicals, cleaning equipment and materials, and additional supplies. The mechanical room is usually separate from the pool area but is still close by. A mechanical room located as close to the pool as possible requires less piping, which reduces the costs and thermal losses during heat recirculation.[1, 2]

Towels and swimsuits are a necessary part of aquatic therapy. Therefore, every pool area needs a place to collect, clean, and store soiled linen and swimsuits.

The Pool

There are many shapes and sizes of therapeutic pools. However, the most common shapes are rectangular or square.[1] A pool may be of any size, but it must be large enough and deep enough for the chosen rehabilitation techniques and walking reeducation programs.

The surface of the pool floor should be nonslip. The color should be light, with a contrasting color marking the entry, the exit, and any changes in water depth.[1–3]

Entering and Exiting the Pool

Both staff and patients should shower with soap before and after pool sessions. Showering before pool sessions ensures a high level of hygiene, and showering afterward removes the harsh pool chemicals from the skin.

There are many methods of entering and exiting a pool. The methods chosen depend on the design of the pool, the number of patients being treated at one time, and the degrees of disabilities being treated in the pool.[3] Ambulant patients should have no trouble using ramps, steps, or even a ladder, so long as these structures are safely secured with handrails and bright, nonslip markings. Nonambulant patients can use wheelchairs specifically designed for use in the water, swivel chairs, or hoists. All patients can benefit from a level deck entry, such as a movable floor, regardless of their ambulatory status.

Hydraulic lift systems, hoists, wheelchairs, and any other pool equipment should be checked, tested, and maintained regularly. Faulty equipment, frayed cables, and any other equipment defects that are discovered during routine maintenance checks must be repaired or replaced immediately to ensure the safety of both patients and staff.

Water pressure is much greater than atmospheric pressure. As the water depth increases, so does the hydrostatic pressure of the water and its effects on the immersed body parts. Respiration is affected because the water resists the walls of the chest during inspiration. This effect is most noticeable in patients with low vital capacity (1500 mL),[6] in cardiac patients, and in frail or older adults. *These patients should enter the pool slowly.*[3]

Water Purity

Health inspectors and authorities require public aquatic facilities with high bather loads to maintain a high standard of water purity. An effective and most commonly used chemical is chlorine. Other options include bromine, which some find gentler on the skin, and ozone, which requires a backup system.

Chlorine can be introduced into the water either automatically with a liquid chlorine injector or manually as a granular compound or chlorine "puck." Chlorine levels must be kept between 1.5 and 3.0 ppm, with free chlorine levels between 0.5 and 1.5 ppm. Chlorine levels must be tested at least twice a day—preferably, once before the first session of the day and once in the late afternoon. This protects all bathers from waterborne bacteria and illnesses. It is important that a complete water turnover occur every 4 hours. This ensures the circulation of any chemicals introduced into the pool during the day, so that the water tests will provide an accurate picture of the actual chemical levels in the pool.

Maintenance of optimal chemical levels is very important. Chlorine levels, for example, are affected by the alkalinity of the water. An optimal pH range is between 7.5 and 8; pH levels below 7.3 are too acidic and may cause skin irritation and burning eyes. If the pH level is frequently on the lower end of the scale, therapists and patients may find that their swimsuits break down much faster. If the pH level of the water is too acidic, soda ash must be added, and if the water is too alkaline, hydrochloric acid must be added to the water.

Other water tests that should be performed regularly include water hardness, copper (if necessary), and bacteriology tests. All test results must be recorded and filed.

Scheduling

It is important to determine the number of people who will be using the pool so that adequate staffing and classes can be calculated. Therapists should not be in the water longer than 2 hours without a break.[7] If the hours of operation are long, scheduled breaks are necessary to combat fatigue.

After the hours of operation have been determined, the schedule of classes is established. Some conditions, such as arthritis, cause morning stiffness. Arthritis classes should therefore be scheduled later in the day, when the joints are more limber. Patients who require medication in order to exercise (eg, painkillers or nonsteroidal anti-inflammatory drugs) may need special considerations in scheduling, especially if they need to see practitioners of other disciplines before or after the pool session.

The facility should keep a file for each patient. The file should contain a letter of consent signed by the patient, a signed referral and medical release from the patient's physician, assessment forms, the program goals, and the aquatic exercise therapy protocols appropriate for the referred condition. No condition should be treated without a referral.

The program card should contain the name, address, and phone number of the patient and the name and number of the patient's physician. Other information on the program card should include any contraindications to pool therapy, medications, the date the program started, the days and dates of each exercise session the patient has participated in, the name and phase of the aquatic exercise therapy (AET) protocol the patient is using, the results of the physical evaluation, and the program goals. The therapist should also record, daily, any quantitative data that is relevant to the patient's performance, including motivational levels, changes in pain patterns or levels during exercise, increases or decreases in repetitions, and so on. There should be enough space for these "progress notes" as well as any "additional comments."

An aquatic class or session can take many forms. The class may include patients with general injuries, such as shoulder or back injuries. It may involve only patients with a specific condition, such as total knee replacement. Or it may be a mixed class. A session can be one-on-one, the patient with the therapist, or the patient can work alone with an assigned protocol. A pool program can have a combination of many class types (Fig. 2–1).

Screening for Contraindications to Pool Therapy

All patients should be screened for any contraindications to pool therapy. Each facility should develop its own set of precautions, with absolute and relative contraindications. The parameters depend on the program and the patient population being treated. Some contraindications to pool therapy include the following:

1. Waterborne diseases such as typhoid, cholera, and dysentery.
2. Fever higher than 100°F (38°C).
3. Cardiac failure.
4. Kidney diseases (where there is an inability to adjust to fluid loss).
5. Gastrointestinal disorders.
6. Infectious diseases.
7. Open wounds.
8. Contagious skin rashes.
9. Perforated eardrums.
10. Incontinence of feces or urine.
11. Menstruation without internal protection.
12. Epilepsy.
13. Abnormal blood pressure (hypotension or hypertension).
14. Current or recent radiation treatment (during last 3 months).
15. Low vital lung capacity (900–1500 mL).

Patients with high or low blood pressure may be treated in the pool for short periods of time. These patients should be given frequent rests between exercises, and they should be encouraged to report any dizziness or lightheadedness to the therapist.

Patients with skin infections such as tinea pedis (athlete's foot) must be cured before starting pool therapy. Precautions must be taken with patients who have acquired immunodeficiency syndrome. These patients should not be treated in the pool if they have any open sores or skin cuts.

Patients who wear hearing aids can still participate in AET classes but must avoid immersing or wetting the device in any way. Patients with severe mental retardation require special supervision and assistance in the water and on land.

THE AQUATIC REHABILITATION PLAN

An effective rehabilitation program begins with gathering enough patient information to accurately assess the severity of the dysfunction presented. After this information has been gathered, the therapist must determine whether AET would be a beneficial modality in restoring function. If aquatic ther-

DATE	POOL THERAPY CLASSES					
NAME OF CLASS (TYPE)	CLASS TIME (DURATION)	PATIENT NAME	BOX TO RECORD UNITS	PATIENT NAME	BOX TO RECORD UNITS	NUMBER OF PATIENTS PER CLASS
Upper extremity	8:15–9:45	John Smith	6/11	Dave Green	6/11	4
		Jane Doe	6/11	Sue Holmes	6/11	
Chronic back	9:45–10:30	[illegible]	[illegible]	[illegible]	[illegible]	3
		[illegible]	[illegible]			
Lower extremity	11:00–11:45	[illegible]	[illegible]	[illegible]	[illegible]	2
Arthritis	2:00–2:30	John Doe	6/11	Mary Bates	6/11	2
TOTAL ATTENDANCE						11

FIGURE 2–1. A sample of an aquatic rehabilitation class schedule.

apy is indicated, the therapist should define the goals and objectives of the treatment.[8, 9] The therapist must develop a clear plan as to how these goals should be implemented.[10] Each goal must have a measurable objective or outcome[8] and be reassessed on a regular basis.

Assessing Dysfunction

It is necessary for the therapist to gather enough information to accurately assess the severity of the patient's dysfunction and determine whether the patient would benefit from AET. This involves both a physical evaluation and the gathering of relatively subjective information.

Physical Evaluation

The physical evaluation of the patient produces the measurable data necessary for evaluation of the program goals and objectives. The aquatic therapist should receive any information regarding the following:

1. Postural abnormalities.
2. Ambulatory status or gait abnormalities.
3. Activities of daily living skills or functional capacity.
4. Joint range of motion (ROM) (active and passive).
5. Resisted muscular tests.
6. Appearance (eg, swelling, atrophy).
7. Pain levels (on a scale of 1 to 10).

Subjective Information

The subjective assessment should provide details that may influence the outcome of the program. The therapist should record the following:

1. Patient information (the program card).
2. General health history.
3. History of the condition and any related history, such as the date of the injury or onset of pain.
4. The behavior or symptoms over a 24-hour period.
5. Postsurgical status.
6. Assessment of water skills or hydrophobic tendency.

The Aquatic Treatment Plan

The aquatic treatment plan is based on program goals derived from the physical evaluation, the subjective assessment, the patient's psychologic status, and the patient's plan to return to work or activity. A plan of care is necessary to determine what therapeutic approaches would best meet the goal of the rehabilitation program. Each goal should include a measurable objective outcome,[8] reproducible tests, and an expected treatment time. The therapist must be able to document the changes that occur (Table 2–1).

A program should include both long-term and short-term goals. The long-term goal is usually the final, measurable outcome expected at the end of a particular phase or at the conclusion of the program. Short-term goals involve all the components necessary to achieve the long-term goal. These may include mastery of each exercise phase or of the required exercise techniques or additional therapeutic modalities necessary for rehabilitation of the patient.

TABLE 2–1. Tests and Measurements Used to Evaluate Patient Progress

Range of motion—Goniometry tests
Muscular tests—Strength grade
Appearance—Circumference measurements
Pain scale and pain diagrams
Functional capacity and activities of daily living skills—Ability to perform specified tasks (eg, comb hair, swing racket, perform gait)

The therapist must determine other details of the plan:

1. The frequency of treatments (usually two to five times per week).
2. The intensity of the program, based on the entry level or phase.
3. When the patient should begin water exercise. This depends on the injury or condition and whether there are any open wounds or movement restrictions.
4. The duration of the aquatic exercise session.

Implementing the Aquatic Treatment Plan

After the aquatic treatment plan has been established, the therapist must determine the specific techniques or the specific exercise phases that are to be employed in the treatment plan to meet the goals of the program. Presurgical patients may enter a program at a higher phase. Physicians often postpone surgery and have patients exercise in the pool to improve muscle tone and joint ROM. Exercising in the pool before surgery helps to improve the outcome of the procedure and motivates the patient to continue exercising after surgery.

Regardless of the patient's status in the water, the progressive aquatic exercise phases are designed to maximize the complete function of a joint or body part. There are five progressive phases: the postsurgical or acute phase; the early exercise phase; the intermediate exercise phase; the advanced exercise phase; and the phase of integration to land.[9]

Phase One—The Postsurgical or Acute Phase

In this phase, there is a lot of pain, inflammation, swelling, and loss of mobility and function. The patient should begin exercising as soon as the incision heals but preferably within the first 24 hours after the injury or procedure.[9] Open wounds can be covered with waterproof bandages, if necessary. Exercising in the warm water reduces the pain, stimulates healing, and prevents further deconditioning. Exercise priorities are as follows:

1. Gentle ROM and strengthening exercises of the joints immediately adjacent, both distally and proximally, to the healing structure, unless this is contraindicated.[9]

2. Mild stretching of the healing structure.
3. Gentle ROM of the healing structure, staying within the limits of pain and using the resistance of the water only.
4. The use of other therapeutic modalities (eg, traction, ice, ultrasound) to help reduce pain and thus make exercising easier.

Phase Two—The Early Exercise Phase

In this phase, there is a general decrease in the severity of the symptoms exhibited. Symptoms still present include minimal to moderate intermittent pain, moderate inflammation and swelling, and a moderate loss of mobility and function in the healing structure. Exercise priorities are as follows:

1. Specific stretching exercises.
2. The use of supportive and assistive exercise equipment to maximize ROM, using resistance of water only.
3. Muscle contraction without a significant increase in pain.
4. Restoration or maintenance of the strength of the muscles surrounding the healing structure.

Phase Three—The Intermediate Exercise Phase

By phase three, there is minimal intermittent pain, and all the other symptoms are minimal. The patient should begin to use resistive devices in order to increase strength and perform pain-free muscle contractions. Neuromuscular coordination should be almost normal, and the surrounding structures should have at least 50% of their strength and ROM restored. Exercise priorities are as follows:

1. Stretching exercises.
2. Moderate progressive resistance exercises using aquatic principles such as speed, turbulence, and surface area.
3. Full-range movements.

Phase Four—The Advanced Exercise Phase

The objective of this phase is to maximize muscular strength, endurance, and ROM to within 90% of normal for the patient. Some patients may never progress past this stage. Exercise priorities are as follows:

1. Flexibility and ROM exercises.
2. Maximal resistive exercise.
3. Muscular endurance (maximal repetitions).
4. Neuromuscular coordination.

Phase Five—The Phase of Integration Onto Land

This phase is for patients who are able to perform both water and land programs. The aquatic program should now include aerobic conditioning. The therapist should begin to plan for discharge into a maintenance, community, or home-based aquatic program.

A maintenance program helps the patient to maintain or improve the functional levels achieved and the present quality of life and level of independence; to avoid institutionalization; and to improve activities of daily living skills.

The land-based program should focus on restoration of muscular strength and endurance of the injured part as well as the entire body. Athletes need to address the speed, power, and agility components. Drills can be performed in the water and progressed onto land.

In general, a patient can progress to the next phase of the program after he or she is able to perform the indicated exercises *three times without a significant increase in pain* and with no aftereffects. For some conditions, however, the patient must stay in a given phase for a specific length of time to ensure that the involved structures have healed well enough to progress to the next phase.

Evaluating the Aquatic Program

The therapist should document the patient's progress throughout the entire program, noting both positive and negative results. Accurate reports aid the evaluation of the program performance according to the goals and objectives established.[8]

The patient's performance should be assessed frequently with reproducible tests and measurements or simply by comparison of admission status with discharge status (see Table 2–1). The therapist should identify goals and relate them to specific tests and measurements. Goals that have been achieved can be dropped, and any new goals that need to be addressed as a result of changes in the patient's condition or lifestyle can be added.[10]

The Rehabilitation Team

The successful rehabilitation of a patient often involves the efforts of an interdisciplinary team.

Each team member may be involved with the patient at specific points of the treatment or in an ongoing fashion. The members of the rehabilitation team should communicate frequently and be made aware of the primary goals of the program, both long-term and short-term (Fig. 2–2).

There are many program models that can operate simply by having a common set of protocols so that each member knows what the others are doing (Fig. 2–3). Treatment techniques may overlap, but this only contributes to the continuity of care for the patient.

The rehabilitation team may include a surgeon or physician; a physiotherapist or occupational or other therapist; a kinesiologist or exercise physiologist; and an aquatic instructor.

The physician or surgeon is responsible for diagnoses and for performing the surgical procedure. Only a licensed physician can make a medical diagnosis. Physicians also can provide information outlining any recommendations or contraindications for treatment.

It is the job of the therapist to assess the patient and to decide on the details of the treatment. All

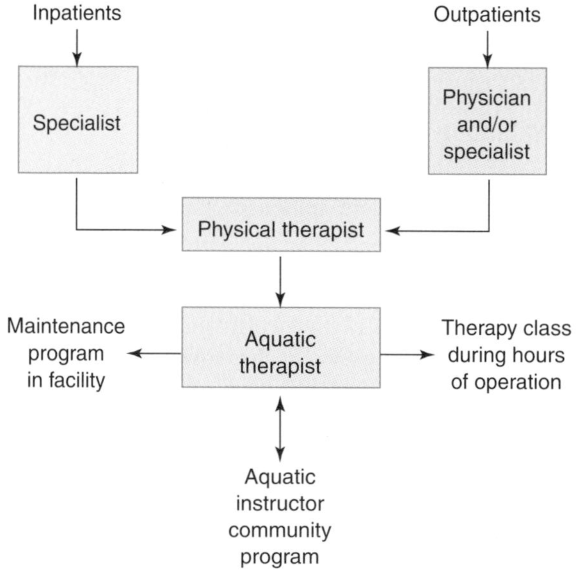

FIGURE 2–2. The lines of communication between the professionals involved in implementing an aquatic therapy program.

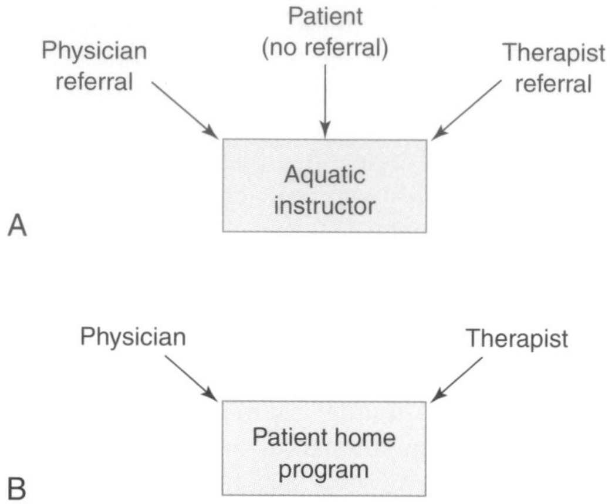

FIGURE 2–3. A common set of protocols allows *(A)* the aquatic exercise instructor to implement the rehabilitation program or *(B)* the patient to follow the orders of the therapist or physician.

professionals involved in treating the patient or implementing the program should become familiar with the patient's health status and medical history. It is important to treat *only* the conditions for which the patient was referred. Patient documents and accurate records of all incidents or occurrences should be kept according to applicable statutes of limitation.[9]

In many facilities, the therapist works with other professionals, such as a kinesiologist or exercise physiologist, to develop and implement the aquatic program. It is important that these team members follow the expressed orders of the referring physician or therapist and that they use only those therapeutic methods that they are qualified to use and that the law states they can use.[9] These team members are responsible for providing reports to the referring therapist, assessing the aquatic skills of the patient, and preparing the patient for a maintenance or community program.

After the patient enters the community, the rehabilitation team may need an aquatic instructor to continue to implement the aquatic program based on the directions or protocols received from the therapist or aquatic professional. The instructor should provide feedback or progress reports to the referring therapist. Again, treatment must be given only for the conditions for which the patient was referred. It is the patient who provides the ultimate feedback as to the effectiveness of the program.

REFERENCES

1. Francis IN. Design of therapeutic pools. Physiotherapy 75:141–142, 1989.
2. Greenlees KR. Hydrotherapy pool design. Physiotherapy 51:315–319, 1965.
3. Golland A. Basic hydrotherapy. Physiotherapy 67:258–260, 1981.
4. Edlich RF. Design of hydrotherapy exercise pools. Burn Rehabil Forum 9:505–509, 1988.
5. Jamison L, Ogden D. Aquatic Therapy Using PNF Patterns. Tucson, Therapy Skill Builders, 1994.
6. Skinner AT, Thomson AM. Duffield's Exercise in Water. 3rd ed. East Sussex, Bailliere Tindall, 1983.
7. Thomson A, Skinner A, Piercy J. Tidy's Physiotherapy. 12th ed. Toronto, Butterworth-Heinemann, 1991.
8. Breckenridge K. Medical rehabilitation program evaluation. Arch Phys Med Rehabil 59:419–423, 1978.
9. Arnheim D. Modern Principles of Athletic Training. 6th ed. St. Louis, Time Mirror/Mosby College Publishing, 1985.
10. Kisner C, Colby L. Therapeutic Exercise: Foundations and Techniques. 2nd ed. Philadelphia, F.A. Davis, 1990.

Chapter 3

The Principles and Properties of Water

WATER AND EXERCISE
RELATIVE DENSITY (SPECIFIC GRAVITY)
BUOYANCY
THE EFFECTS OF BUOYANCY ON WEIGHT BEARING
FLUID RESISTANCE
MOVEMENT THROUGH WATER
HYDROSTATIC PRESSURE
SPECIFIC HEAT OF WATER
REFRACTION

WATER AND EXERCISE

Although both air and water are fluids, they possess different properties and have unique roles in the rehabilitative environment. Water is a fluid medium that can exist as a solid below 32°F (0°C), as a liquid between 32°F and 212°F (0°–100°C), or as a gas above 212°F (100°C). As its molecular structure changes, so do its fluid characteristics.

As an exercise medium, water can be very beneficial for those who understand its principles and properties. All aquatic exercise therapy (AET) routines must address two important factors: the body's physiologic response to being immersed in water and the physical properties of water. The first point was addressed in Chapter 1. This chapter deals with several basic principles of physics that must be considered when water is used as a medium for exercise.

The program designer must have a sound understanding of these principles because they dramatically affect each exercise. For example, we rarely consider the resistance of air when we do a leg lift on land. We assume that all of the resistance is provided by the effect of gravity on the leg. When this exercise is performed in water, however, the effect of gravity is opposed by the force of buoyancy. Therefore, most of the resistance to movement actually comes from the fluid resistance of the water and not the weight of the leg. By considering the physical properties of water to be discussed in this chapter, the program designer should be able to logically plan a safe and effective exercise routine.

RELATIVE DENSITY (SPECIFIC GRAVITY)

The relative density of an object is the property that determines whether the object will float. The terms relative density and specific gravity are synonymous. The relative density of an object is the ratio of the weight of the object to the weight of an equal volume of water.[1] If this value is greater than 1, the object will sink; if it is less than 1, the object will float. If the value is exactly 1, the object will float just below the surface of the water.[2] The specific gravity also indicates the portion of an object's volume that will be floating underwater.[3] For example, if a floating person's specific gravity is 0.96, 4% of the body will be above the surface of the water and 96% will be below the surface.

The relative density of a body depends on its composition. The specific gravities of fat, bone, and lean muscle are 0.8, 1.5 to 2.0, and 1.0, respectively.[4] Consequently, lean people tend to sink, and obese people tend to float. The specific gravity of a lean person can be as high as 1.10, and that of an obese person can be as low as 0.93.[2] Generally speaking, women have more body fat than men, so they tend to float better. As people age, their bone density tends to decrease, their percent of body fat tends to increase, and their muscle mass tends to decrease. Therefore, people usually float more easily as they age.[2, 4]

The relative density of individual limbs also varies. The specific gravity of a limb is usually 1.0, but this varies with the ratio of adipose to muscle tissue.[1] There may even be a difference between the right and left side. For example, people with congenital and traumatic loss of limbs have unequal relative densities between the two sides of the body. The side with the higher relative density tends to sink and the other side to float, producing instability in the water. Flotation devices can be used to alter the position of the center of buoyancy and maintain a vertical position. Because paralyzed or weak limbs have much less muscle mass, their specific gravity is less than that of the uninvolved side.[5]

BUOYANCY

Buoyancy and relative density are very closely related. Archimedes' principle states that when a body is fully or partially submerged in a fluid at rest, it experiences an upward thrust equal to the weight of the fluid displaced.[1, 2, 5] Thus, an object with a relative density less than 1 will float because the weight of the object is less than the weight of the water displaced.[4, 6]

As previously mentioned, specific gravity indicates the portion of an object's volume that will be floating below the surface of the water. If a floating person's specific gravity is 0.96, 96% of the body must be submerged to displace enough water so that the upward force of buoyancy will equal the downward force of gravity[6] (Fig. 3–1).

Buoyancy can be assistive, resistive, or supportive. This force assists any movement toward the surface of the water and resists any movement away from the surface of the water. When buoyancy equals the force of gravity, any horizontal movement is said to be supported.[1, 5] These three attributes of buoyancy can be enhanced through the use of flotation devices. These are particularly effective for exercising the arms or legs. For example, shoulder abduction can be assisted by the addition of a handheld flotation device, but shoulder adduction would be resisted by the same device. If the flotation device is used only to keep the arm floating on the surface of the water during shoulder horizontal abduction, it is classed as a "supportive" device (Fig. 3–2).

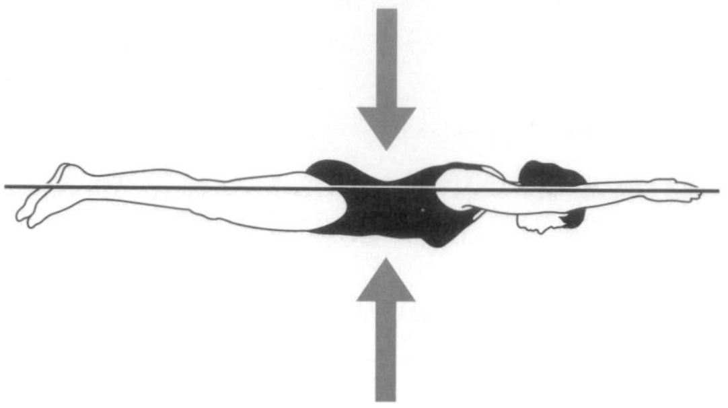

FIGURE 3–1. The buoyant force is equal to the weight of the water displaced by the swimmer (force of gravity).

The point through which the buoyant force acts is called the *center of buoyancy* (the center of gravity of the displaced fluid). It is an upward thrust that acts in the direction opposite to that of the force of gravity. A body in water, therefore, is subject to two opposing forces: gravity, acting through the center of gravity; and buoyancy, acting through the center of buoyancy.[4] If the floating body is equal to the weight of the displaced fluid, the center of buoyancy and the center of gravity are in vertical alignment.

However, if the weight of the submerged part of the body is not equal to the weight of the fluid displaced, the center of buoyancy and the center of gravity are not in the same vertical line (Fig. 3–3). This may happen, for example, with the use of flotation devices. As a result, the forces of gravity and buoyancy acting on the body will cause it to roll over or turn until it reaches equilibrium. This has obvious implications for a person exercising in

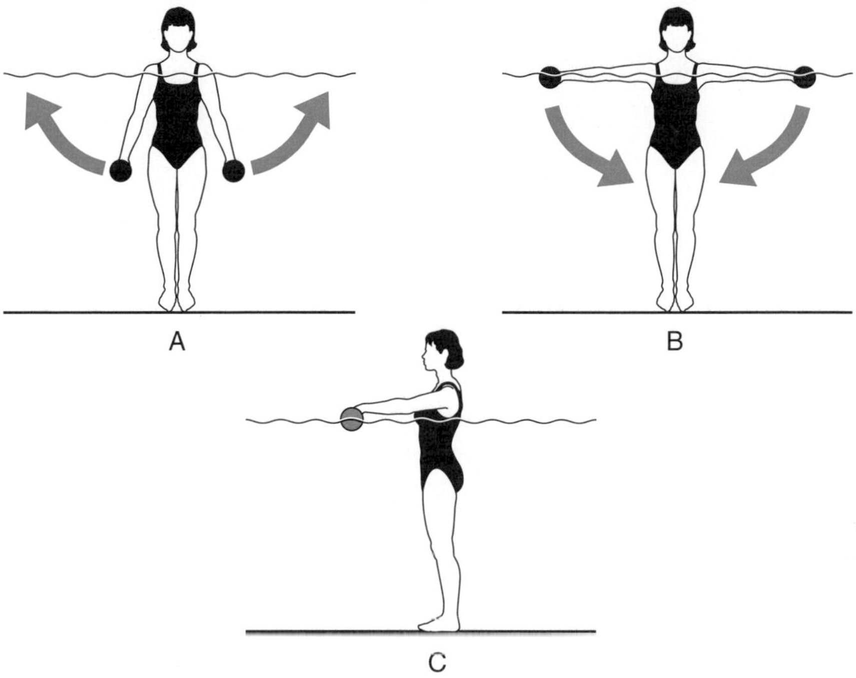

FIGURE 3–2. A hand-held flotation device can be *(A)* assistive during shoulder abduction, *(B)* resistive during shoulder adduction, or *(C)* supportive during horizontal abduction and adduction on the surface of the water.

water, especially if flotation devices are added to the lower extremities. This turning effect can cause a person's feet to float up to the surface of the water so that the body is in a horizontal position. The therapist should be alert to prevent this from happening.

When considering the amount of assistance or resistance that a flotation device provides to a given movement, buoyancy must be considered as a moment of force. A moment of force is defined as a force that pivots something around a point.[1] If the force is buoyancy, it is referred to as the moment of buoyancy.[1, 4] It can be calculated using the formula

$$m = Fd$$

where m is the moment of force, F is the upward force applied by buoyancy, and d is the horizontal distance from the vertical to the center of buoyancy.

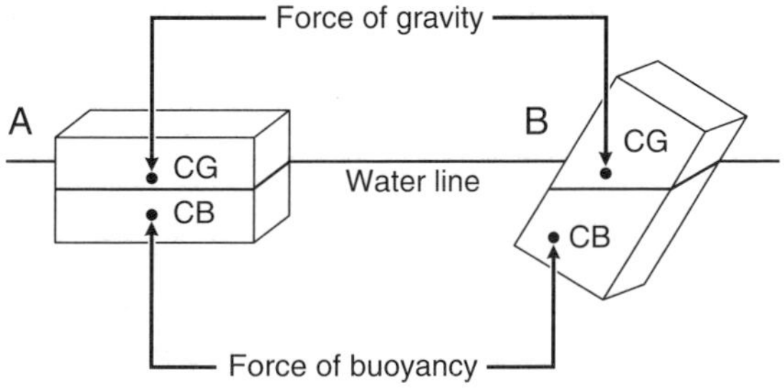

FIGURE 3–3. The forces acting on *(A)* a floating body in equilibrium and *(B)* a floating body not in equilibrium. CB = center of buoyancy; CG = center of gravity.

Figure 3–4 demonstrates how the horizontal distance varies during shoulder abduction. As the limb moves closer to the surface of the water, the effect of buoyancy becomes greater. If the segment is shortened, the center of buoyancy moves closer to the pivot point and the distance (d) is shortened; as a result, the moment of buoyancy is less.

In reality, it is not practical to precisely measure the moment of force for each exercise to be performed. It is, however, important to keep this principle in mind when modifying an exercise for a specific person. Two methods can be used to change the size of the moment of buoyancy: the size of the flotation device can be changed, and the horizontal distance (d) can be altered, either by changing the

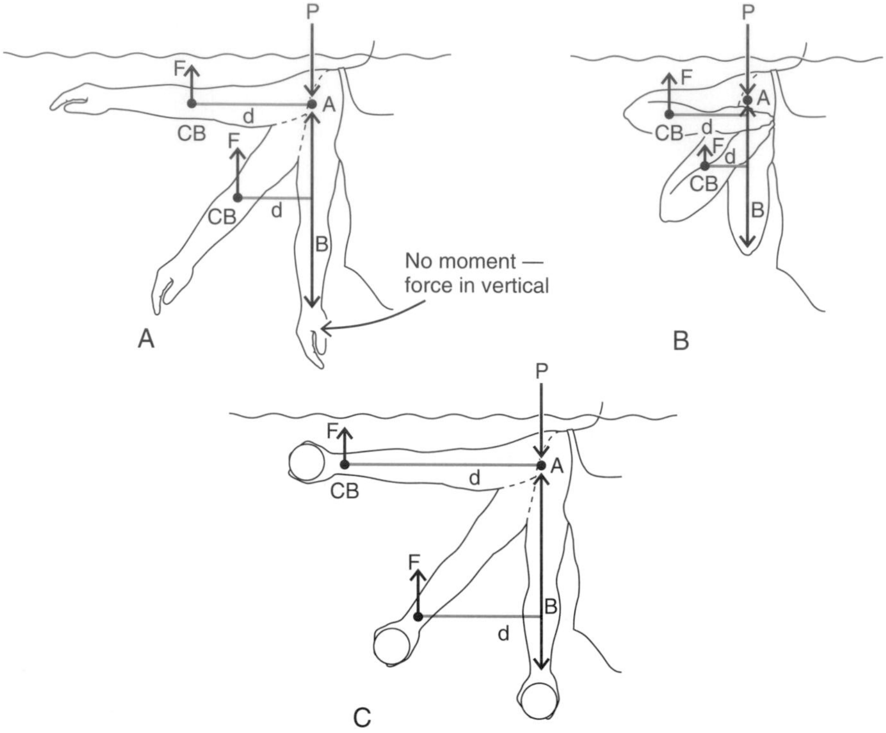

FIGURE 3–4. The turning effect of buoyancy on the arm *(A)* with the arm extended (long lever), *(B)* with the elbow bent (short lever), and *(C)* holding a float. P is the pivot point, F is the upward force of buoyancy, and d is the horizontal distance from the vertical (AB) to the center of buoyancy (CB).

position of the flotation device on the limb or by flexing the limb (effectively changing the length of the lever arm).[3, 7] The moment of buoyancy can be decreased by using a smaller flotation device, by positioning the device more proximally on the limb, or by holding the knee or elbow flexed during the movement. If a larger moment of buoyancy is desired, a larger flotation device should be placed on the distal end of a fully extended limb.

THE EFFECTS OF BUOYANCY ON WEIGHT BEARING

One of the main advantages of AET is the reduction in weight-bearing forces. Patients exercising in water feel lighter, move more easily, and feel less weight on their joints because of buoyancy. On land, the center of gravity of a body is just in front of the sacrum (S2 level). In the water, the center of gravity is located at the level of the lungs. Hence, the degree of partial weight bearing varies with pool depth[8] (Fig. 3–5).

FLUID RESISTANCE

The resistance to movement through a fluid that is caused by friction between the molecules of the fluid is known as *viscosity.* This resistance is negligible and is usually ignored when the medium is air. In water, however, there are several forces that come into play. Cohesion is the force of attraction between neighboring molecules of the same type of matter. Adhesion is the force of attraction between neighboring molecules of different types of matter. Surface tension is the force of attraction between the surface molecules of a fluid (this is not a factor if the moving body part is completely submerged in water, but it is a significant factor when a limb

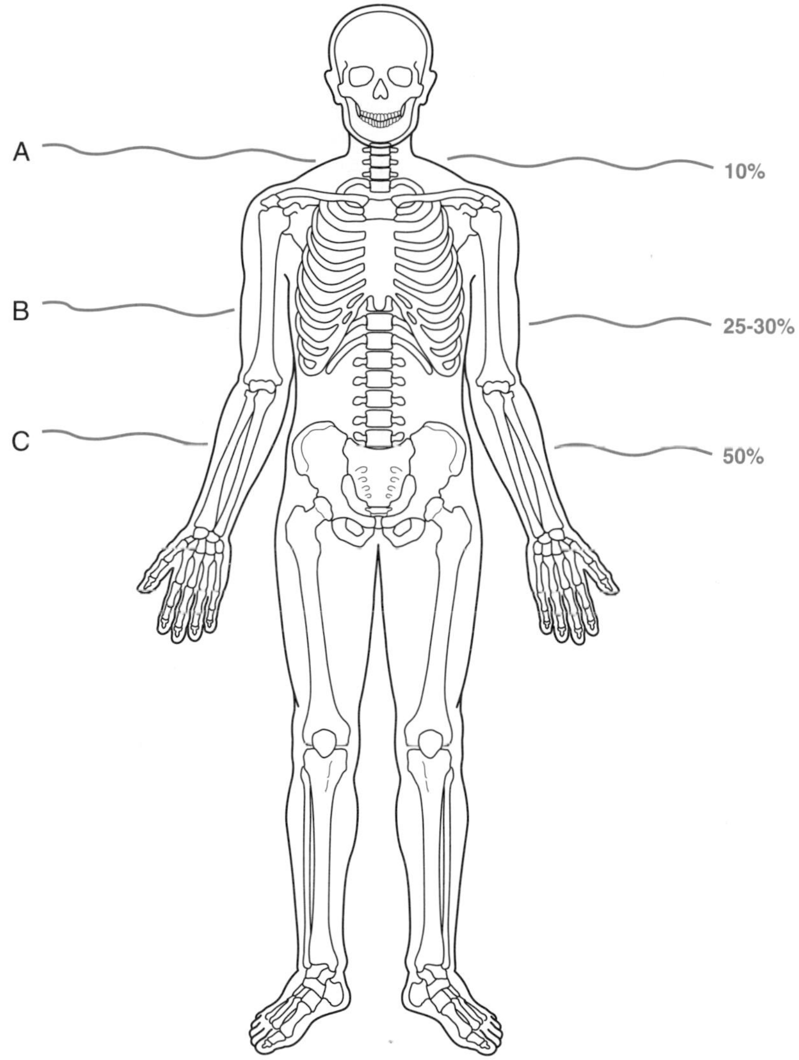

FIGURE 3–5. Percentage of body weight supported by the lower limbs at various water depths: A, the neck (C7); B, the chest (xiphisternum); and C, the pelvis (anterior superior iliac spine).

breaks the surface of the water).[5] As water temperature increases, viscosity decreases because the molecules are farther apart. This is beneficial for small, weak muscles. However, viscosity acts as a resistance to movement because molecules of a fluid tend to adhere to the surface of a body moving through it. This force of resistance is known as *drag,* and it should be considered during development of an AET program.

MOVEMENT THROUGH WATER

The amount of drag that an object experiences as it moves through water depends on a number of factors. The first factor that must be considered is that the movement can be either streamlined or turbulent. Movements are often described in terms of the fluid's moving around the object rather than the object's moving through the fluid (Fig. 3–6).

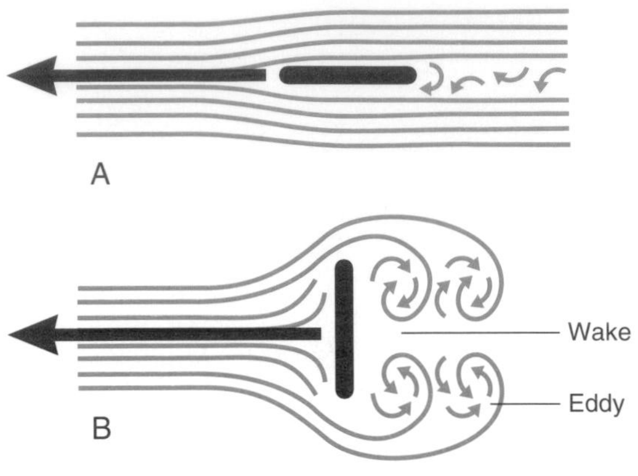

FIGURE 3–6. The movement of a paddle through the water *(A)* parallel to the flow of water, producing a streamline flow, and *(B)* perpendicular to the flow of water, producing turbulence.

During streamline flow, there is a continuous, steady movement of the fluid.[1] There is little friction between the layers of the fluid because they separate to move around the object and smoothly rejoin behind it.[6] During turbulent flow, there is an irregular movement of the layers of the fluid.[1, 6] Irregular movement produces an increase in friction between the molecules of the fluid and between the object and the fluid.[6] Instead of rejoining smoothly behind the object, the layers of the fluid move in circular patterns, which are called eddies[6] (see Fig. 3–6). This results in an area of low pressure behind the moving object, which tends to hold the object back.[3, 6] The resistance to turbulent flow is obviously greater than the resistance to streamline flow.

Turbulence occurs when an unstreamlined object moves through a fluid or when a streamlined object moves through fluid at a speed greater than its "critical velocity." This relation between the object's shape, its velocity, and the amount of drag it experiences can be calculated from the following formula:

$$F_D = PCV^2A/2G$$

where F_D is the force of drag, P is the fluid density, C is the coefficient of drag, V is the velocity of the object, A is the frontal area of the object (the limb plus the resistance device), and G is a gravitational constant.[2] This equation also applies to land exercises, but the density of air is so low that it makes the drag force insignificant. Because neither the fluid density of water nor the gravitational constant changes appreciably, changes in the force of drag can be attributed to the other three variables.

The coefficient of drag is related to how streamlined an object is. The more streamlined the object, the lower the coefficient. The coefficient is 1.0 for a square, 1.17 for a circular plate, 0.38 for the convex surface of a half sphere, and 1.42 for the concave surface.[9] In terms of exercising in the water, this means that a cupped hand moving through water experiences more than 30% more drag than a flat hand.

The velocity at which the object is moving through the water and the frontal area are also important variables. From the equation, it can be seen that the drag force is proportional to the square of the velocity. Therefore, if the velocity of a moving limb is doubled, the drag force is multiplied by a factor of four. The fact that frontal area is directly proportional to drag force means that it has a significant effect on the resistance of a given aquatic exercise; for example, doubling the frontal area doubles the drag. With upper limb exercises, the area of the hand can be effectively increased simply by separating the fingers slightly. This occurs because the "boundary layer" of fluid moving around an object (such as a finger) is greater in water than in air. When the fingers are slightly separated, their boundary layers overlap.[3]

As with the moment of buoyancy calculation, it is not practical to precisely determine the drag force for each exercise. It is important to understand, however, how small changes in the size, shape, and velocity of a resistance device can affect an exercise performed in the water. One must also consider how these and other forces can combine to have an effect on movement through water. For example, a given flotation device may have both assistive and resistive qualities. The fact that an object is buoyant implies that it will assist movement, but its size and shape may produce a drag force that resists movement. It is the net effect of the device on the limb's movement that must be considered.

The combined total of a moving limb's velocity, the body's velocity, and the water's velocity also affects the drag force during exercise.[5] If the patient is walking forward and also moving the arm forward, the two velocities must be added together to determine the arm's velocity relative to the water.

Any movement of the water, such as that produced during alternating reciprocal movements, also affects the drag. For example, abduction of the arm causes the water to move in the same direction as the arm. If the arm movement is suddenly reversed, the arm will be moving against the flow of water. This results in a dramatic increase in drag and increases the resistance of the exercise. Conversely, any movement that occurs in the same direction as moving water will encounter less drag than if it were occurring in stationary water.

In addition to increasing the drag forces, reversing the direction of movement also adds the work of having to overcome inertia.[5] In order to stop a moving limb, the appropriate muscles must produce the force necessary to decelerate both the mass of the limb and the mass of the water that is moving in behind it. The classic formula, $a = F/m$ (where a is acceleration or deceleration, F is force, and m is mass), deals with mass and not weight. This means that although the force of drag plays a role in acceleration underwater, buoyancy does not, because buoyancy does not affect an object's mass.[2]

The last force that must be considered when dealing with aquatic exercise is that of impact. It can be calculated from the following formula:

$$F_I = m\,E(V_1 - V_2)/t$$

where F_I is the impact force, m is the mass of the body, E is the modulus of elasticity of the floor, V_1 is the velocity when leaving the floor, V_2 is the velocity when landing on the floor, and t is the time in contact with the floor. Once again it can be seen that weight and buoyancy are not the major factors. The primary reason that aquatic exercise is "low impact" compared with land exercise is that aquatic exercise is performed at a lower velocity. Both V_1 and V_2 are much lower than if the exercise were performed on land.[9]

HYDROSTATIC PRESSURE

Pascal's law states that fluid pressure is exerted equally on all surfaces of an immersed body at a given depth (Fig. 3–7). The pressure is directly

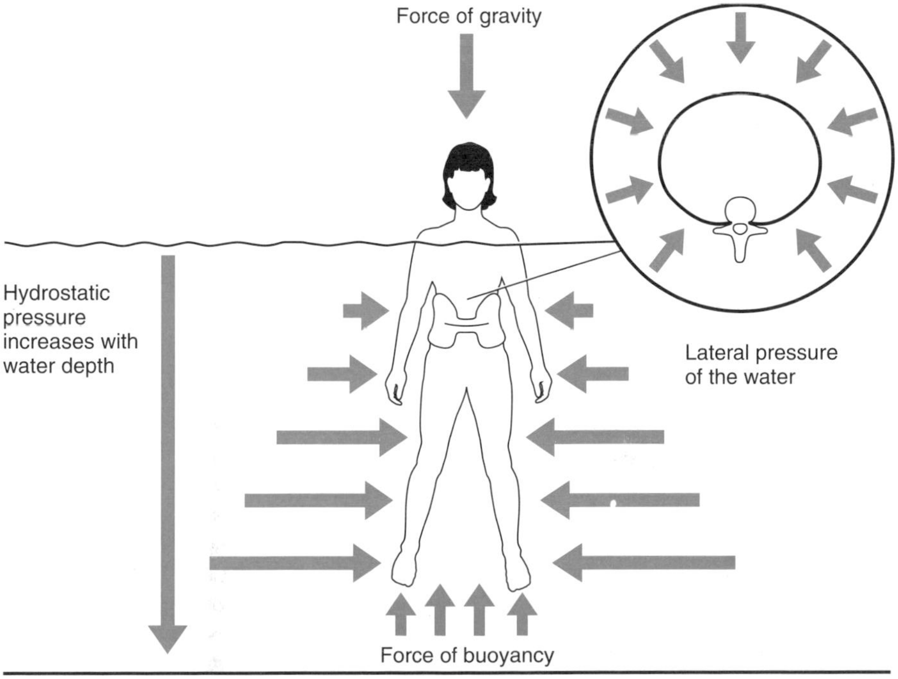

FIGURE 3–7. The pressures exerted on the body during immersion with the head out of water.

proportional to both the depth and the density of the fluid.[2] From a baseline of 14.7 psi (atmospheric pressure) at the surface, fluid pressure of water increases by 0.43 psi per foot of depth.[2] For this reason, it is not advisable to put patients with a vital capacity below 1500 mL (such as patients with chronic obstructive pulmonary disease) into a pool at 85% immersion.[10] Such patients may have difficulty breathing because the pressure of the water resists chest wall expansion. Hydrostatic pressure opposes the tendency of blood to pool in the lower portions of the body, which helps to reduce unnecessary swelling. Hydrostatic pressure also helps stabilize unstable joints.

SPECIFIC HEAT OF WATER

One often overlooked physical property of water is that of its specific heat. This is defined as the amount of energy required to raise the temperature of 1 g of water by 1°C. The specific heat of water is several thousand times that of air, and heat loss to water is 25 times that to air at a given temperature.[2] This heat loss can occur either by conduction (movement of thermal energy from something warm to something cool) or by convection (heat loss caused by movement of water against a body even if the water and the body are the same temperature). If more heat is lost to water than is produced by the muscles, the patient will feel cold.

Consequently, both the temperature of the water and the amount of heat produced by the body must be considered when determining a comfortable water temperature in which to exercise. Vigorous exercise performed in warm water (91°F, or 33°C) results in an increase in core temperature (to 103°F, or 39.4°C) and premature fatigue.[2] Vigorous exercise in cold water (65°F, or 18°C) leads to a drop in core temperature (to 96.8°F, or 36°C) and an inability to contract muscles.[2] The ideal temperature for vigorous exercise is 82° to 86°F (28°–30°C). Because therapeutic exercises such as those described in this book are not vigorous, they produce little body heat, and it is suggested that the temperature of the therapeutic pool be kept between 91° and 95°F (33°–35°C).

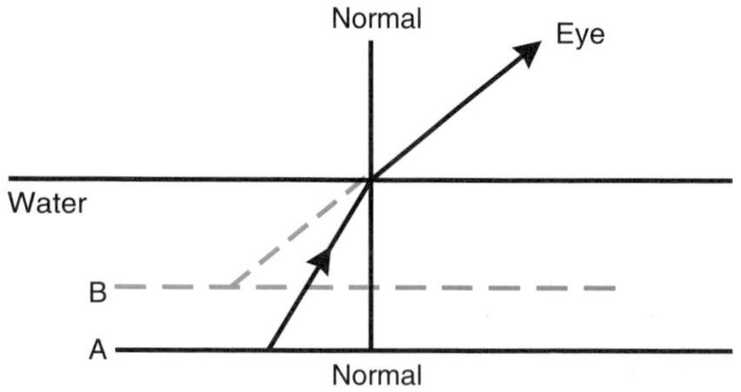

FIGURE 3–8. Refraction of light causes rays reflected from the true bottom of the pool (A) to appear at a false bottom (B).

REFRACTION

Refraction is the bending of a ray of light as it moves from one medium into another medium of different density. Figure 3–8 shows how a ray bends away from the normal when it moves from the water (greater density) into the air (lesser density). Refraction is the reason pools appear to be shallower than they truly are.[6] The limbs of people exercising in water also appear distorted. The parts that are submerged seem to bend away from the normal at water level. As a result, visual feedback, monitoring of joint position, and postural education are very difficult. Instructors often find it easiest to simply stand on the pool deck and demonstrate from there. Nevertheless, whenever a patient is in an upright position, correct posture should always be reinforced.

REFERENCES

1. Haralson KM. Therapeutic pool programs. J Clin Manage 5:510–513, 1988.
2. Edlich RF, Towler MA, Goitz RJ, et al. Bioengineering principles of hydrotherapy. J Burn Care Rehabil 8:579–584, 1987.
3. Bolton E, Goodwin D. An Introduction to Pool Exercises. 2nd ed. London, E. & S. Livingstone, 1962.
4. Hay J. The Biomechanics of Sports Techniques. Englewood Cliffs, N.J., Prentice-Hall, 1978.
5. Jamison L, Ogden D. Aquatic Therapy Using PNF Patterns. Tucson, Therapy Skill Builders, 1994.
6. Skinner AT, Thomson AM, eds. Duffield's Exercise in Water. 3rd ed. London, Bailliere Tindall, 1983.
7. Kinder T, See J. Aqua Aerobics: A Scientific Approach. Dubuque, Iowa, Eddie Bowers Publishing, 1992.
8. Johnson C. Backstrokes: An Aquatic Rehabilitation Program for People with Back Pain. Haverton, Pa., Occupational Therapy Associates, 1989.
9. Lenk M. Aquaphysics: The 1993 Aquatic Therapy Symposium Syllabus. Port Washington, Wis., Aquatic Exercise Association, 1993.
10. McDonald G. The benefits of water therapy: An overview. Aquatic Exercise Association, AKWA Newsletter, 1991.

AQUATIC EQUIPMENT

CHAPTER 4

There are many types of equipment used in an aquatic therapy setting, including safety equipment, therapeutic equipment, and exercise equipment.

SAFETY EQUIPMENT

All safety equipment should be located in a place that is visible and easily accessible to the therapists. Staff members should be trained in the emergency action plan of the facility and any related policies and procedures. Emergency alarms should also be easily accessible and should be tested frequently. Therapists working in the pool area should be trained in cardiopulmonary resuscitation, basic water safety, and first aid. First aid kits should include waterproof bandages, ear plugs, nose plugs, and standard items. If the therapy class is large or held in a public facility, the therapist may want to hire a lifeguard for the duration of the class.

Therapists need to know the correct use and application of all safety equipment in the pool area. This includes buoyant towing aids, shepherd's crooks or poles, spinal boards, and any other pieces of safety equipment.

THERAPEUTIC EQUIPMENT

In the pool area, there are many types of therapeutic equipment. These include such items as lifts, steps, parallel bars, handrails or holds, and aquatic stools, wheelchairs, and stretchers.

Lifts and steps provide a method of entry into the pool and may be either fixed or movable. All lift equipment should be well maintained and tested frequently if it is not used on a regular basis. Steps should be wide (approximately 3 ft, or 91 cm) and should have handrails on both sides. The edge of each step should be marked with a contrasting color.

Parallel bars are long, stainless steel bars that are anchored to the bottom of the pool; they are either fixed or movable. The ends should be rounded or have rubber tips to prevent injury. They are used mostly for ambulation and to provide safety and comfort in the water during non–weight-bearing or partial weight-bearing exercise.

Handrails, bars, or holds, which are fixed to the pool wall, are beneficial because they allow patients who are unstable in the water to perform their exercises and move around more freely. Weighted stools are also beneficial in pools with a set depth to provide stability during upper extremity exercises performed while seated.

EXERCISE EQUIPMENT

Aquatic therapy equipment includes supportive, assistive, and resistive devices.

Supportive equipment is used to maintain the trunk in an upright, supine (on the back), or prone (on the stomach) position. The therapist can use this type of equipment to comfortably and safely position a patient.

Assistive equipment includes buoyant devices used in a manner that assists a motion. If joint mobility is the primary concern, the therapist can use assistive equipment to increase the range of motion (ROM). For example, to increase knee flexion and extension, a movement toward the surface can be buoyed, or a movement toward the bottom of the pool can be weighted. Both of these are assistive adjustments.

Resistive equipment provides some form of resistance, by tension (eg, stretch bands), by increased surface area, or by added buoyancy or weights that increase the intensity of the exercise.

Some pieces of equipment, such as floats, have multiple functions. Such equipment can assist some motions (eg, hip abduction) and resist others (eg, hip adduction).

Using Aquatic Equipment to Vary Exercise Intensity

The progressive overload method for increasing muscular strength and endurance is equally effective in the water and on land. The therapist can vary the number of times a particular movement is performed and the degree of resistance or intensity for each exercise. Aquatic equipment can be used to alter the intensity of an exercise by increasing the ROM, changing the length of the lever arm, increasing the surface area of resistance, changing the speed of motion, increasing the effects of gravity, or creating tension.

Range of Motion

Buoyant devices can be used to increase the ROM of a joint from functional to maximal efficiency. After a knee replacement, for example, the capsule is very stiff, and knee flexion is often impaired. The therapist can use a flotation device to gently assist knee flexion and extension by simply changing the position of the patient. The amount of assistance provided can be altered by changing the size of the float or the amount of air in the flotation device. This allows the therapist to gradually increase the effects of buoyancy acting on the knee joint. Exercising through a full ROM helps to prevent muscle shortening.

Lever Arms

Movement is performed by the contraction of skeletal muscle. The body can be viewed as a system of levers that help increase the efficiency of muscle action. All levers have a fulcrum or point of rotation (the *joint*), a point of effort or application of force (the *muscle*), and a point of resistance application (the *weight*). The relative positions of these three points determine the type of lever.

There are three types of levers: first-class, second-class, and third-class (Fig. 4–1). In a first-class lever, the fulcrum (joint) always lies between the effort (muscle) and the resistance (weight). A good

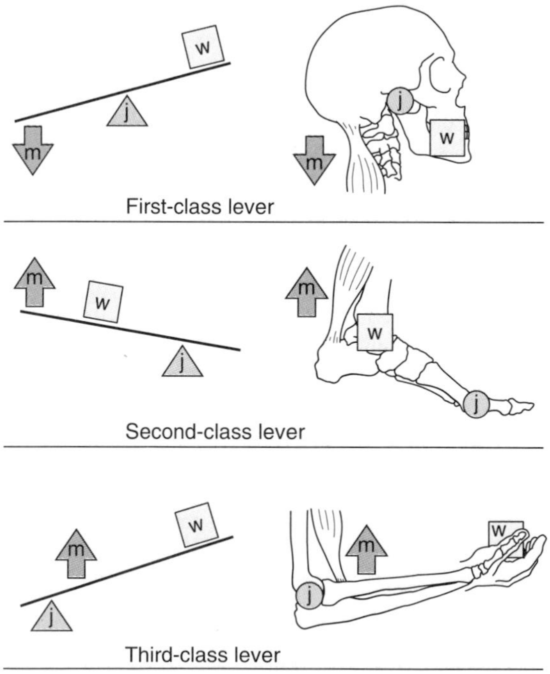

FIGURE 4–1. The three types of levers. j = joint, m = muscle, w = weight. (Modified from Kapit W, and Elson L. The Anatomy Coloring Book. Copyright © 1977 by Wynn Kapit and Lawrence M. Elson. Reprinted by permission of HarperCollins Publishers, Inc.)

example of this type of lever is a seesaw. This is the most efficient class of lever. In a second-class lever, the resistance (weight) always lies between the fulcrum (joint) and the effort (muscle). A good example of this type of a lever is a wheelbarrow.

Most of the levers of the body are third-class levers, in which the effort (muscle) is located between the resistance (weight) and the fulcrum (joint). In the water, the resistance is equal to the amount of water displaced during exercise.

When exercising in the water, it is best to start with short levers and progress to longer levers, because flexed limbs offer less resistance or assistance than straight limbs.

Surface Area of Resistance

Walking through the water sideways is much easier than walking through the water forward, because a greater surface area of the body is exposed to the direction of motion. Aquatic equipment can be used in a similar manner. A flat hand produces a streamlined movement with little frontal surface area and hence little intensity or resistance. Placing the hand at right angles to the direction of motion increases the intensity of the movement. By gradually increasing the surface area of resistance, the therapist can increase the intensity of the exercise in a controlled manner.[1, 2]

Speed of Movement

Water has a greater density than air. For this reason, water provides more resistance to motion and reduces the speed of each movement. When the body begins to move, the muscles contract to overcome first inertia, and then the resistance of the water. Once in motion, it is easier for a body to continue moving in one direction than it is to change directions or work against a current.

Moving against resistance requires a considerable amount of effort from the muscles. With increased speed and range of movement, the patient must increase the amount of force applied to perform a given movement. Consequently, the effort required from the working muscles also increases. Therefore, changing the speed changes the amount of effort required by the muscles to overcome the encountered resistance. The addition of resistive equipment further increases the required effort. Changing the speed of a movement is a way to vary the intensity of an exercise without changing the exercise.

The Effects of Gravity

As discussed in Chapter 3, the more submerged the body is, the less are the effects of gravity. By slowly reducing the depth of the water, the therapist can gradually train various muscles to respond favorably to the effects of the force of gravity.

Tension

Certain pieces of equipment, such as stretch bands, can provide resistance through tension. The tension of the bands can gradually be increased without changing the exercise.

Precautions

Certain precautions should be taken when using aquatic exercise equipment.

1. The patient should maintain correct postural alignment. It is important not to let resistance compromise posture. The body should be stabilized and abdominals should be tight throughout the execution of an exercise.
2. The patient should never lock a hinge joint. Joints should remain "soft." Resistance should not put unnecessary stress on a joint. Full extension of the elbows and knees should be avoided.
3. The patient should always stretch what will be strengthened. Before working with equipment, the patient should perform a warm-up. This will prepare the joints and muscles to be stretched.
4. The patient should start with short levers, and progress to longer ones.
5. The patient should maximize the range of motion of a joint before using resistive exercise equipment for strengthening muscles.
6. The type of equipment used should suit the purpose or objectives of the exercise.

Types of Aquatic Exercise Equipment

The equipment used in the pool area should be well constructed and resistant to bacterial growth. There should be adequate storage and drainage for all equipment in the pool area. Aquatic exercise equipment should be used only for the purpose of which it was designed. Safety should always be the primary concern.

INNER TUBES. These are donut-shaped rubber tubes that are available in a variety of thicknesses and diameters. *Purpose:* supportive devices used to aid in flotation and to increase safety and comfort in the water. The patient may be supported in a vertical, supine, or prone position by use of an inner tube.

THE DEEP WATER FLOAT BELT. This is a long foam belt with an adjustable strap and buckle. *Purpose:* a deep water supportive device worn around the waist. It may also be used whenever increased buoyancy is required.

WATER EXERCISE DUMBBELLS. These are strong bars made of polyvinyl chloride with closed cell foam caps on each end. The dumbbells for use by people with arthritis have grip sponge over the bar, which makes handling much easier. *Purpose:* flotation devices that provides resistance against buoyancy. Dumbbells can also provide support under the arms or knees.

THE KICKBOARD. This is a high-density, closed-cell ethylene vinyl acetate foam board. It is flat and has a large surface area. Although the size and shape may vary, most are rectangular. *Purpose:* a flotation device used to support the body in a prone position with arms extended. When held under the water, it provides great resistance during walking or other exercises.

THE WAND. This is a plastic, hollow stick approximately 2 ft (61 cm) in length and open at both ends. *Purpose:* an assistive device to increase upper body ROM and provide mild resistance.

THE RESISTIVE PADDLE. This is a plastic paddle with thick Velcro straps. It provides an increased surface area during the performance of various movements. *Purpose:* a resistive device that may be strapped to the ankles or held by the hands to work various muscle groups. Paddles must be secured properly and speed must be regulated to maintain the integrity of the exercise. Resistive paddles can uniquely provide equal resistance during opposing exercise movements.[1, 2]

WRIST AND ANKLE WEIGHTS. These come in various sizes and have Velcro straps to secure them safely to wrist or ankle during exercise. *Purpose:* resistive devices that may be used on land or in the water. Weights provide resistance and stability during exercise through various ROMs.

ANKLE CUFFS. These are made from closed-cell ethylene vinyl acetate foam. They are three-sided and have a belt with an adjustable strap, a buckle, and an added adjustable heel strap to prevent the cuff from sliding up the leg during exercise. *Purpose:* flotation devices that can be used to support the legs in a supine or prone position. They can be used as resistive or assistive devices while working through the various ROMs.

STRETCH BANDS. These are bands used for toning that come in various levels of resistance. *Purpose:* resistive devices that can be used to strengthen various parts of the body. Correct placement and use of the bands is critical in a therapeutic setting. Stretch bands should not be used unless the purpose of the exercise is understood and any possible contraindications have been resolved.

THE STEP. This is a large, stable surface area of varying height that can be placed at the bottom of the pool. *Purpose:* a supportive device used to step onto repeatedly. It may also be used for shorter patients to stand upright during upper body exercises, or it may act as an assistive device during stretching of the lower body.

REFERENCES

1. Abidin MR, Thacker JG, Becker DG, et al.: Hydrofitness devices for strengthening upper extremity muscles. J Burn Care Rehab 9:199–202, 1988.
2. Goitz RJ, Towler MA, Buschbacher LP, et al.: A new hydrofitness device for leg musculoskeletal conditioning. J Burn Care Rehab 9:203–206, 1988.

CHAPTER 5

Introduction to Aquatic Rehabilitative Exercises

Leg Exchange
Jogging
Bicycle
Pelvic Movements

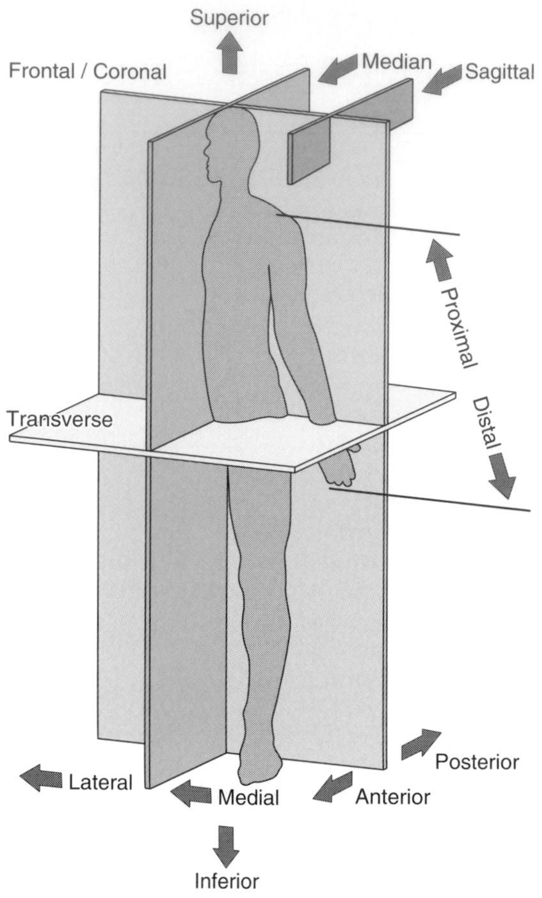

FIGURE 5–1. The planes of movement and anatomic directions.

REVIEW OF MOVEMENT TERMINOLOGY

The Anatomic Position

The anatomic position is a universally accepted position in which the trunk is erect, the arms are at the sides, the palms face forward, and the legs are straight. It is considered the "zero position" for defining and measuring joint motion.[1]

Planes of Movement

The basic planes of movement are derived from the dimensions in space and are at right angles to each other[2] (Fig. 5–1).

The **median plane** is a midline plane that divides the body into right and left halves.

The **sagittal plane** is vertical and extends from front to back (anteroposterior), dividing the body into right and left halves.

The **frontal or coronal plane** is vertical and extends from side to side at right angles to the sagittal plane, dividing the body into front and back portions.

The **transverse plane** is horizontal and divides the body into upper (cranial) and lower (caudal) portions.

Anatomic Directions

Directional terms are used to describe the positions of body structures relative to one another. These terms are always used with reference to a body in the anatomic position[2] (see Fig. 5–1).

Superior (cranial): toward the head or higher than another structure in the body; upper.

Inferior (caudal): away from the head; closer to the feet or lower than another structure in the body; lower.

Anterior: situated in front of, or in the forward part of, the body.

Posterior: situated behind, or toward the rear of, the body.

Medial: toward the midline of the body.

Lateral: away or farther from the midline of the body.

Proximal: closer to the midline of the body or point of origin (refers to the limbs only).

Distal: farther away from the midline of the body or point of origin (refers to the limbs only).

Axes of Motion

The axes of motion are lines, real or imaginary, about which movement takes place. The three basic types of axes are at right angles to each other and are related to the planes of movement.[2]

Sagittal axis lies in the sagittal plane and extends horizontally from front to back; the movements of abduction and adduction take place about this axis in a frontal or coronal plane.

Coronal (frontal) axis lies in the coronal plane and extends horizontally from side to side; the movements of flexion and extension take place about this axis in a sagittal plane.

Longitudinal axis is a vertical axis extending in a cranial-caudal direction; the movements of medial and lateral rotation take place about this axis in a transverse plane.

JOINT MOVEMENT

Types of Joints

A joint is formed whenever two or more bones meet or bones and cartilage meet. Some joints are highly movable, and others are virtually fixed. There are three types of joints: fibrous, cartilaginous, and synovial.

Fibrous Joints

An example of a fibrous or immovable joint is a suture of the skull. In fibrous joints, the bones fit tightly together. They are bound to one another by more-or-less inextensible connective tissue and permit little or no movement (Fig. 5–2).

Cartilaginous Joints

An example of a cartilaginous or slightly movable joint is the intervertebral disc. In cartilaginous joints, the bones are separated by cartilage, either fibrous or hyaline. Slight movement occurs with fibrocartilage; usually, no movement occurs with hyaline cartilage (Fig. 5–3).

Synovial Joints

An example of a synovial or freely movable joint is the knee. There are six subcategories of synovial joints.

HINGE OR GINGLYMUS JOINTS. The bones fit together like the two parts of a hinge (Fig. 5–4). Hinge joints are uniaxial, and typically collateral ligaments support each side of the joint. *Example:* knee.

CONDYLOID OR ELLIPSOID JOINTS. A biconvex surface fits into a biconcave surface (Fig. 5–5). This arrangement allows back-to-front and side-to-side motion but denies any twisting or rotation. *Example:* radiocarpal joint of the wrist.

BALL-AND-SOCKET JOINTS. A ball-shaped end of one bone fits into a socket offered by a

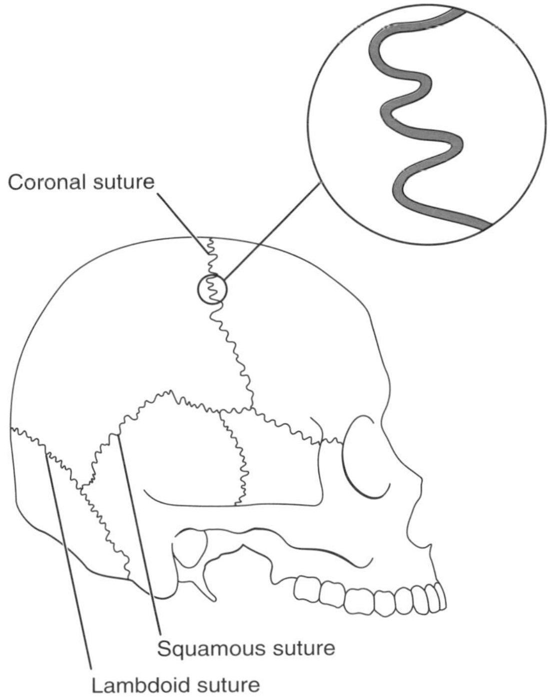

FIGURE 5–2. A fibrous joint: a skull suture.

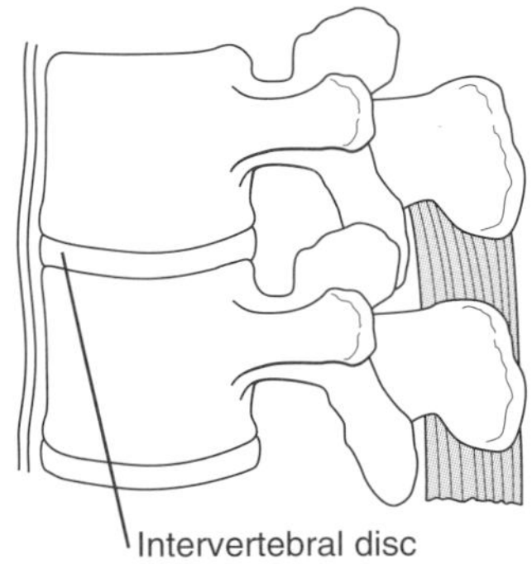

FIGURE 5–3. A cartilaginous joint: an intervertebral disc.

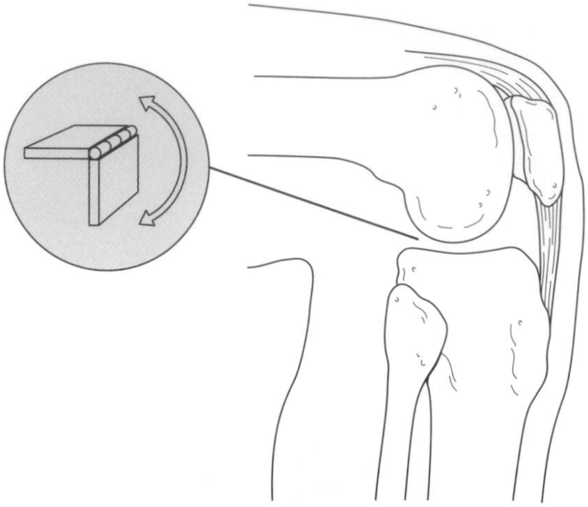

FIGURE 5–4. A hinge joint: the knee.

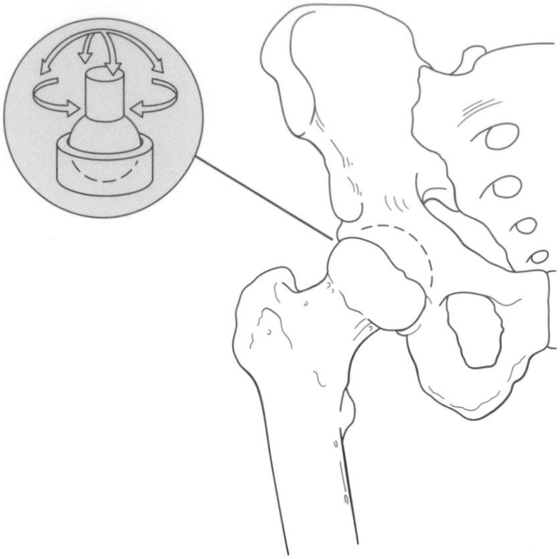

FIGURE 5–6. A ball-and-socket joint: the hip.

second bone (Fig. 5–6). Joints of this type are the most freely movable joints in the body. For this reason, they are supported by muscles rather than tight ligaments, and consequently they are more prone to dislocation. *Example:* hip and shoulder.

GLIDING JOINTS. The articulating surfaces are more-or-less flat and permit sliding movements in two planes, back-to-front and side-to-side (Fig. 5–7). *Example:* carpal bones.

PIVOT JOINTS. One bone pivots on another, allowing a rotational movement (Fig. 5–8). *Example:* proximal radioulnar joint.

SADDLE JOINTS. This joint articulates such that the bones can move back-and-forth or side-to-side but cannot twist (Fig. 5–9). *Example:* carpometacarpal thumb joint.

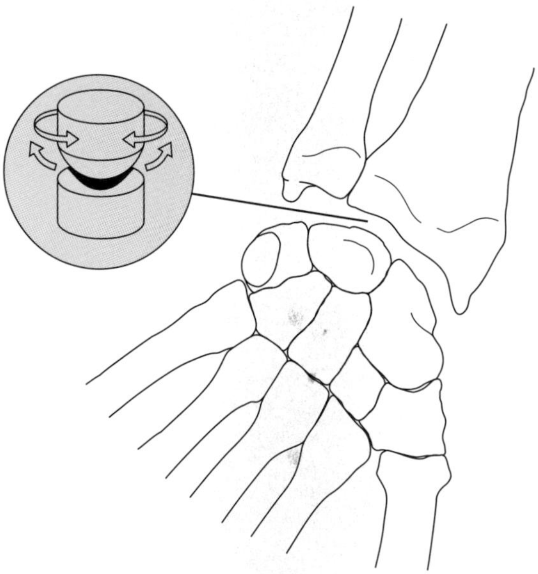

FIGURE 5–5. A condyloid (ellipsoid) joint: the radiocarpal joint of the wrist.

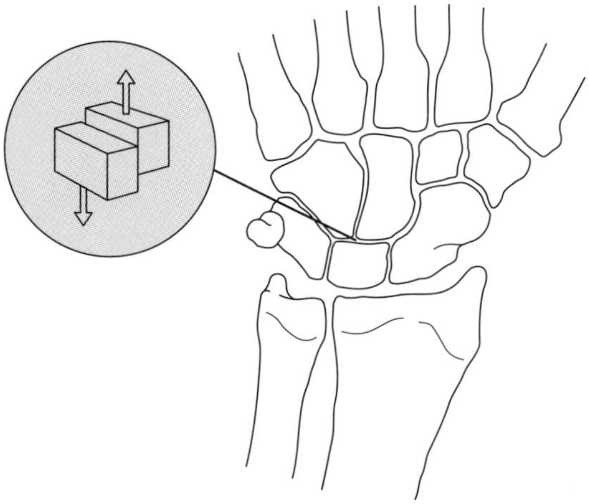

FIGURE 5–7. A gliding joint: an intercarpal joint.

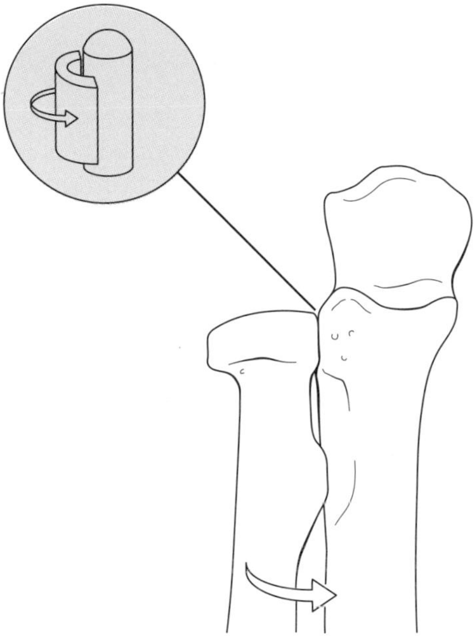

FIGURE 5–8. A pivot joint: the proximal radioulnar joint.

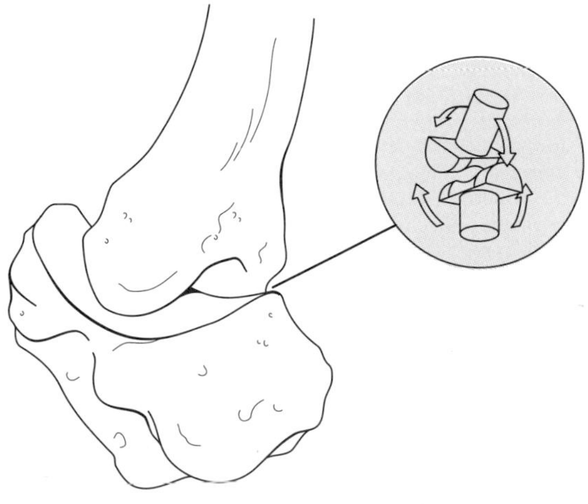

FIGURE 5–9. A saddle joint: the carpometacarpal joint of the thumb.

A Typical Synovial Joint

Synovial joints have certain features that are necessary to any free-moving bony articulation (Fig. 5–10). These features are as follows:

1. A joint cavity.
2. A capsule that encloses the joint cavity. The capsule is usually attached close to the articulating end of each bone involved.
3. A synovial membrane that lines the inside of the capsule and covers that part of the bone inside the joint cavity, except for the articular surfaces.
4. Synovial fluid secreted by the membrane to lubricate the joint.
5. Hyaline cartilage covering the articulating surfaces.
6. Ligaments binding and supporting the joint and its capsule.

There are some additional structures that are not always present. For example, some joints have fibrocartilage pads that help to lubricate the joint by reducing shock and increasing the surface contact areas. Also, many synovial joints have bursae, which are small, synovium-lined sacs that help to reduce friction between the moving surfaces (eg, tendon and bone, muscle and bone).

Joint Definitions

Table 5–1 gives the definitions of joint motions for synovial joints. These anatomic movements are always described in reference to the anatomic position.

Range of Motion

One of the most beneficial effects of exercising in the water is the ability to maintain or increase the range of joint movement. Movement at a joint is caused by muscle contraction or an external force. However, the way a segment moves depends on the bony structure of the articulating surfaces and the integrity and flexibility of the soft tissues surrounding the joint (Fig. 5–11). The complete scope of movement that is possible at the joint is referred to as the range of motion (ROM). When describing the ROM about a joint, we use terms such as flexion and extension. Movement of the various body segments can be achieved through passive, active or active-assistive ROM.[3]

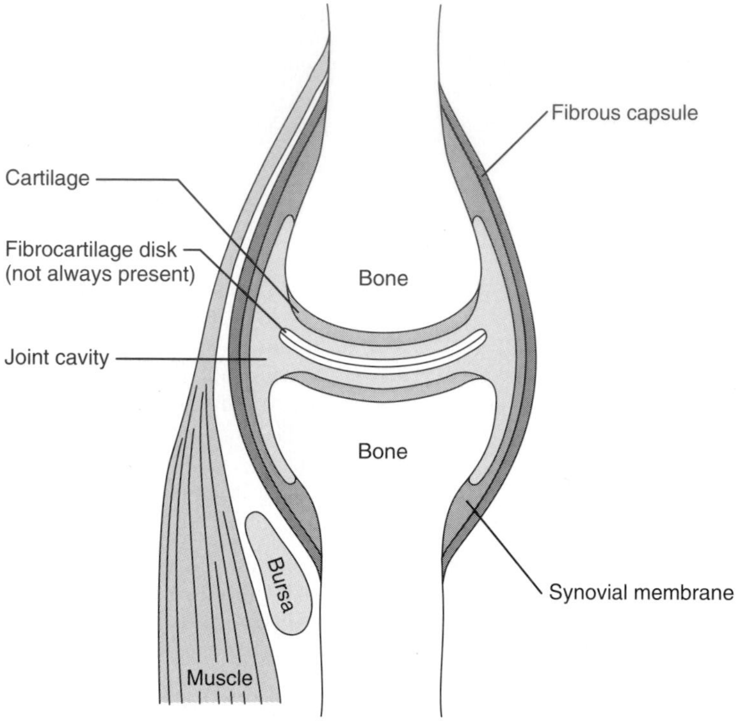

FIGURE 5–10. The structure of a typical synovial joint.

TABLE 5–1. Description of Joint Movements

Joint Movement	Description
Flexion	A movement in the anterior direction, toward the head, by the joints of the arms or the hip. Flexion of the knee or toe refers to movement in the posterior direction.
Extension	The opposite of flexion; movement in the posterior direction by the arms or hip. Extension of the knee or toe refers to movement in the anterior direction.
Abduction	Movement away from the midline of the body.
Adduction	Movement toward the midline of the body.
Lateral flexion	Lateral movement of the spine (ie, movement from left to right).
Rotation	A movement rotary about the longitudinal axis.
Circumduction	A movement that combines flexion, abduction, extension, and adduction whereby the trace of the moving part resembles a cone.
Hyperextension	An excessive amount of extension past normal range.
Horizontal abduction	Movement with the arms extended at shoulder level by which the arms move posteriorly away from the midline of the body.
Supination	A rotational movement of the forearm whereby the palm of the hand is turned upward (anteriorly).
Pronation	The opposite of supination; a movement of the forearm whereby the palm of the hand is turned downward (posteriorly).
Radial deviation	A lateral movement of the wrist toward the radial side of the forearm.

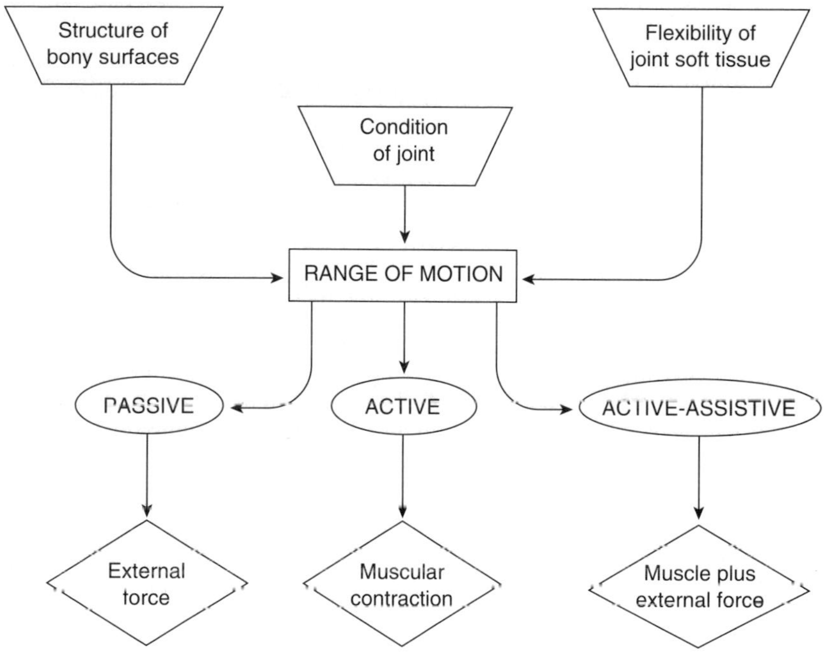

FIGURE 5–11. Summary of factors influencing joint range of motion. (Modified from Kendall EP, McCreary EK. Muscle: Testing and Function. 3rd ed. Baltimore, Williams & Wilkins, 1993.)

TABLE 5–1. Description of Joint Movements *Continued*

Joint Movement	Description
Ulnar deviation	The opposite of radial deviation; a lateral movement of the wrist toward the ulnar side of the forearm.
Dorsiflexion	A movement of the ankle whereby the dorsal surface (top) of the foot is moved toward the head.
Plantar flexion	The opposite of dorsiflexion; a movement of the ankle whereby the plantar (bottom) surface of the foot is moved toward the ground.
Inversion	A movement whereby the foot is turned inward (supinated and abducted).
Eversion	The opposite of inversion; a movement whereby the foot is turned outward (pronated and abducted).
Posterior tilt	A backward tilt of the pelvis.
Anterior tilt	A forward tilt of the pelvis.
Internal (medial) rotation	The rotation of a segment toward the midline of the body.
External (lateral) rotation	The rotation of a segment away from the midline of the body.
Protraction	A forward movement of the neck or the shoulder girdle.
Retraction	A backward movement of the neck or the shoulder girdle.
Elevation	A superior or upward movement of the shoulder girdle.
Depression	An inferior or downward movement of the shoulder girdle.

PASSIVE RANGE OF MOTION. Movement of a segment is produced entirely by an external force; there is no voluntary muscle contraction.

ACTIVE RANGE OF MOTION. Movement of a segment is produced by an active contraction of the muscles crossing the joint.

ACTIVE-ASSISTIVE RANGE OF MOTION. Assistance is provided by an outside force during active ROM because the prime mover (muscle) requires help to complete the motion.

The indications for ROM exercises in the water are similar to those on land. Warm water immersion, however, provides unique treatment opportunities not possible on land.

Assessing Joint Range of Motion

Joint ROM is usually measured with a goniometer. There are many types of goniometers, but the ones most commonly used are those that measure 0° to 180° and have one arm that is stationary and one that is fully movable.

Standardized body positions and anatomic landmarks ensure that the results of the test are accurate and reliable. Joint ROM is usually described in terms of degrees (0°–180°). The anatomic position is usually considered the "zero position" when defining and measuring joint motion.[4–6]

THE PRINCIPLES AND PHILOSOPHY OF AQUATIC EXERCISE THERAPY

The Principles

The member of the rehabilitation team who is responsible for implementing the aquatic program or teaching the therapeutic exercises plays a vital role in the patient's recovery. In order to ensure a successful outcome, it is critical to obtain accurate information regarding the status of each patient and his or her condition. As discussed in Chapter 1, the data obtained must first define the anatomic structures involved, the functional limitations, and any contraindications to pool therapy. The next step is to determine the exercise goals for the patient and develop a treatment plan to achieve those goals.

The proper selection of aquatic exercises is critical. Water is an effective medium in which to exercise, provided that the instructor has adequate knowledge of the injury being treated and how the physical properties of the water influence movement. As discussed in Chapter 2, it is important to consider the responsibilities and limitations of each member of the rehabilitation team. Regardless of who is implementing the aquatic therapy program, there are some basic principles that must be followed.

1. The patient should not be afraid of the water.
2. The patient should be able to maintain a comfortable position throughout the execution of exercise. The position must be safe and involve the least amount of strain possible.
3. The therapist must securely stabilize the joints that are adjacent to the injured part during exercise of a specific body segment.
4. All movements in the water should be performed slowly and smoothly to start, or until correct mechanics is achieved.
5. For exercises performed with the head out of the water, ensure that the patient remembers to breathe; breath holding only creates tension and inhibits the relaxing benefits of warm water exercise.
6. All movements should be performed within a pain-free range or within the restraints of a given condition.
7. Each exercise must be taught carefully and demonstrated by the instructor, then repeated by the patient, to ensure biomechanical accuracy. Exercises involving the lower limbs are sometimes best demonstrated initially on the deck of the pool, so that the refraction of the water does not inhibit vision.
8. The patient must fully understand the purpose of each exercise and which muscles and body regions are primarily involved.[7]

The Philosophy

The ultimate goal of the aquatic exercises presented in this manual is to prevent dysfunction and to aid in the development, improvement, restoration, or maintenance of normal function including muscular strength and endurance, flexibility and mobility, relaxation, coordination, and, at the appropriate time, cardiovascular endurance.

Warm water immersion provides unique treatment opportunities not possible on land. Exercise can be divided into two basic categories—active and passive.

Active Exercise

Active exercises require the contraction of skeletal muscle. They may be isotonic, isometric, or isokinetic.

Isotonic exercise involves movement through a full or partial ROM during which the resistance is kept constant but the speed of movement is allowed to vary. For example, the surface area of a resistive device remains the same throughout the exercise.

Isometric exercise involves a buildup of tone in a muscle or group of muscles without movement of the body part through any part of the ROM. This is also known as a static contraction.

Isokinetic exercise is a method of exercising in which the speed is held constant throughout the movement. This is achieved by matching the resistance encountered to the force applied by the moving limb. Although the resistance encountered during movement through water does increase as the force applied by the limb increases, the speed of movement is not assured to be constant.[7, 8]

Benefits of Active and Active-Assistive Range of Motion Exercise

1. This type of exercise helps to maintain or increase the flexibility of involved muscles, promotes muscular relaxation, and increases peripheral circulation.[9]
2. Muscles can begin strengthening without the pain of active movement against gravity. In the water, buoyancy assists joint ROM and simultaneously resists movement in all directions.
3. The patient is able to strengthen the muscles without the compression forces of gravity.
4. This type of exercise helps to improve the coordination and motor skills of the patient. It provides sensory feedback from the contracting muscles.
5. Therapists can replicate athletic movements such as a soccer kick, simulate work tasks such as lifting, and practice active daily living skills. Achieving functional strength and endurance levels in the water may help the patient to maintain independence or avoid institutionalization.
6. Exercising in the water helps to reduce edema because of the hydrostatic force of water.

Passive Exercise

Passive exercises require an external force, either manual or mechanical, to perform a given action.[10] Passive movements may be physiologic or accessory. Passive physiologic movements require an outside force to create the movement and take the joint through its full ROM. Passive accessory movements are those movements that occur between the articulating surfaces of a joint during physiologic motion. These accessory movements cannot be produced actively.[3, 11] Terms such as "glide," "spin," and "roll" are used to describe accessory movements.

Benefits of Passive Range of Motion Exercise

1. Passive ROM exercises help maintain the integrity and flexibility of the joint and surrounding soft tissues. In the water, gravity is eliminated and buoyancy assists movement, making it easier.
2. This type of exercise helps to prevent or minimize muscle tightness or shortening (contracture).
3. It can promote muscular relaxation, and it helps to stimulate circulation in the submerged body parts. This is possible because the body stays warm throughout the entire session.
4. Pain is inhibited. Passive ROM exercises in the water eliminate the compression forces exerted on painful joints. In addition, the sensory input caused by warm water immersion competes with the pain input, thus reducing pain levels.
5. Patients are able to begin the rehabilitative process earlier than would be possible on land.
6. Passive ROM exercises help to improve body and movement awareness.
7. The therapist is able to comfortably position awkward patients or those with a lot of pain in the water in order to achieve a variety of movements.
8. Passive ROM exercise helps to reduce spasticity and tone.
9. Passive ROM exercise, however, can neither stop muscle wasting, increase muscular strength and endurance, nor benefit circulation as well as active motion does.[5]

Exercise Protocols

Many therapeutic pools are not used to their full capacity because they are not seen to be cost-effective. It is often thought that it takes too much of a therapist's time to treat a patient in a pool. In order to survive, a rehabilitation facility must provide quick and effective treatment. The rehabilitative protocols outlined in this book are designed to assist the health care professional in prescribing effective aquatic programs that encourage patient independence. This is accomplished, in part, by having set protocols for common conditions. There are many benefits of having a set protocol for the treatment of a common condition:

1. The therapist saves time by not having to write out a given patient's routine.
2. Treatment can be individualized by making minor additions to or deletions from the set routine.
3. Another health care professional can implement the prescribed protocol, leaving time for the therapist to see other patients.
4. The therapist has control over how and when the patient progresses (by prescribing more difficult phases of a set protocol). Even if there is no therapeutic pool located in the rehabilitation facility, the patient can perform the clearly outlined exercise routines in a pool outside the facility and then return to the therapist for reassessment and progression to the next phase or level.
5. The therapist saves time in the documentation of a patient's progress by simply stating which phase of a given protocol the patient is working in.
6. The therapist can prescribe home aquatic exercise programs that are understandable and easy to increase in difficulty.
7. Community aquatic instructors can understand the types of exercises the patient should be doing.
8. Set protocols help to facilitate communications between members of the rehabilitation team.

Set protocols also encourage patient independence during the rehabilitation process. Independent programs can benefit both the therapist and the patient because they allow the therapist to treat a greater number of patients at the same time, therefore increasing profit and making programs more economically feasible; to assign aquatic exercises as part of a patient's home program; and to use the benefits of aquatic exercise therapy even if there is no pool within the rehabilitation facility. The patient also benefits from independent and class aquatic therapy programs. Such programs encourage the patient to take an active role in recovery and help to improve the patient's social interaction during a class or scheduled outing to the pool.

AQUATIC ORTHOPEDIC REHABILITATION AND EXERCISE

The aquatic exercises presented in this chapter represent an innovative approach to aquatic rehabilitation. Each exercise makes use of the physical properties and warmth unique to therapeutic waters. Progressive protocols are provided for each condition to help return the patient to land-based exercises, if possible. The descriptions are worded for the benefit of the therapist, but therapists are encouraged to use their own teaching styles to convey the essence of the exercises to patients.

Each of the exercises in this chapter is described in terms of joint movements (see Table 5–1). Anatomic terms of reference are given for some exercises to provide further clarity. The prime movers for each exercise are given, and the progressive phases can be applied to increase the difficulty of each exercise with respect to the patient's condition.

The Warm-up

The warm-up has an accepted role in almost all exercise programs. The warm-up usually occupies 20% to 30% of the total exercise period and should be performed at a low intensity. A gradual beginning to any exercise program helps to reduce the risk of muscular injuries.[12]

In a rehabilitative setting, the benefits of a warm-up cannot be ignored. One of the most significant physiologic changes that occurs during the warm-up is an increase in temperature within the cells of the involved muscles. This is accompanied by an increase in metabolic rate of these cells. The rate of metabolic change is temperature sensitive. That is, for each degree of internal temperature rise, there is a corresponding rise in the rate of metabolism of about 13%.[13, 14]

The higher the temperature, the greater the rates of biologic or enzymatic reactions at a cellular level. This leads to faster and more complete dissociation of oxygen from hemoglobin and myoglobin, which improves the transportation and utilization of oxygen during exercise.[13, 15] Therefore, warm-up exercises in warm water help make the muscles ready to perform sooner and more efficient at transporting and utilizing the available oxygen.

Upper Body Warm-up Exercises

Bent Arm Pull (Fig. 5–12)

Prime movers: anterior deltoid, pectoralis minor, latissimus dorsi, teres major, rhomboids, trapezius, biceps, brachialis, triceps, and brachioradialis.

- Reach forward with the involved arm
- Pull the arm back with a bent elbow, extending the arm only at the shoulder

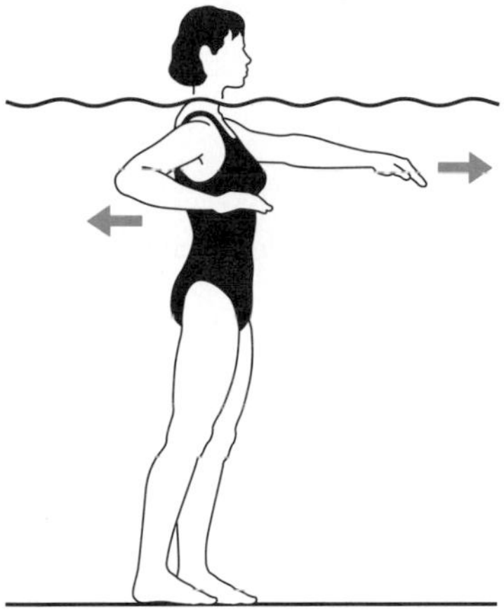

FIGURE 5–12. Bent arm pull.

Straight Arm Pull (Fig. 5 13)

Prime movers: deltoids, supinator, pronator quadratus, latissimus dorsi, pectoralis minor, rhomboids, and trapezius triceps.

- Keeping the elbow straight, supinate one hand (turn palm up) and push the arm in front of the body
- At the same time, pronate the other hand (turn palm down) and push the arm behind the body
- Repeat, switching arms

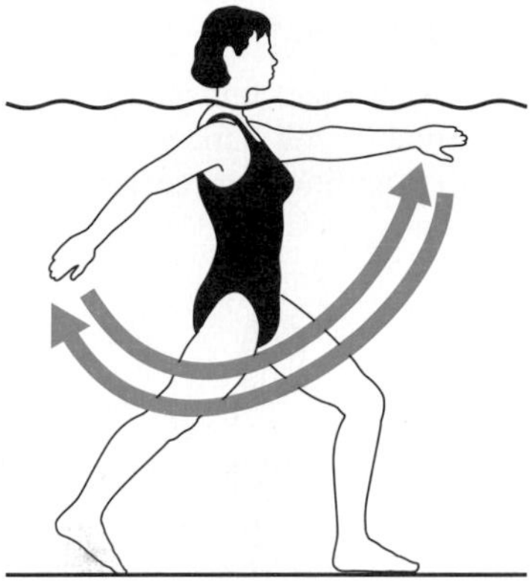

FIGURE 5–13. Straight arm pull.

Breast Stroke (Fig. 5–14)

Prime movers: deltoids, pectoralis major, pectoralis minor, coracobrachialis, infraspinatus, teres minor, rhomboids, and trapezius.

- Reach forward with both arms
- Horizontally abduct the arms until they are in the same plane as the body
- Bend the elbows to 90° and adduct the arms to the midline

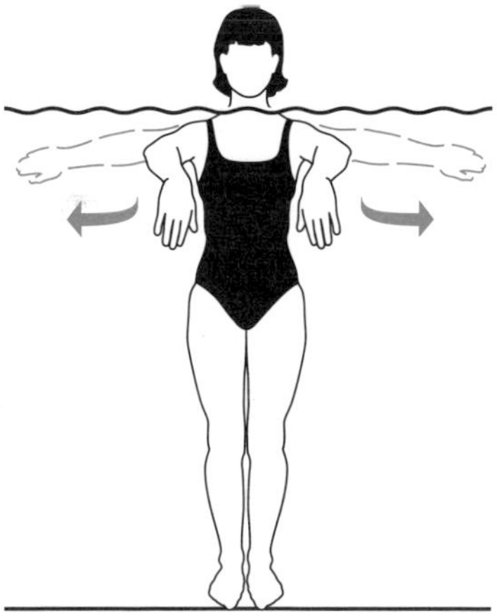

FIGURE 5–14. Breast stroke.

Cross-Body Pull (Fig. 5–15)

Similar to Breast Stroke, but perform the exercise one arm at a time (other hand on hip). Rotate the trunk toward the midline and reach across the body during adduction

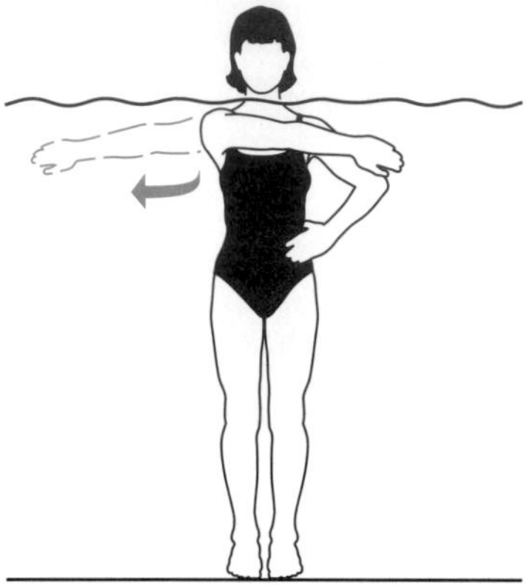

FIGURE 5–15. Cross-body pull.

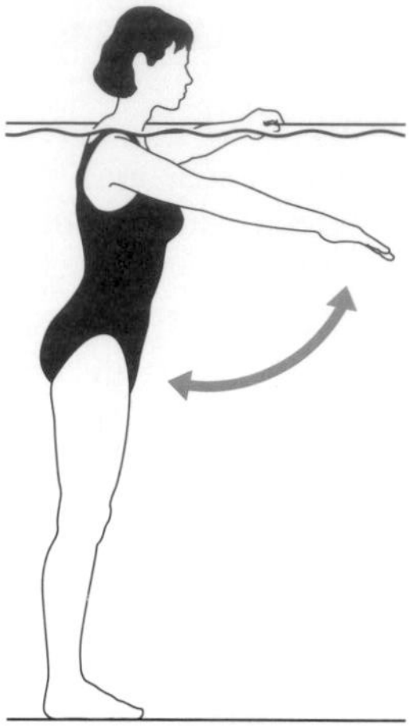

FIGURE 5–16. Pendulum exercise, front to back.

Pendulum Exercises

For this group of exercises, wrist weights may be used if the therapist wishes to create a manipulative effect on the involved joint, if the limb is too flaccid (floats easily) and the patient is having difficulty performing the pendulum movements, or if the therapist wants to increase the difficulty of the exercise by increasing the effect of gravity.

Pendulum Front to Back (Fig. 5–16)

Prime movers: anterior deltoid, pectoralis minor, latissimus dorsi, and teres minor.

- Stand straight with the uninvolved hand on the hip or on the edge of the pool
- Swing the opposite arm forward and back by flexing and then extending at the shoulder

Pendulum Circles (Fig. 5–17)

Prime movers: deltoids, pectoralis, supraspinatus, latissimus dorsi, and teres major.

- Stand straight with the uninvolved hand on the hip or on the edge of the pool
- Move the opposite arm in a circle clockwise, then counterclockwise

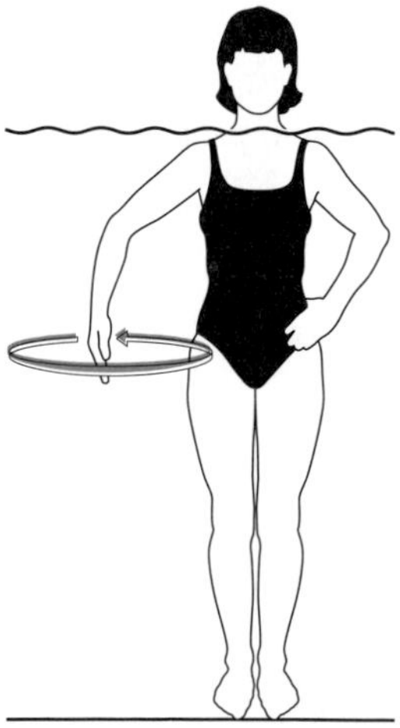

FIGURE 5–17. Pendulum exercise, circles.

Pendulum Pulls (Fig. 5–18)

Prime movers: rhomboids, deltoids, teres major, trapezius, latissimus dorsi, pectoralis, biceps, brachialis, and brachioradialis. *Action performed:* shoulder protraction and retraction.

- Stand straight with the uninvolved hand on the hip or on the edge of the pool
- Reach out in front of the body with the opposite arm
- Pull the arm back, retracting the shoulder blades and flexing the elbow

Pendulum Crisscross (Fig. 5–19)

Prime movers: for abduction, medial and posterior deltoids, infraspinatus, teres minor, latissimus dorsi, and teres major; for adduction, anterior deltoid, pectoralis major, pectoralis minor, coracobrachialis, and biceps brachii. *Action performed:* horizontal abduction and adduction.

- Stand straight with the uninvolved hand on the hip or on the edge of the pool
- Horizontally abduct and then adduct the opposite arm, swinging the arm from side to side in front of the body

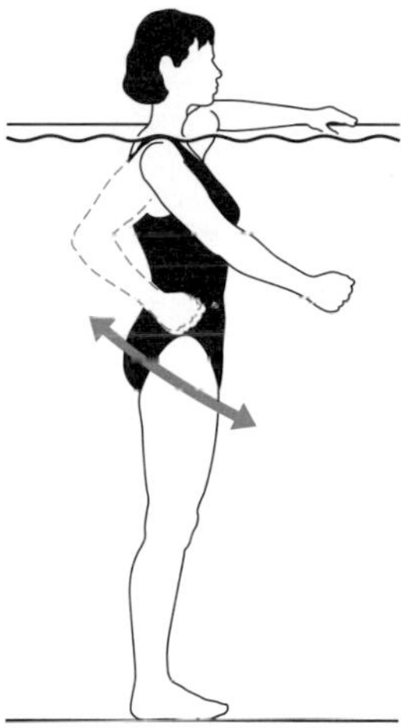

FIGURE 5–18. Pendulum exercise, pulls.

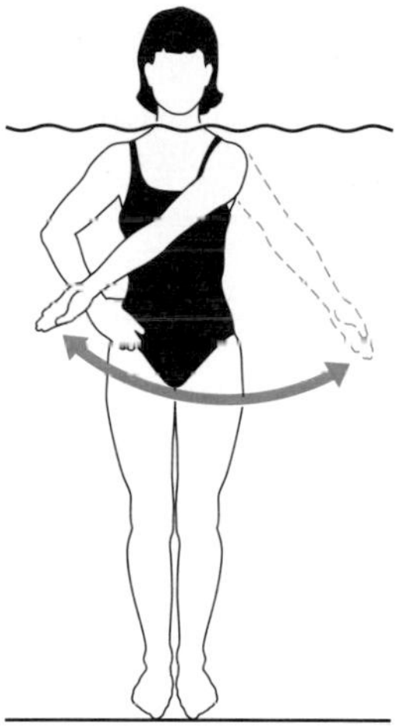

FIGURE 5–19. Pendulum exercise, crisscross.

Combination Arm Movements (Fig. 5–20)

This exercise consists of three parts performed in sequence.

Part A

Prime movers: deltoids, pectoralis, and trapezius.

- Extend the arms at the sides, parallel to the floor but slightly below 90°

Part B

Prime movers: deltoids, rhomboids, trapezius, latissimus dorsi, and teres major.

- Circle the arms backward four times
- Join the hands behind the back
- Straighten the arms and gently pull upward, then extend the arms to the original position

Part C

Prime movers: biceps brachii, brachialis, brachioradialis, triceps, pectoralis major, pectoralis minor, rhomboids, and trapezius.

- Circle the arms forward four times
- Join the hands in front of the chest
- Push forward, straightening the elbows and protracting the shoulder blades

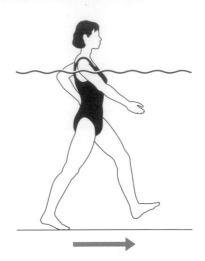

FIGURE 5–21. Forward walking.

Lower Body Warm-up Exercises

Forward Walking (Fig. 5–21)

Prime movers: iliopsoas, rectus femoris, pectineus, gluteus maximus, hamstrings, quadriceps, gastrocnemius, and soleus.

- Standing upright, flex one hip and knee
- Extend the leg and dorsiflex the ankle, landing on the heel
- Roll forward onto the toes and push off
- Repeat with the opposite leg

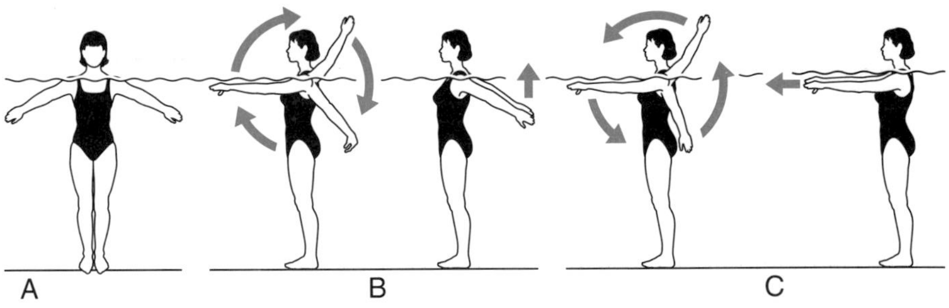

FIGURE 5–20. Combination arm movements done in three steps (A–C).

Backward Walking (Fig. 5–22)

Prime movers: iliopsoas, rectus femoris, pectineus, gluteus maximus, hamstrings, quadriceps, gastrocnemius, and soleus.

- Standing upright, flex one hip and knee
- Extend the leg posteriorly, behind the body
- Plantar flex the ankle, landing on the toes
- Gently roll onto the heel
- Repeat with the opposite leg

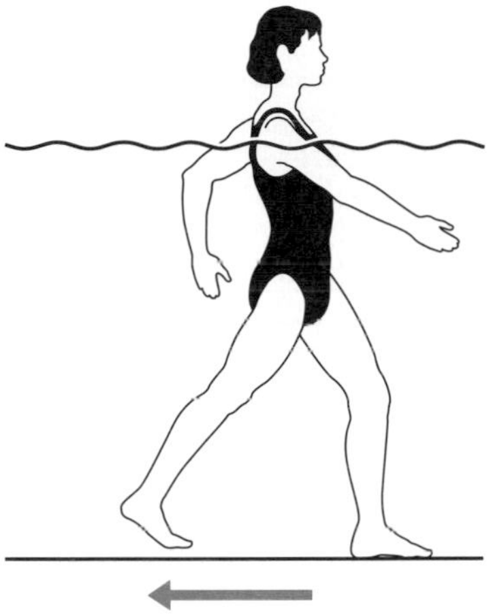

FIGURE 5–22. Backward walking.

Side Stepping (Fig. 5–23)

Prime movers: gluteus medius, iliopsoas, sartorius, rectus femoris, tensor fasciae latae, gluteus minimus, pectineus, gracilis, adductor longus, adductor brevis, and adductor magnus.

- Stand upright with the legs straight
- Abduct one leg and contact the foot to the floor
- Adduct the opposite leg to the midline, returning to a standing position
- Repeat in the opposite direction

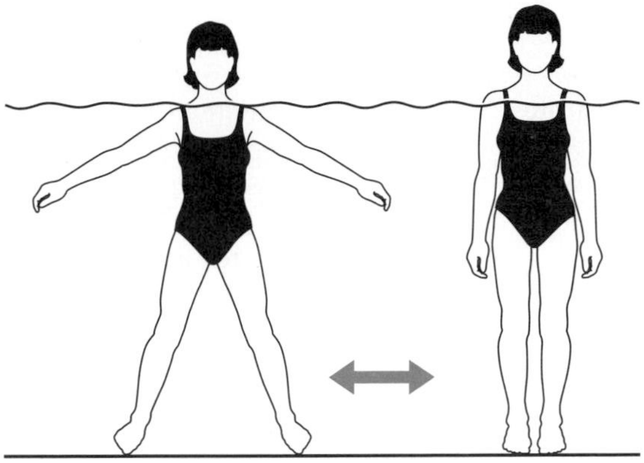

FIGURE 5–23. Side stepping.

Crossover Stepping (Fig. 5–24)

Prime movers: gluteus medius, iliopsoas, sartorius, rectus femoris, tensor fasciae latae, gluteus minimus, pectineus, gracilis, adductor longus, adductor brevis, and adductor magnus.

- Standing upright, adduct one leg, crossing the midline, and contacting the foot to the floor
- Abduct the opposite leg to return to a standing position

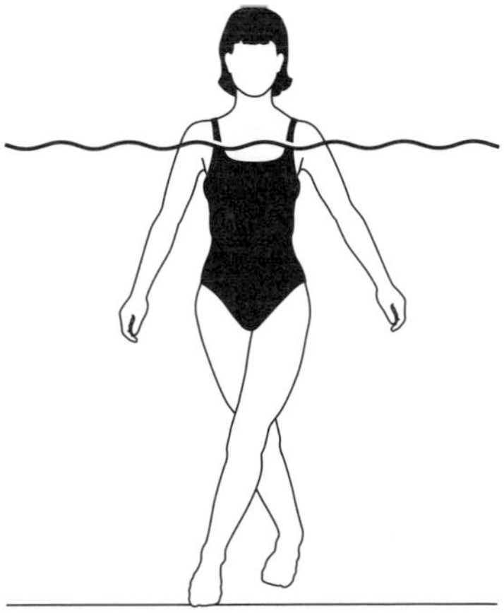

FIGURE 5–24. Crossover stepping.

Stiff Leg Walking (Fig. 5–25)

Prime movers: hip flexors, gluteus maximus, and hamstrings. There are three variations of this exercise.

- Variation 1: Stand upright and walk forward with little or no knee flexion, with a slight heel-toe action
- Variation 2: Perform the exercise on the toes, maintaining plantar flexion (no heel contact with floor)
- Variation 3: Perform the exercise on the heels, maintaining dorsiflexion (no toe contact with floor)

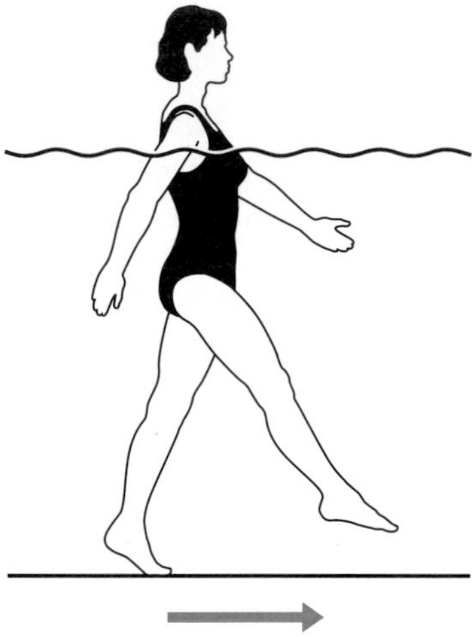

FIGURE 5–25. Stiff leg walking (variation 2).

Lunge Walking (Fig. 5–26)

Prime movers: same as for Forward Walking.

- Keeping the trunk upright, walk forward using large steps
- Flex the knee of the leading leg while keeping the knee of the trailing leg straight
- Keep the trunk upright and the abdominals tight

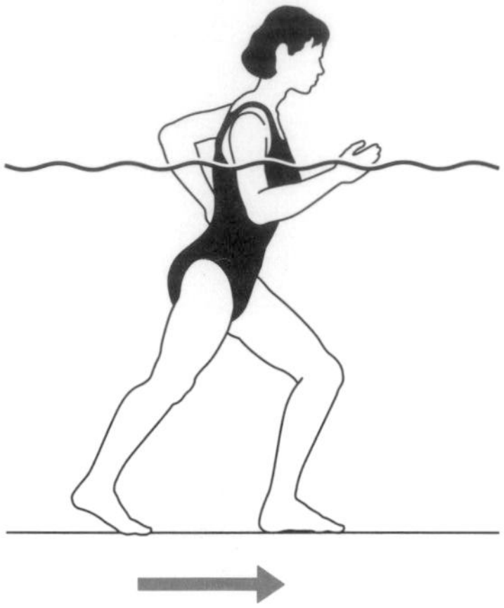

FIGURE 5–26. Lunge walking.

Walking with Tray (Fig. 5–27)

Prime movers: same as for Forward Walking. Use of the tray increases the resistance during performance of the lower body exercises already described (see Figs. 5–21 through 5–26). Some pointers:

- Hold the tray in front of the body during forward or backward walking
- Maintain a pelvic tilt and correct postural alignment
- When walking sideways, hold the tray under the water and over the hip on the leading side

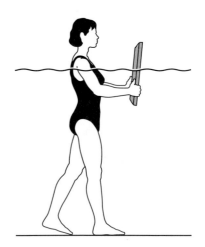

FIGURE 5–27. Walking with tray.

Marching (Fig. 5–28)

Prime movers: hip flexors, gluteus maximus, sartorius, quadriceps, hamstrings, hip abductors, gastrocnemius, soleus, deltoids, pectoralis, rhomboids, and biceps.

- Standing upright, flex one hip and knee to 90°
- Bring the leg down and flex the opposite hip and knee in a marching action
- Emphasize a comfortable arm action

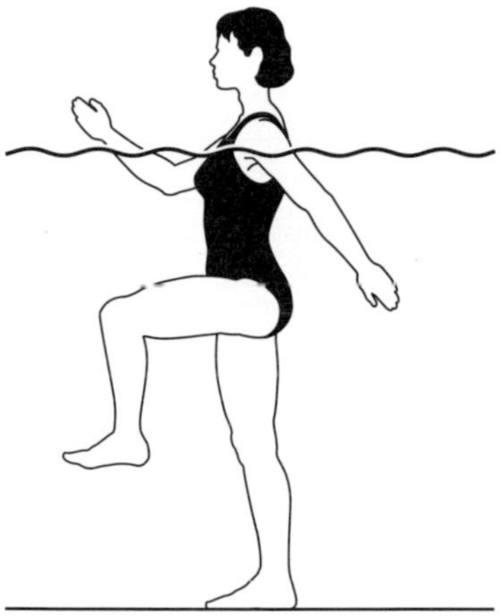

FIGURE 5–28. Marching.

Leg Exchange (Fig. 5–29)

Prime movers: hip flexors, gluteus maximus, and hamstrings.

- Start with the right arm and left leg forward and the left arm and right leg back
- Perform a cross-country ski action, jumping up in order to switch the leg and arm positions
- Bend the knees to absorb the impact (the deeper the water, the less the impact)

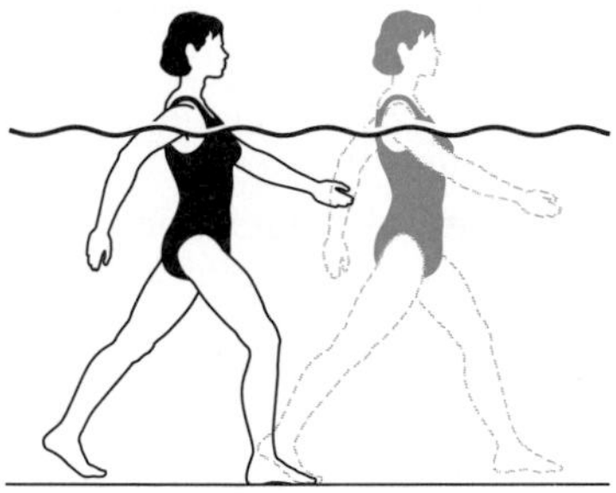

FIGURE 5–29. Leg exchange.

Jogging (Fig. 5–30)

Prime movers: same as for Forward Walking.

- Standing upright, alternately flex and extend one and then the other hip and knee, performing a jogging action in one spot
- The deeper the water, the less the impact on the spine and joints of the lower extremity
- The exercise should be performed at a speed that is comfortable for the patient; at this stage, the correct movement sequence is more important than an aerobic response

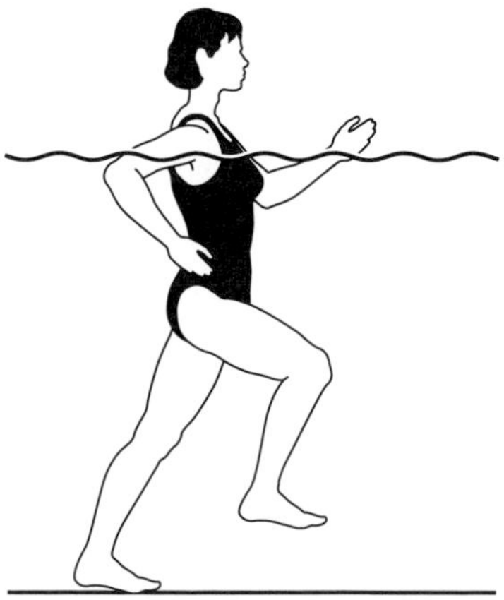

FIGURE 5–30. Jogging.

Bicycle (Fig. 5–31)

Prime movers: hip flexors, gluteus maximus, quadriceps, and hamstrings.

- Use a tube or flotation device for support, and keep the spine straight by tightening the abdominals
- Alternately flex and extend one and then the other hip and knee, reaching out with the leg to perform a vertical cycling action

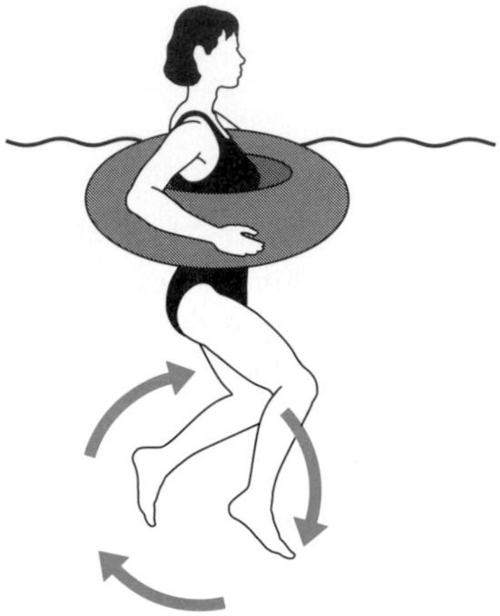

FIGURE 5–31. Bicycle.

Pelvic Movements (Fig. 5–32)

Prime movers: rectus abdominis, sacrospinalis, and quadratus lumborum.

- Stand with the feet shoulder-width apart and arms extended parallel to the floor (neutral position)
- Focus the eyes forward and slightly bend the knees
- Move the hips in sequence forward, to the neutral position, backward, to the neutral position, to the right side, to the left side, and back to the neutral position

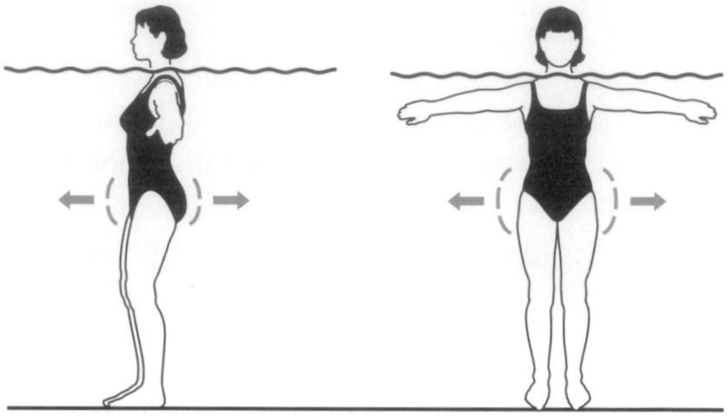

FIGURE 5–32. Pelvic movements.

REFERENCES

1. Hollinshead W, Jenkins D. Functional Anatomy of the Limbs and Back. Philadelphia, W.B. Saunders, 1981.
2. Rasch P, Burke R. Kinesiology and Applied Anatomy. Philadelphia, Lea & Febiger, 1972.
3. Gould J, Davis G. Orthopaedic and Sports Physical Therapy. Toronto, C.V. Mosby, 1985.
4. Green W, Heckman J. The Clinical Measurement of Joint Motion. Rosemont, IL: American Academy of Orthopaedic Surgeons, 1994.
5. Norkin CC, White DJ. Measurement of Joint Motion: A Guide to Goniometry. Philadelphia, F.A. Davis, 1985.
6. Arnheim D. Modern Principles of Athletic Training. Toronto, Times Mirror/Mosby College Publishing, 1985.
7. Kisner C, Colby L. Therapeutic Exercise: Foundations and Techniques. 2nd ed. Philadelphia, F.A. Davis, 1990.
8. McCarthey P, Knopf K. Adapted Physical Education for Adults with Disabilities. 3rd ed. Iowa, Eddie Bowers, 1992.
9. Hoppenfeld S. Physical Examination of the Spine and Extremities. New York, Appleton-Century-Crofts, 1976.
10. Magee D. Orthopaedic Physical Assessment. Philadelphia, W.B. Saunders, 1987.
11. Nafziger N, Lee S, Huang S: Passive exercise system: Effect on muscle activity, strength, and lean body mass. Arch Phys Med Rehabil 73:184–189, 1981.
12. Krejci V, Koch P. Muscle and Tendon Injuries in Athletes. Chicago, Year Book Medical Publishers, 1976.
13. Brooks G, Fahey T. Exercise Physiology. Toronto, John Wiley & Sons, 1984.
14. Licht S, ed. Medical Climatology. Baltimore, Waverly Press, 1964.
15. Martin BJ, Robinson S, Wiegman DL, Anlik LH. Effects of warm-up on metabolic responses to strenuous exercise. Med Sci Sports Exer 7:146, 1975.

Chapter 6

Exercising in Deep Water

THE BENEFICIAL PROPERTIES OF DEEP WATER EXERCISE

Deep water exercise can play an important role in aquatic rehabilitation. The versatility of the movements and the fact that the patient does not need to know how to swim allow deep water exercise programs to be implemented in a variety of settings for a number of conditions. The therapeutic benefits of exercising in deep water accentuate several characteristics associated with aquatic exercise.

The most obvious benefit of deep water exercise is that there is no impact or contact with the pool floor or walls. The movement of a given body part stops when the end of range of motion is reached or when the patient willingly stops the movement.

In either case, there is no impact force placed on the body because it is not working against a fixed resistance. Deep water exercise therefore can be referred to as an open kinetic chain. In contrast, when a given body part or joint moves against a fixed resistance, such as the pool floor, a closed kinetic chain is formed. Shallow water exercises performed in a vertical position are an example of a closed kinetic chain.[1] Repetitive strain injuries, such as stress fractures, benefit tremendously from the zero impact aspect of deep water exercise.

Because gravity works in opposition to buoyancy, in the water its effect is hardly noticeable. When a person is in contact with the earth (either sitting or standing), gravity has a compressive effect on the joints of the lower extremities and spine. During deep water exercise, buoyancy supports the body and protects the weight-bearing joints. Because the amount of loading experienced by the body is a function of immersion, there is no pain from impact forces during exercise.[2]

In deep water, the patient's spine experiences a mild traction effect. This occurs primarily because the compressive force of gravity is counteracted by the buoyant effect of water. The effect can be increased by the use of weights on the hips or ankles along with a flotation tube held at chest level. Gravity pulls the feet toward the floor while the chest flotation maintains the position of the upper body (Fig. 6–1). During this traction, intradiscal pressure decreases, foraminal size may increase, and there may be some gapping of the facet joints. This effect often allows patients with low back problems to exercise with considerably less discomfort. It is important to remember, however, that the spine should be loaded gradually at the end of the session.

USING DEEP WATER IN REHABILITATION

Maintaining Muscular Strength and Endurance

The literature documenting increases in muscular strength and endurance with deep water exercise is sparse and is generally limited to specific populations such as patients with multiple sclerosis.[3] Water running has been found to be effective in maintaining leg strength in runners.[4] Based on our clinical observations, deep water exercise is also beneficial for sedentary patients who want to maintain or increase their strength level while recovering from an injury. Those with weaker muscles exhibit greater observed strength gains. Because all body parts from the neck down are submerged under the water, there is a greater surface area of resistance

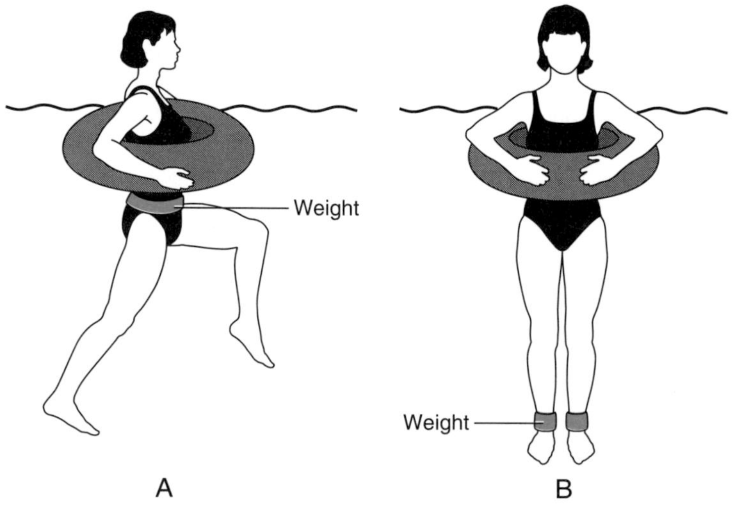

FIGURE 6–1. Floating traction using a flotation tube with (*A*) a diving weight belt around the hips or (*B*) weights suspended from the ankles.

during exercise. The movements use all the major muscle groups, working the prime movers and antagonistic muscles alternately. This reciprocal strengthening provides muscular balance through the full range of motion and helps to reveal any imbalances that may exist. Because the hydrostatic pressure that acts on the submerged parts is equal and constant, imbalances may be identified and corrected. Hydrostatic pressure also provides resistance to chest expansion in deep water. The intercostals and diaphragm must work harder, thereby strengthening the muscles involved in breathing.

The resistance experienced by the body or its parts also depends on the amount of force exerted in the water. Resistance increases in response to the force exerted and stops instantly when the force is removed. This allows maximum control so that the patient can exercise within a manageable pain range.[5]

During aquatic exercise, there is essentially no eccentric muscle activity. The resistance of the water slows the movement of a limb so that the patient's muscles don't have to. During water walking and running, only one-half to one-third the speed is required to produce the same metabolic intensity observed on land.[6] This reduces risk of muscle or bone microtrauma, which may occur during the eccentric component of land-based exercise. Shin splints are a good example of this type of overuse injury. By not stressing the injured tissue, patients are actually resting the injury while they continue to exercise. Because many athletes do not like to "rest" anything, deep water exercise can be an important part of their rehabilitation.

Improving Fitness Level

Deep water exercises can be used to maintain or improve aerobic conditioning during the healing process. They can also be used as a progression to more difficult levels of exercise. As the patient progresses in recovery from injury, a general fitness program may be indicated.

The metabolic responses observed in deep water running are significantly different from those in land-based running.[7] During deep water running, maximum oxygen uptake (Vo_2max) and maximal heat rate tend to be lower than during treadmill running.[8] The principles and guidelines for aerobic conditioning are discussed in further detail in Chapter 17. High-intensity, long-duration activities should not be performed in warm water. Ideally, aerobic activities should be performed in water that is between 82° and 86°F (28°–30°C) in order to prevent the body from storing heat during exercise.[8]

Correct Body Alignment

A deep water belt or vest helps the patient maintain a correct vertical alignment during exercise. The water line should be at shoulder level with the head comfortably out of the water even when the neck is slightly flexed. When exercises are performed in deep water, the body should be held vertically, the chest should be lifted, and the abdominals and gluteal muscles should be contracted slightly (Fig. 6–2). On land, the center of gravity is located at the symphysis pubis (about S1 or S2); during immersion in water from the neck down, the center of gravity shifts to the chest (pleural cavity). This difference creates a turning effect (or buoyancy torque) that causes the body to rotate around the chest if the body is not floating in a neutral position. During water exercise, the patient must actively counteract this torque. Severely weak or deconditioned patients (eg, those with accelerated amyotrophic lateral sclerosis) should not perform water exercise because it could pose a safety hazard if they were unable to return to a standing position.

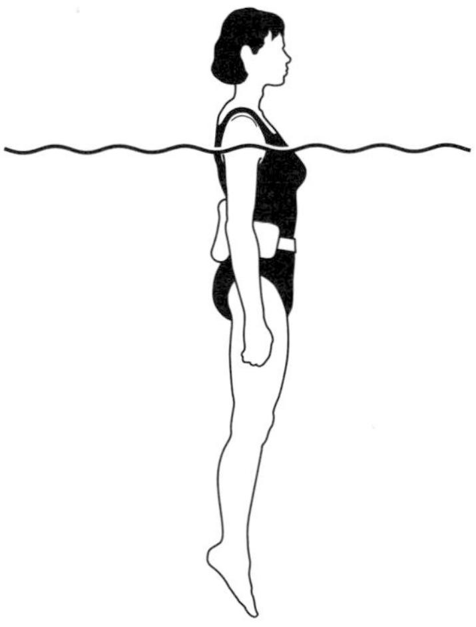

FIGURE 6–2. Correct vertical alignment (starting position) for deep water exercises.

During deep water running, the body is tilted slightly forward, approximately 5° past the vertical, with the spine in neutral position (Fig. 6–3). This bend should occur at the hips, not at the waist. The biomechanical movement pattern of water running resembles that used on land. Proper form requires the following:

1. The head is held comfortably out of the water, facing forward; avoid neck extension.
2. The spine is in neutral position, slightly forward of the vertical.
3. The arm action is the same as for land running, with the primary movement occurring at the shoulder and with the hands relaxed but lightly closed.
4. Hip flexion reaches approximately 60° to 80° at the same time the knees flex or extend.
5. The ankle undergoes plantar flexion and dorsiflexion.[8]

Symmetry is necessary during all exercises. If one side of the body is working harder than the other, it will be impossible to maintain a correct vertical position, and any muscular imbalances will therefore become evident. During execution of an exercise, correct body position is critical. Leaning too far forward or too far back creates a turning effect or torque in the water. Because there is no contact with the pool floor, the patient's trunk muscles must act to stabilize the body as the limbs are moved. This does not build strength and power in these muscles, but it does improve coordination and proprioception. This is particularly beneficial to the patient with a hypermobile spine (eg, in spondylolisthesis).

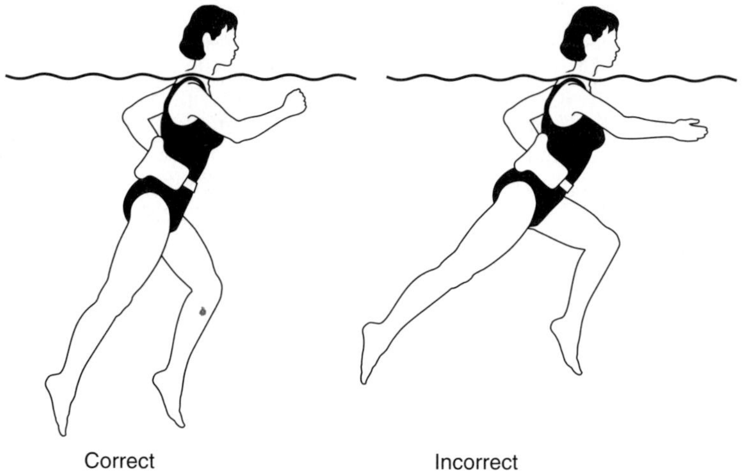

FIGURE 6–3. Correct position for deep water running.

DEEP WATER EXERCISES FOR THE UPPER BODY

Bent Arm Pull (Fig. 6–4)

- Assume vertical position
- Reach forward with one arm
- Pull the arm back with a bent elbow as other arm comes forward
- Repeat with the other arm

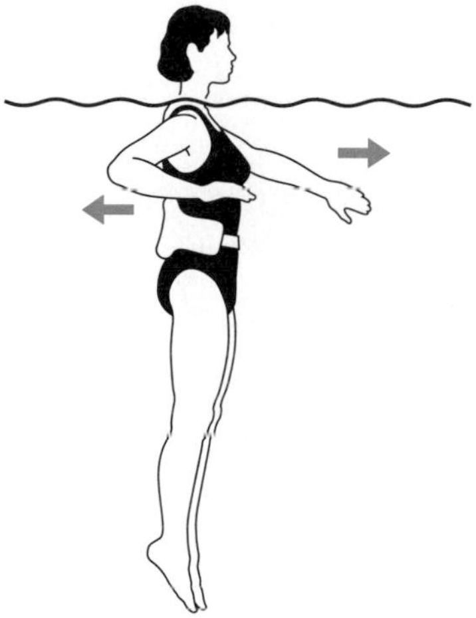

FIGURE 6–4. Deep water bent arm pull.

Straight Arm Pull (Fig. 6–5)

- Assume vertical position
- Keeping the elbow straight, supinate one hand (turn palm up) and push the arm in front of the body
- At the same time, pronate the other hand (turn palm down) and push the arm behind the body
- Repeat, switching arms

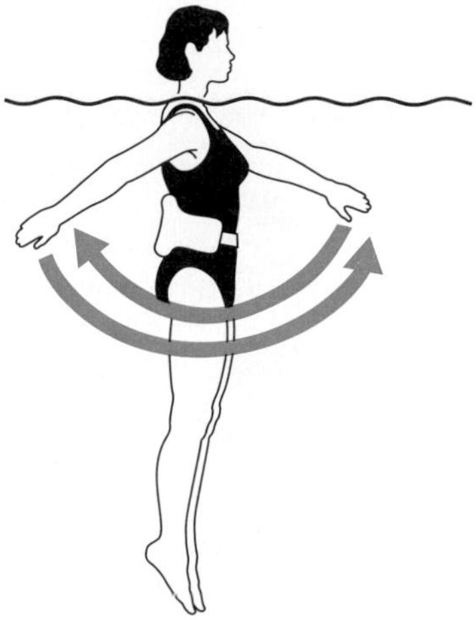

FIGURE 6–5. Deep water straight arm pull.

Shoulder Circles (Fig. 6 6)

- Assume vertical position
- Reach the arms out to the sides 45° below the surface of the water
- Keeping the elbows straight, move the arms in circles
- Continue the circular movement, varying the size

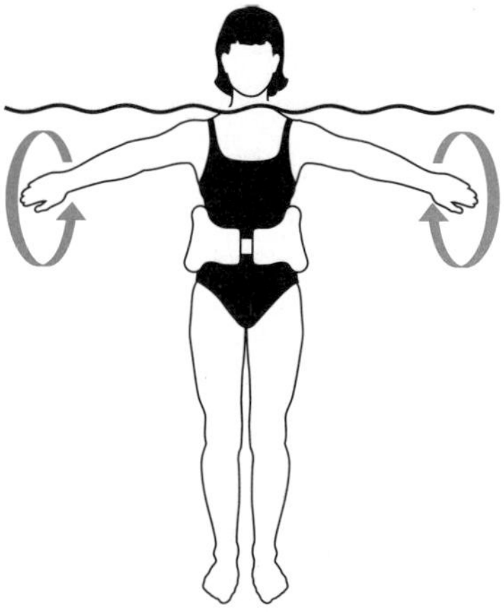

FIGURE 6–6. Deep water shoulder circles.

Breast Stroke (Fig. 6–7)

- Perform Breast Stroke as described in Chapter 5 (see Fig. 5–14)

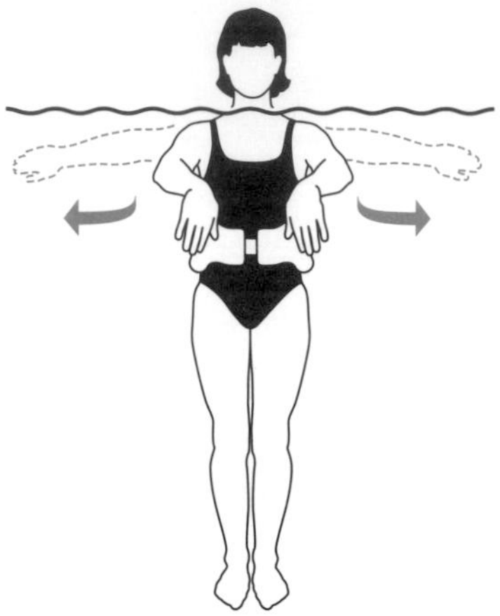

FIGURE 6–7. Deep water breast stroke.

Shoulder Press (Fig. 6–8)

- Assume vertical position
- Simultaneously press both hands forward from the chest

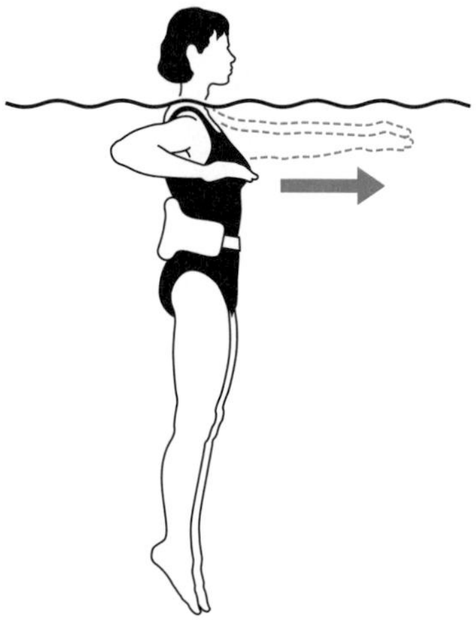

FIGURE 6–8. Deep water shoulder press.

Elbow Press (Fig. 6–9)

- Assume vertical position
- Alternately flex one elbow and extend the other, so that the lower arms move up and down in front of the body

VARIATION. Perform movement with both arms simultaneously

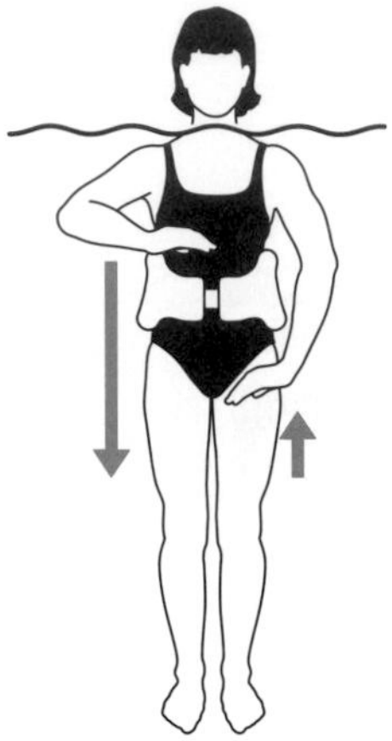

FIGURE 6–9. Deep water elbow press.

Wave (Fig. 6–10)

- Assume vertical position
- Extend the arms out horizontally to the sides
- Keep the elbows straight
- Alternately flex one wrist while extending the other

VARIATION. Perform movement with both wrists simultaneously

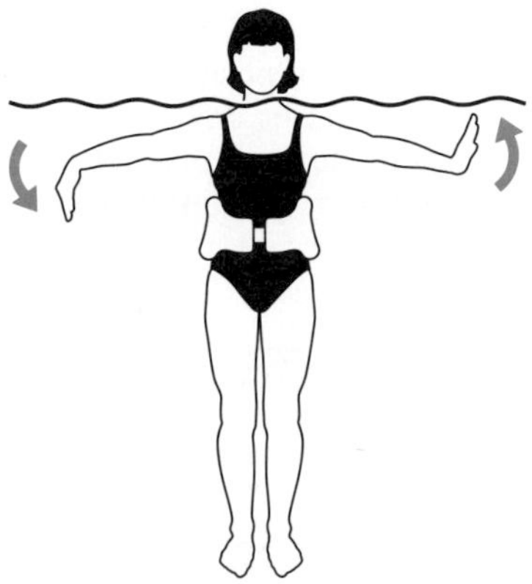

FIGURE 6–10. Deep water wave.

Wrist Side Press (Fig. 6–11)

- Assume vertical position
- Flex the elbows and wrists
- Straighten the elbows, keeping the wrists flexed

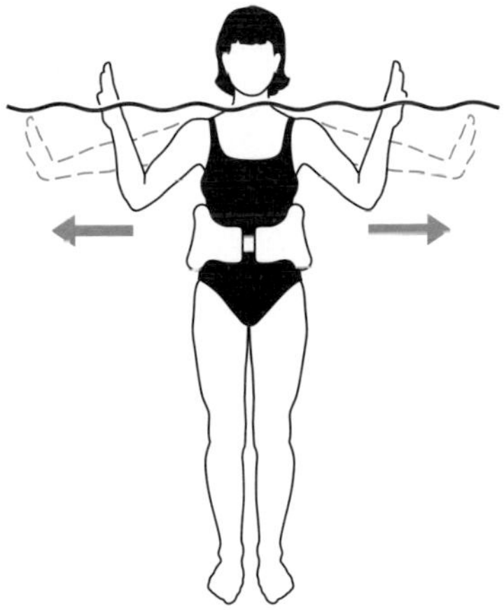

FIGURE 6–11. Deep water wrist side press.

DEEP WATER EXERCISES FOR THE LOWER BODY

Many of these exercises may be performed with handheld floats for greater stability and reduced arm involvement. Exercises that are suitable for this variation are marked with an asterisk.

Running (Fig. 6–12)

- Assume vertical position with the abdominals contracted
- Tilt the torso forward 5°
- Perform a running action, using both arm and leg movements

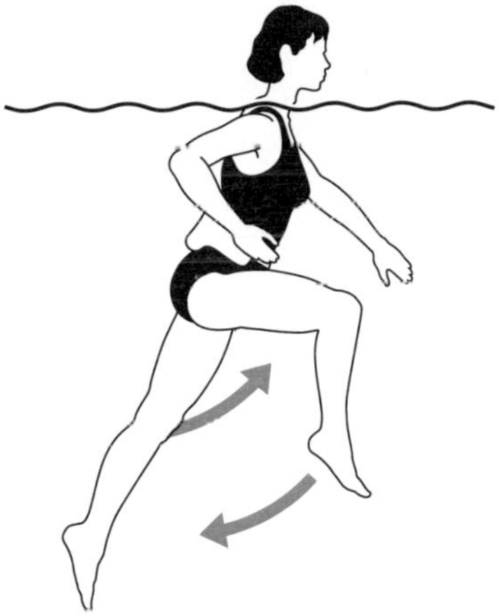

FIGURE 6–12. Deep water running.

Walking (Fig. 6–13)

- Assume vertical position
- Alternately flex and extend the hips and knees, performing a walking action
- Allow the arms to swing opposite from the legs

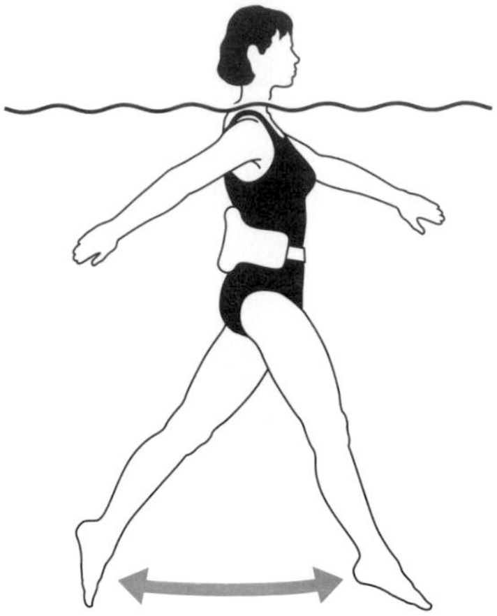

FIGURE 6–13. Deep water walking.

Sit Cycle (Fig. 6–14)

- Assume vertical position
- Flex the hips to 90° (seated position)
- Perform a cycling action with the legs, keeping the trunk vertical and the legs in front of the body

VARIATION. Perform cycling motion in vertical position

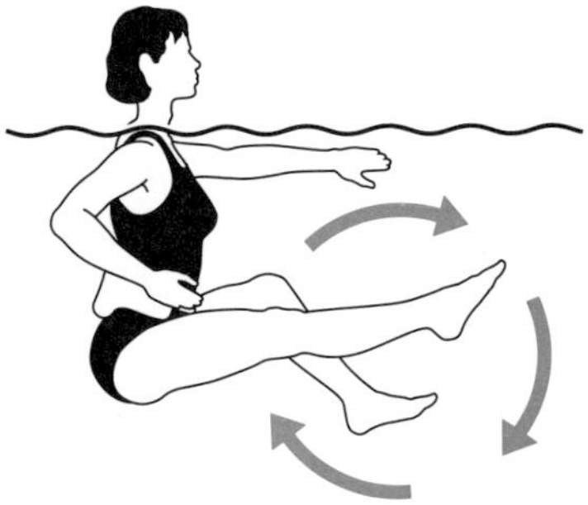

FIGURE 6–14. Deep water sit cycle.

Cross-Country Skiing (Fig. 6–15)

- Assume vertical position
- Keeping the arms and legs straight, alternately flex and extend the hips and shoulders, performing a cross-country ski action

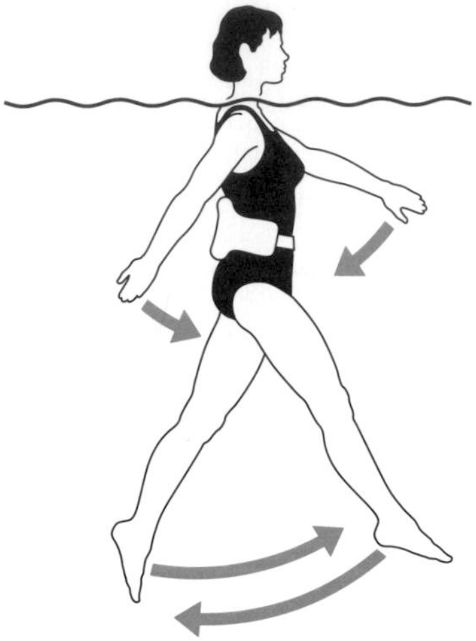

FIGURE 6–15. Deep water cross-country skiing.

Stride Jump (Fig. 6–16)

- Assume vertical position
- Keep the elbows and knees straight
- Simultaneously abduct both hips and adduct the shoulders
- Then simultaneously adduct both hips to the midline while abducting the shoulders

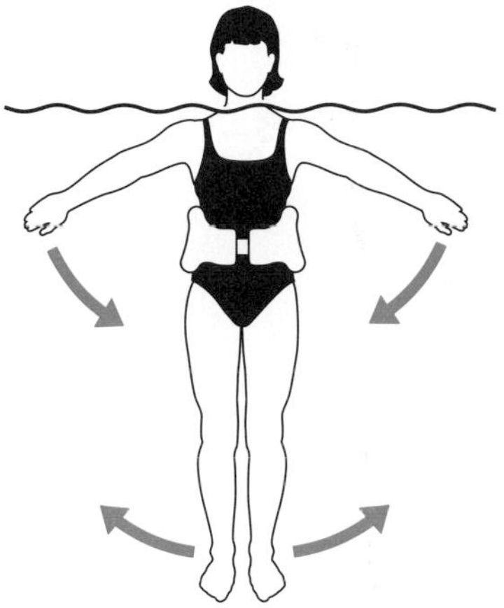

FIGURE 6–16. Deep water stride jump.

Cross-Stride Jump (Fig. 6–17)

- Perform Stride Jump, but abduct the hips past the midline (legs cross)

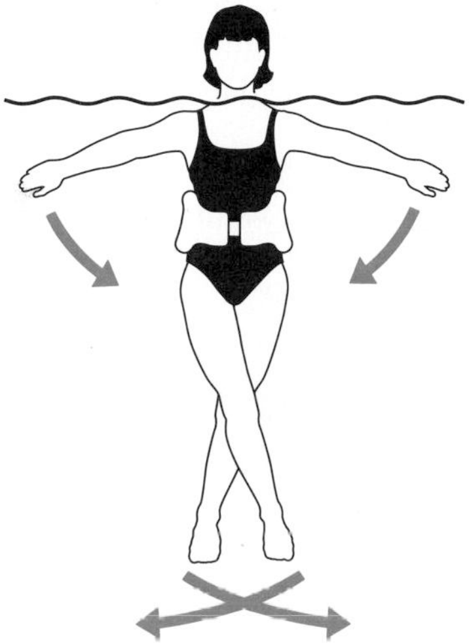

FIGURE 6–17. Deep water cross-stride jump.

Double Knee Lift (Fig. 6–18)

- Assume vertical position
- Keeping the legs together, bring both knees toward the chest
- Lower the legs and repeat

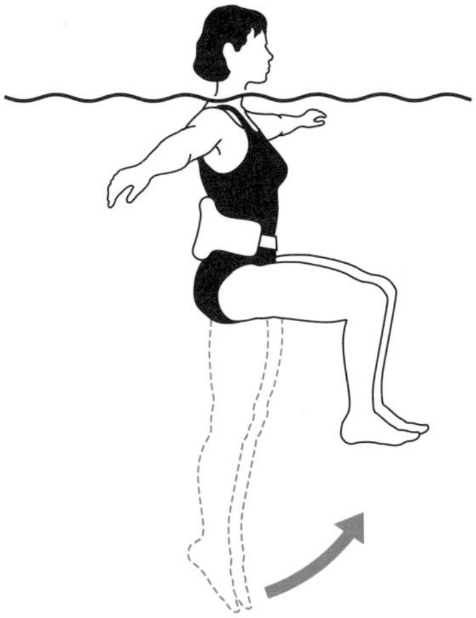

FIGURE 6–18. Deep water double knee lift.

Flutter Kick (Fig. 6–19)

- Assume vertical position
- Keep the hips and knees extended
- Plantar flex the ankle
- Alternately flex and extend the hips, creating a quick, "fluttering" motion with the feet

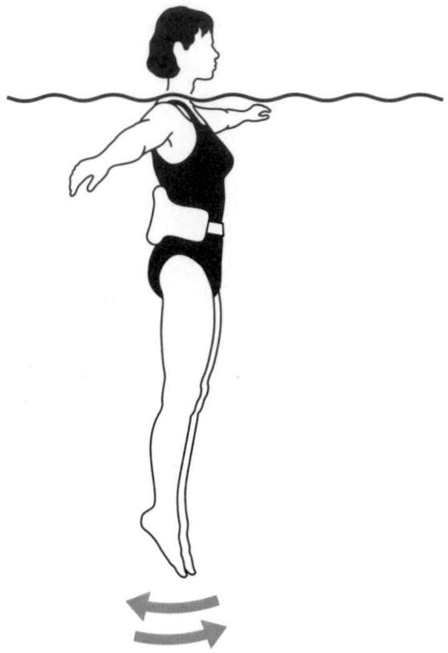

FIGURE 6–19. Deep water flutter kick.

Hip Flexion and Extension (Fig. 6–20)

- Assume vertical position
- Keeping the knees straight, alternately flex and extend the legs from the hips

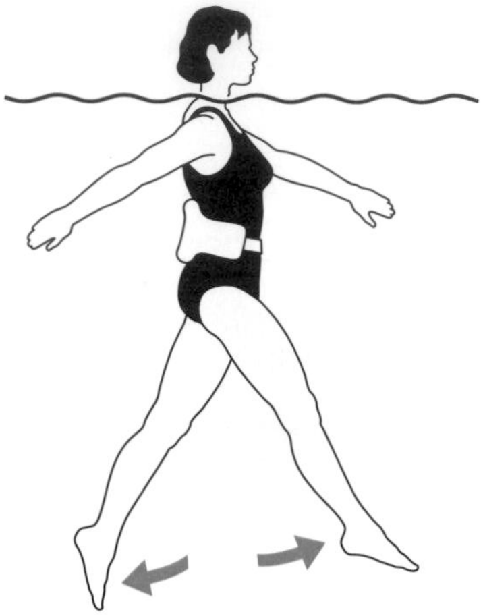

FIGURE 6–20. Deep water hip flexion and extension.

Double Knee Bend (Fig. 6–21)

- Assume vertical position
- Flex both knees, lifting the heels toward the surface of the water
- Extend the knees

VARIATION. Perform movement with each knee alternately

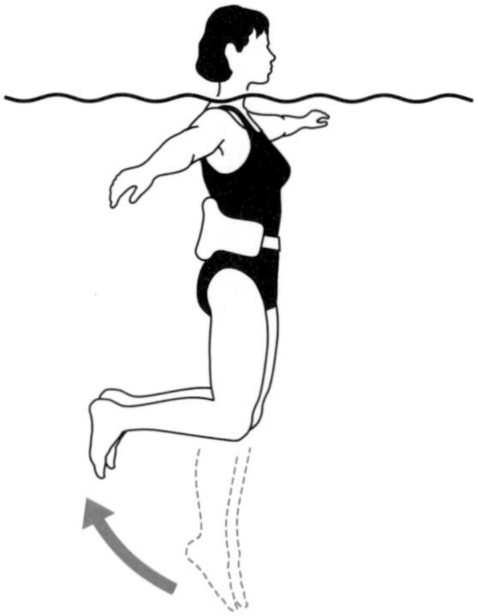

FIGURE 6–21. Deep water double knee bend.

Seated Leg Extension (Fig. 6–22)

- Assume vertical position
- Flex the hips to 90° (seated position)
- Keeping the thighs together, alternately flex and extend the knees

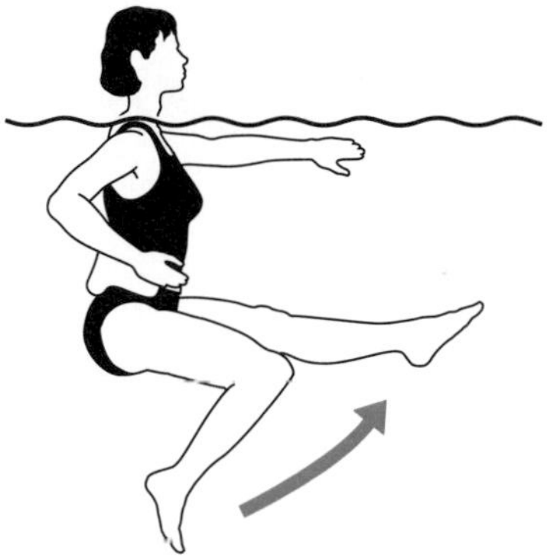

FIGURE 6–22. Deep water seated leg extension.

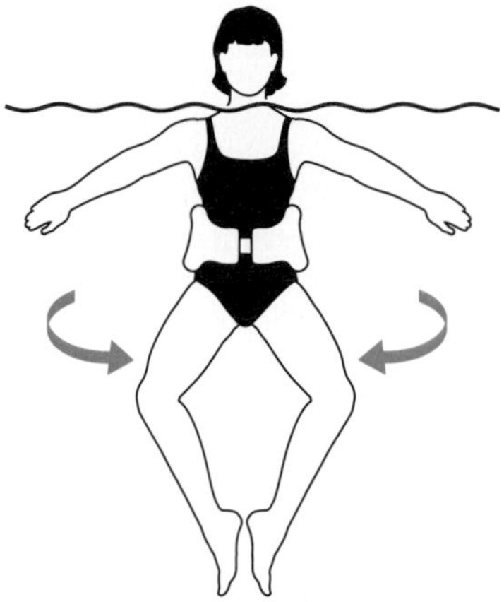

FIGURE 6–24. Deep water diamond.

Diamond (Fig. 6–24)

- Assume vertical position
- Flex the hips, placing the plantar surfaces of the feet together
- Keeping the feet together and the hips slightly flexed, bring the knees together and then apart

Seated Hip Abduction (Fig. 6–23)

- Assume vertical position
- Flex the hips to 90° (seated position)
- Keeping the knees straight, abduct the legs, then adduct the legs

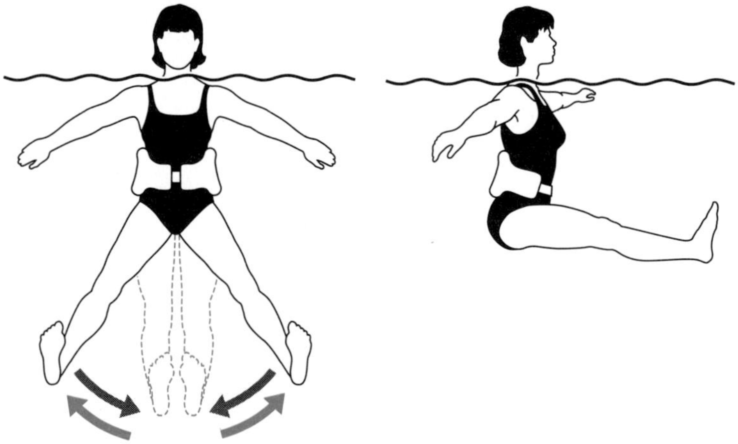

FIGURE 6–23. Deep water seated hip abduction.

Bum Squeeze (Fig. 6–25)

- Assume vertical position
- Flex the hips, placing the plantar surfaces of the feet together with the knees externally rotated (turned out)
- Lift the heels upward toward the groin while squeezing the buttocks together
- Straighten legs, keeping the knees externally rotated

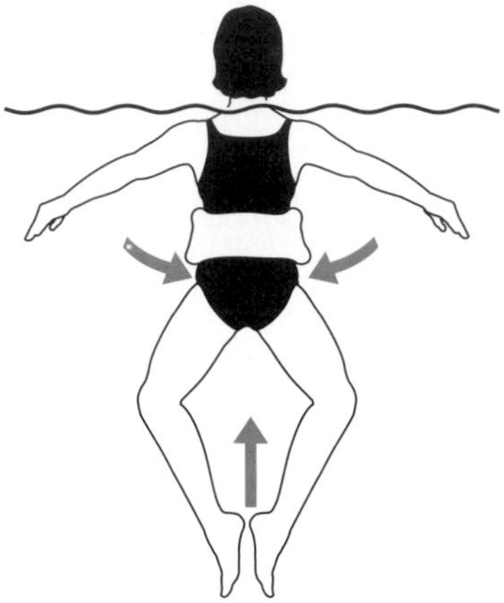

FIGURE 6–25. Deep water bum squeeze.

Hip Flexion with External Rotation
(Fig. 6–26)

- Assume vertical position
- Simultaneously flex both hips and knees with external rotation
- Lower the legs, returning to vertical position

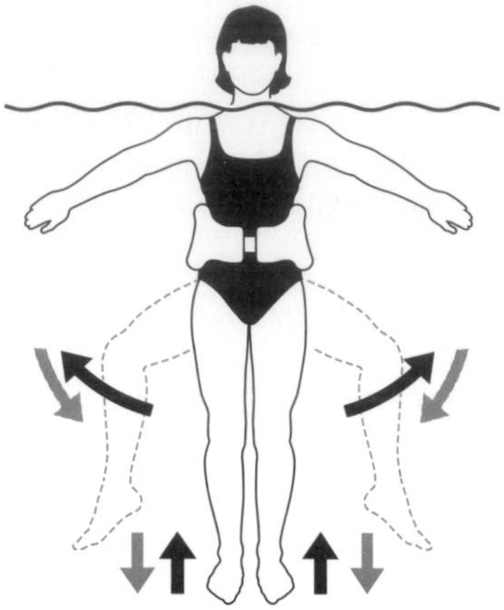

FIGURE 6–26. Deep water hip flexion with external rotation.

Stag (Fig. 6–27)

- Assume vertical position
- Keep one leg straight while flexing and abducting the opposite hip and knee
- Return to vertical position, then repeat movement with the opposite leg

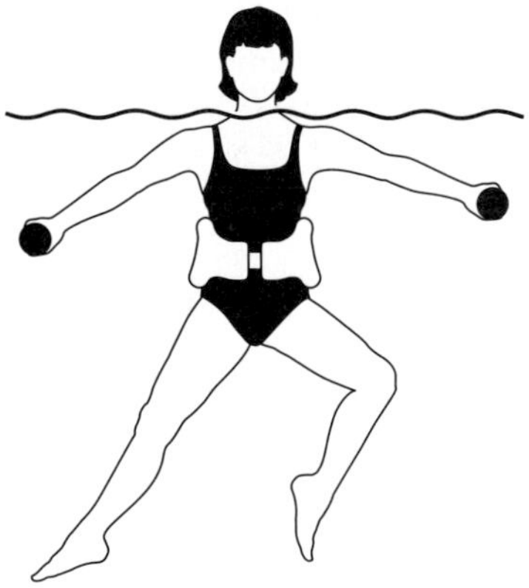

FIGURE 6–27. Deep water stag.

Tuck and Roll (Fig. 6–28)

- Assume vertical position
- Bring the knees to the chest, then lean and roll back, extending both legs forward
- Tuck the knees to the chest again and lean forward, extending both legs backward

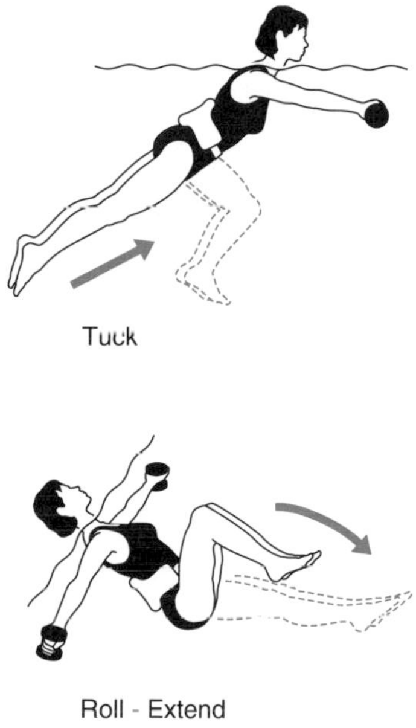

FIGURE 6–28. Deep water tuck and roll.

Hip Abduction and Adduction (Fig. 6–29)

- Assume vertical position
- Keeping the knees straight, simultaneously abduct both legs
- Simultaneously adduct the legs to the original position

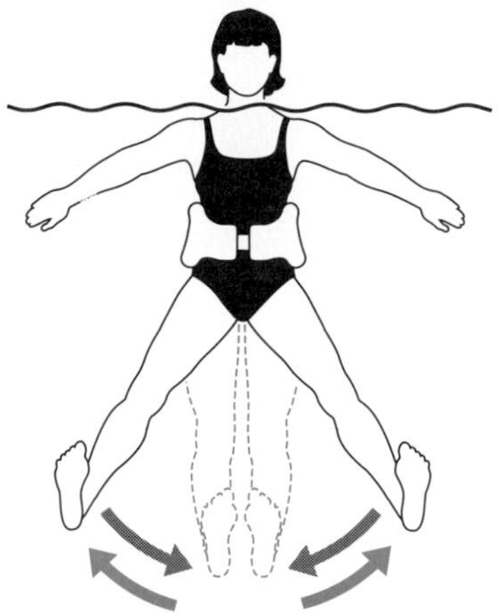

FIGURE 6–29. Deep water hip abduction and adduction.

REFERENCES

1. Becker BE. The Biologic Aspects of Hydrotherapy. J Back Musculoskel Rchabil 4:255–264, 1994.
2. Harrison RA, Hillman M, Bulstrode S. Loading of the lower limb when walking partially immersed. Physiotherapy 78:165–166, 1992.
3. Gehlsen GM, Grigsby S, Winant D. The effects of an aquatic fitness program on the muscular strength and endurance of patients with multiple sclerosis. Phys Ther 64:653–657, 1984.
4. Henker L, Provast CM, Sestili P, et al. Water running and the maintenance of maximum oxygen consumption and leg strength in runners. Med Sci Sports Exerc 24(Suppl. S23 136):3, 1991.
5. Ruoti RG. Overview of non-swimming aquatic research. J Back Musculoskel Rehabil 4:315–318, 1994.
6. Evans BW, Cureton KJ, Purvis JW. Metabolic and circulatory responses to walking and jogging in water. Res Q 49:442–449, 1978.
7. Wilder RP, Brennan DK. Physiologic responses to deep water running in athletes. Sports Med 16:374–380, 1993.
8. Wilder RP, Brennan DK. Fundamentals and techniques of aqua running for athletic rehabilitation. J Back Musculoskel Rehabil 4:287–296, 1994.

Common Orthopedic Conditions

CHAPTER 7

A large number of orthopedic conditions can be classified into a small number of pathologic groups. Each of these groups represents a similar type of defect, regardless of where it presents in the body. For example, osteoarthritis of the knee and osteoarthritis of the elbow have similar origins, pathologies, and signs and symptoms. Consequently, the treatment goals for these two conditions are similar. This chapter outlines the broad topics of arthritis, soft tissue healing, and fractures.

Posture is also discussed, because it is an element of rehabilitation that extends beyond the treatment of an isolated acute injury. If an injury alters posture in one area of the body, other areas are affected. One example of this is the effect that a hip flexion contracture has on the spine. It increases the lumbar lordosis, which increases the thoracic kyphosis, which in turn increases the cervical lordosis. Therefore, treatment of poor neck posture may start with treatment of the hip. Relations such as this must always be considered when analyzing posture.

ARTHRITIS

The term "arthritis" simply refers to any inflammation of a joint. It is most commonly thought of as a chronic inflammatory condition with a significant degree of joint degeneration. Typically, all structures of the joint are affected: bones, articular cartilage, synovial membrane, and joint capsule. The condition is characterized by pain, decreased range of motion, and synovial thickening. When the arthritis is in its active stage, the joint is often warm. The joint also may be swollen and may produce a clicking sensation when it is moved through its range of motion.

Types of Arthritis

PYOGENIC ARTHRITIS. This type of arthritis is caused by a bacterial infection of the involved joint. In its acute phase, it is characterized by pain, swelling, and warmth of the joint. Before any rehabilitation can begin, the infection must be treated medically. Figure 7–1 demonstrates the kind of joint degeneration that may result with this type of arthritis.

TUBERCULOUS ARTHRITIS. As the name implies, this form of arthritis is caused by a tubercle bacilli infection. It most commonly involves the thoracic and lumbar regions of the spine. Figure 7–2 depicts the synovial thickening that is often seen in this type of arthritis and the destruction of the joint that may occur.

GONORRHEAL ARTHRITIS. This manifestation of gonorrhea usually involves the knee joint. In its acute stage, however, several joints may be affected. Its treatment must begin with medical treatment of the disease.

SYPHILITIC ARTHRITIS. As with gonorrheal arthritis, this form of arthritis occurs in the late stages of the venereal disease.

GOUTY ARTHRITIS. Gouty arthritis is caused by a malfunction in the metabolism of purine. This defect results in deposition of uric acid salts in the connective tissues of a joint (ie, cartilage, bursa, or ligaments). It usually involves the hands and feet, and its onset can be sudden. Chronic gout may simulate rheumatoid arthritis.

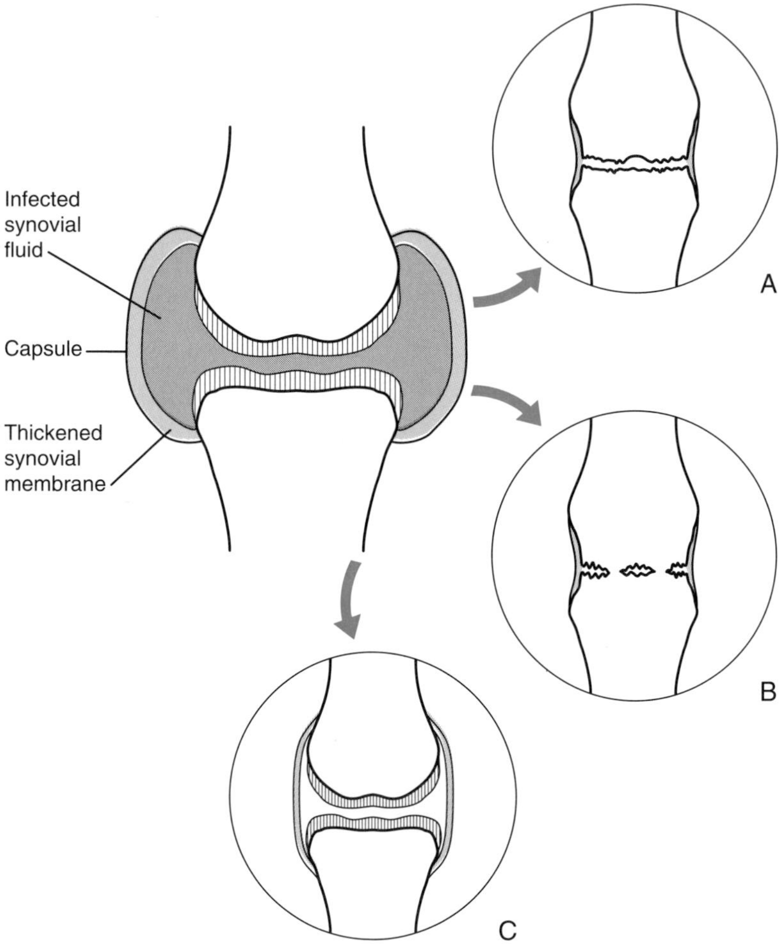

FIGURE 7–1. A joint affected with pyogenic arthritis can undergo *(A)* fibrous ankylosis or *(B)* bony ankylosis or *(C)* return to normal. (Adapted from Adams JC. Outline of Orthopedics. New York, Churchill Livingstone, 1981.)

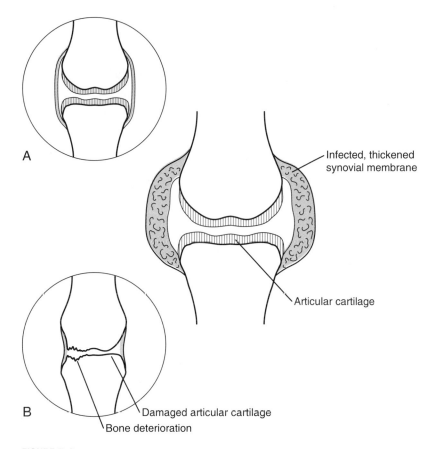

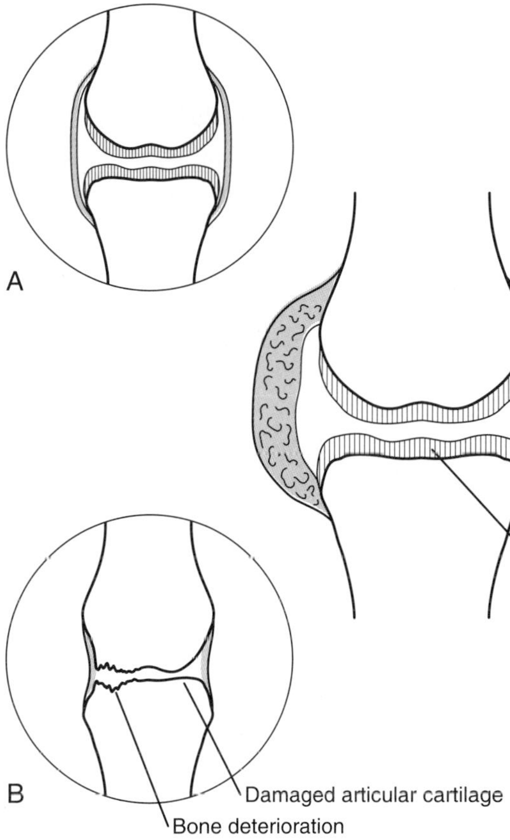

FIGURE 7–2. A joint affected with tuberculous arthritis experiences a synovial infection and will either *(A)* return to normal or *(B)* become fibrous and ankylosed. (Adapted from Adams JC. Outline of Orthopedics. New York, Churchill Livingstone, 1981.)

NEUROTROPHIC ARTHRITIS. This form of arthritis accompanies or is secondary to a disease of the nervous system. These diseases leave the patient with reduced pain sensation. Consequently, the patient may not feel pain when the joint is being injured. Neurotrophic arthritis may be seen with conditions such as cauda equina or diabetes.

HEMOPHILIC ARTHRITIS. This type of arthritis is associated with hemophilia. It is caused by bleeding into a joint. If bleeding becomes a recurrent problem, it may lead to degeneration of the articular cartilage and fibrosis of the synovial membrane.

ARTHRITIS OF RHEUMATIC FEVER. This complication of rheumatic fever involves an acute inflammation of the synovial membrane. Such inflammation may lead to thickening of the synovial membrane and increased production of synovial fluid.

ANKYLOSING SPONDYLITIS. This disease is characterized by a chronic inflammation of the joints and ligaments of the spine. It starts in the sacroiliac joints and progressively moves up the spine. It eventually leads to "ankylosis" (stiffening) of the affected joints. In severe cases, the spine has practically no mobility.

RHEUMATOID ARTHRITIS. Although it appears that this systemic disease results from a problem in the immune system, its exact cause is unknown. It is a progressive disease that starts with synovial membrane thickening and a softening of the articular cartilage. The cartilage gradually erodes until the joint is "bone on bone." If the disease is left to progress, the bone may start to erode. In addition to the joint degeneration, nodules may form in the soft tissues surrounding the joint. Tendon sheaths can become inflamed as tendons become thicker and softer, which may cause the tendons to rupture (Fig. 7–3).

OSTEOARTHRITIS. This is the most common form of arthritis. It is essentially caused by wear and tear on the affected joint. It can be precipitated by a congenital defect, vascular insufficiency, previous injury or disease, obesity, or old age. On X-ray examination, an osteoarthritic joint shows a decrease in "joint space" (the space between the articulating bones) because the cartilage is progressively wearing away. If all of the cartilage wears away, the joint is "bone on bone." After this occurs, the bone on the margins of the joint thickens to form spurs or osteophytes. Figure 7–4 depicts advanced osteoarthritis.

Signs and Symptoms

Although there are several different types of arthritis, the joint degeneration that occurs produces many common signs and symptoms. The most obvious of these are pain and stiffness. These are often most severe when the joint is moved after having been in one position for an extended period. These symptoms occur because the joint has had limited lubrication and nutrition during the period of static position.

Arthritic joints also may be more painful if they have had too much activity. The joints are not healthy enough to cope with that level of activity.

The stiffness present in arthritic joints may result from pain, joint deterioration, or secondary soft tissue shortening. Aquatic exercise will not change

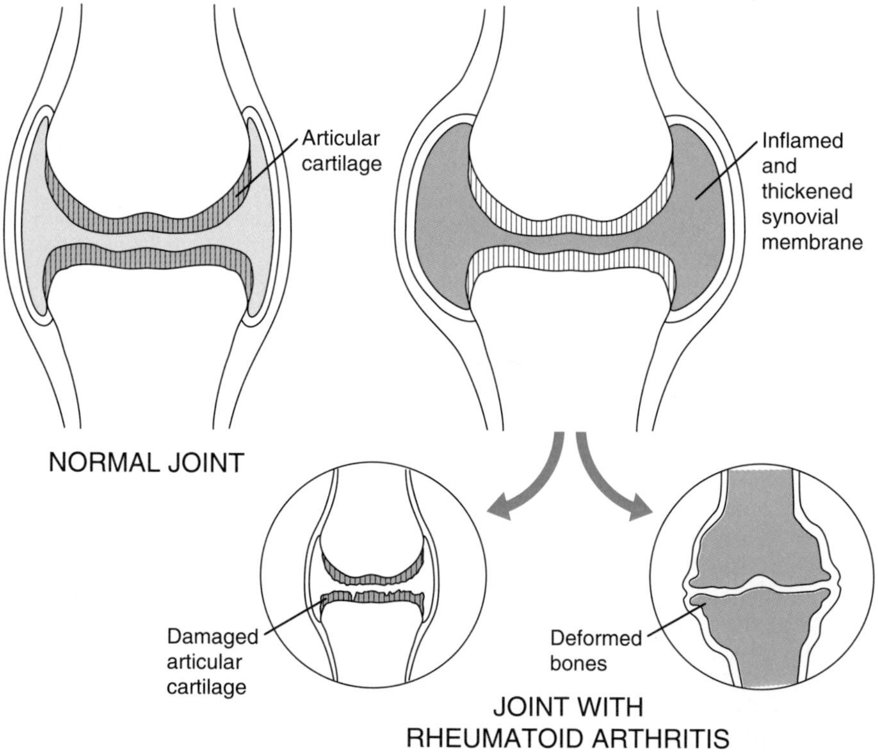

FIGURE 7–3. Pathologic changes in rheumatoid arthritis.

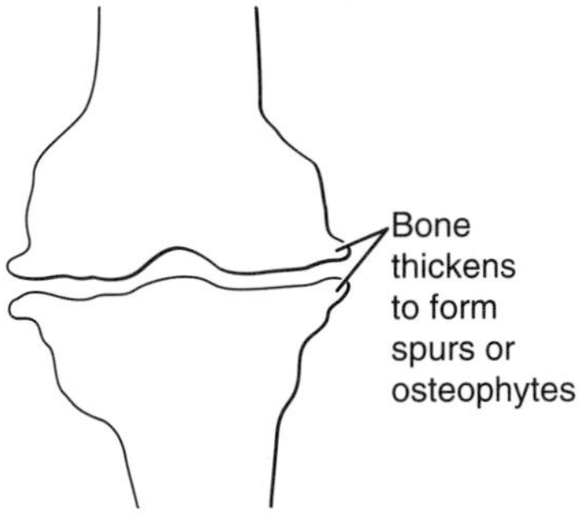

FIGURE 7–4. Advanced osteoarthritis.

the joint deterioration, and it may only temporarily reduce the pain, but it is an excellent environment in which to reverse secondary soft tissue shortening. Aquatic exercise helps maintain or increase the joint's range of motion.

Decreased strength and endurance are also problems for patients with arthritis. Because these factors are directly related to lack of use of muscles, a graduated strengthening program can help maintain a functional level of strength. Many patients with arthritis prefer an aquatic environment because exercise in the water is considerably more comfortable than a land-based strengthening program, especially on weight-bearing joints.

SOFT TISSUE INJURIES

Soft tissue injuries fall into one of three categories: bursitis, sprains, and strains. This section describes the origin, pathology, signs and symptoms, and exercise priorities for these types of injuries.

Bursitis

A bursa is a sac filled with lubricating fluid. This fluid is used to reduce friction between two different types of tissue, such as tendon and bone. Inflammation of a bursa is known as bursitis.

Origin

Bursitis may be caused by trauma, overuse, infection, or calcium deposits. Often, no precipitating incident can be recalled.

Pathology

Bursitis is an inflammation of the bursa. If the condition becomes chronic, there may be some thickening of the walls of the bursa. The epithelial lining may degenerate, and scar tissue may form.

Signs and Symptoms

The classic signs of acute inflammation are pain, heat, redness, and swelling. Pain may be referred to a nearby area of the body, or it may result in "empty end-feel"—that is, pain rather than tightening of soft tissues becomes the limiting factor for measurement of range of motion. If the condition becomes chronic, crepitus may develop, and surrounding soft tissues may become stiffer.

Sprains

A sprain is an injury of a ligament. It can vary from a mild stretch to a complete tear.

Origin

A sprain occurs as the result of trauma to a joint. The joint is twisted or bent in a way that causes excessive stretch on one or more ligaments.

Pathology

Sprains are graded based on the degree of injury that has occurred. Figure 7–5 depicts the three grades of sprains.

Types of Sprains

FIRST-DEGREE SPRAIN. A first-degree sprain is a mild stretch of a ligament. A few fibers may be torn as well. The patient experiences pain when the ligament is stressed.

SECOND-DEGREE SPRAIN. A second-degree sprain involves the partial tear of a ligament. There is more swelling and bruising than there is for a first-degree sprain. Stressing of the ligament produces pain.

THIRD-DEGREE SPRAIN. A third-degree sprain occurs if there is a complete tear of the ligament or if the ligament has pulled completely away from the bone. There is no increase in pain when the ligament is stressed, because there are no intact fibers left to pull on. Such a severe sprain rarely heals without leaving the patient with some degree of joint laxity.

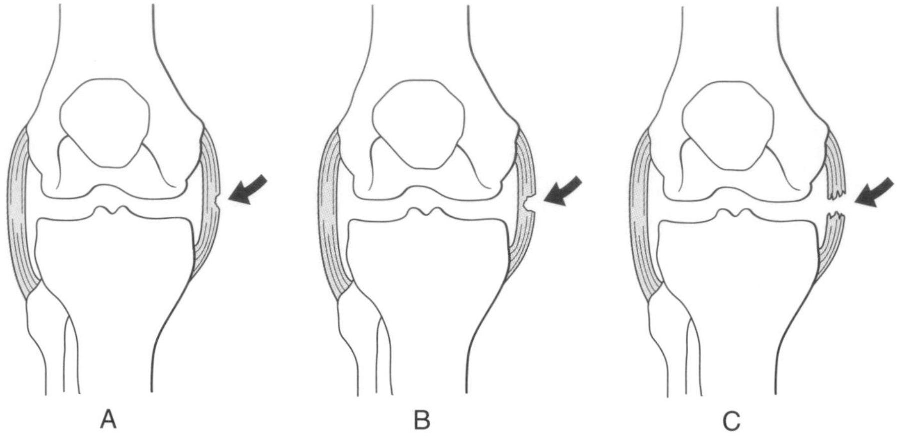

FIGURE 7–5. Knee ligament sprain. *A*, First-degree. *B*, Second-degree. *C*, Third-degree.

The healing of a ligament can be seen as a race between fibroplasia (scarring) and the laying down of collagen (which later turns into ligament). The course of this race is influenced by the amount of tissue damage, the size of the gap, the timing of early treatment, and the prevention of early reinjury. Obviously, the larger the tear, the more scarring takes place.

Exercise can also influence the healing process. The proper exercises, applied in a controlled fashion, provide the right stresses to stimulate healing: the collagen fibers line up along the lines of stress, and crosslinks form between them to add strength. Too much activity increases inflammation, increases scarring, and leads to joint laxity. Because it takes between 3 and 12 months for immature collagen to be replaced by mature collagen, it is important that rehabilitation exercises be continued for months after the injury to ensure maximum recovery.

Signs and Symptoms

Sprains cause varying degrees of pain, swelling, and decreased range of motion. Pain is worse when the injured ligament is stressed. Secondary problems, such as weakness, muscle contractures, and poor posture, may develop as the patient guards against pain.

Strains

A strain is an injury of a muscle or a tendon. A strain is referred to as tendonitis if it involves the inflammation of a tendon, the muscle-tendon junction, or the tendon-bone junction. Related to tendonitis is the condition known as tenosynovitis, which refers to inflammation of the tendon sheath.

Origin

The most common mechanism of a muscle or tendon strain is overuse (repetitive strain). However, what is "overuse" for one person may not cause any problem for a different person. These injuries actually occur because the muscle-tendon unit is too weak or too inflexible for the demands placed on it. Therefore, a lack of conditioning may be just as much to blame as the repetitive activity itself. Other causes of strain include infection, ischemia, and contusion. A violent overstretching can also cause tearing of the muscle or tendon.

Pathology

Strains are graded in the same fashion as sprains (Fig. 7–6). The grading is based on the amount of tearing of the muscle or tendon.

Types of Strains

FIRST-DEGREE STRAIN. This degree of strain involves a muscle pull or a mild stretch of a tendon. Most cases of tendonitis fall into this category. When the tendon is stretched, small vessels within the tendon are damaged. This compromises the blood supply to the tendon, resulting in an inflammatory response.

SECOND-DEGREE STRAIN. Partial tears of muscle or tendon are designated second-degree

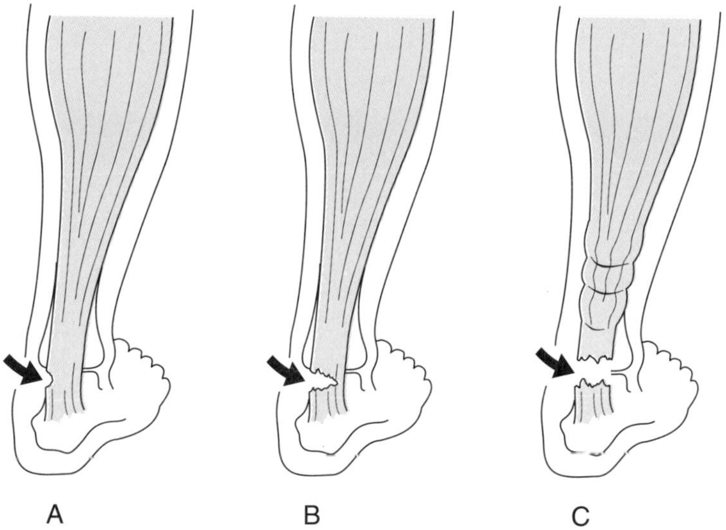

FIGURE 7–6. Achilles tendon strain. *A*, First-degree. *B*, Second-degree. *C*, Third-degree (rupture).

strains. This tearing leads to significant bruising and swelling.

THIRD-DEGREE STRAIN. As with sprains, third-degree strains involve complete tears. In an avulsion injury, the tendon pulls a piece of bone from its attachment. Because the muscle is then attached at only one end, it usually coils up, leaving a visible defect in the muscle. Factors that influence the rate of healing for this type of injury include severity of the injury, blood supply, and presence of any nerve damage. As with ligament injuries, there is a race between the formation of scar tissue and the formation of new muscle tissue. The appropriate amount of exercise, performed early in rehabilitation, facilitates the healing process. Because it takes 6 to 24 months for an injured tendon to return to full strength, it is important that strengthening exercises be continued even after the pain has subsided.

Signs and Symptoms

First- and second-degree strains show an increase in pain with active movement, isometric contraction, or stretch of the involved muscle. Swelling and bruising vary with the amount of tissue damage. Third-degree strains may actually be less painful than other strains in the early stage of injury. As with third-degree sprains, this occurs because there are no remaining intact fibers to pull on.

FRACTURES

The human skeleton supports the body and protects the organs. Bones of the skeleton are divided into four categories: long bones (eg, femur, humerus), short bones (eg, scaphoid, talus), flat bones (eg, ribs), and irregular bones (eg, vertebrae). Some bones are protective, forming body cavities. Other bones, such as those of the arms and legs, act as levers for muscles.

Bones have both rigid and elastic qualities. The rigidity is a result of the mineral content, and the elasticity comes from the protein in bones. The relative amounts of these two components change with age. As a result, bones become more brittle and fracture more easily as a person ages.

Fractures are most often the result of a single traumatic incident. They can be partial, or they can go completely through the bone. Some fractures may even puncture the skin.

Types of Fractures

AVULSION FRACTURE. A small portion of bone is pulled away at the point at which the tendon or ligament attaches to the bone (Fig. 7–7).

COMMINUTED FRACTURE. The bone is fractured into three or more segments. This type of

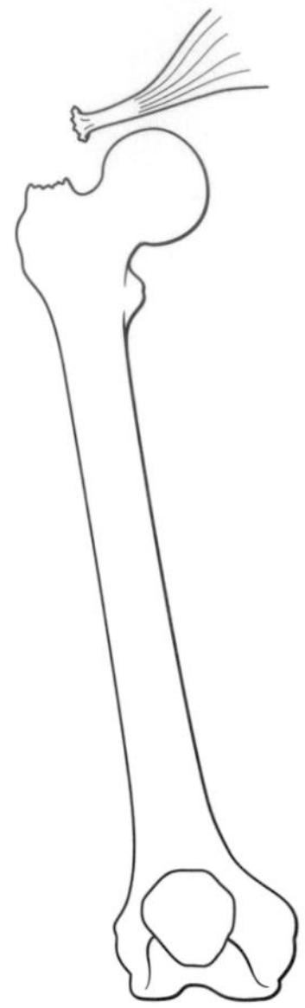

FIGURE 7–7. Avulsion fracture.

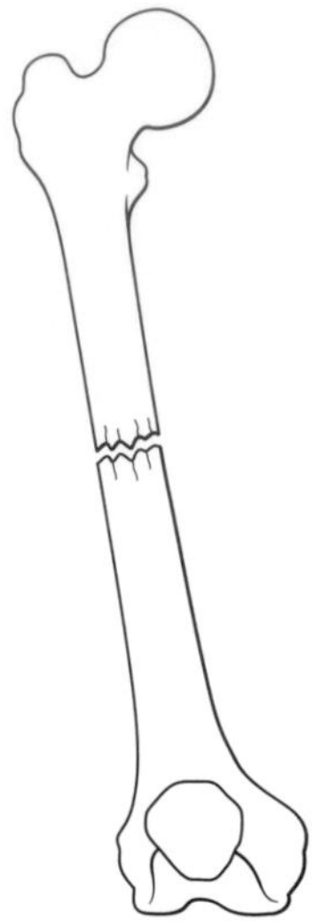

FIGURE 7–9. Complete fracture.

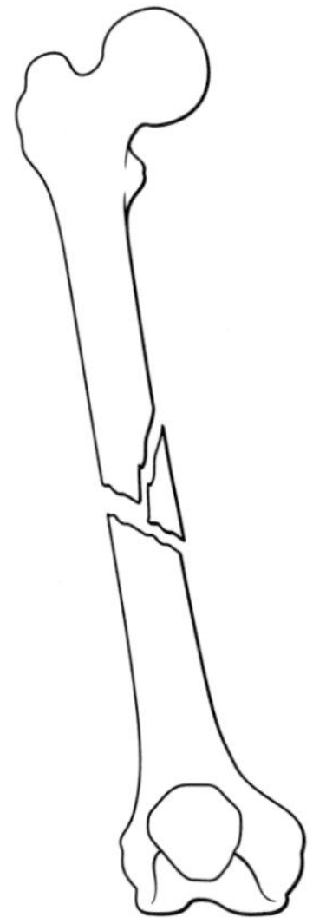

FIGURE 7–8. Comminuted fracture.

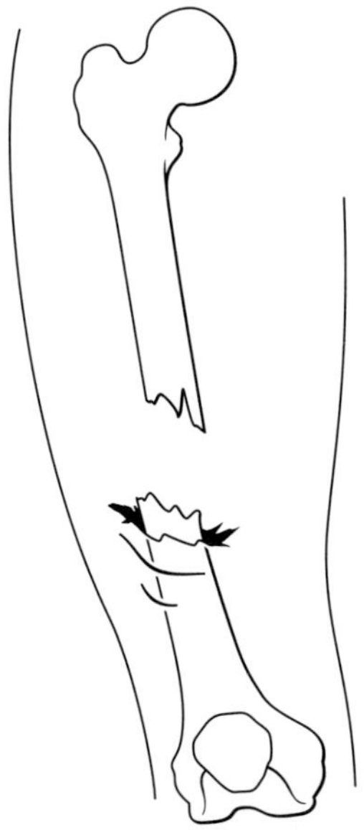

FIGURE 7–10. Compound fracture.

fracture often must be held together with some kind of fixation device (Fig. 7–8).

COMPLETE FRACTURE. The fractured bone segments are completely separated. A clean break usually heals relatively quickly (Fig. 7–9).

COMPOUND (OPEN) FRACTURE. At least one bone fragment punctures the skin. The risk of complicating infection rises dramatically with this type of fracture (Fig. 7–10).

GREENSTICK FRACTURE. This is an incomplete fracture with the fragments joined by at least some bone. As the name implies, the fracture resembles a partially broken stick (Fig. 7–11).

SPIRAL FRACTURE. Shearing forces cause the fractured segments to separate in a spiral fashion (Fig. 7–12).

TRANSVERSE FRACTURE (WITH DISPLACEMENT). The fractured bone segments are displaced and are not in normal alignment. An open or closed reduction is necessary to align the pieces (Fig. 7–13).

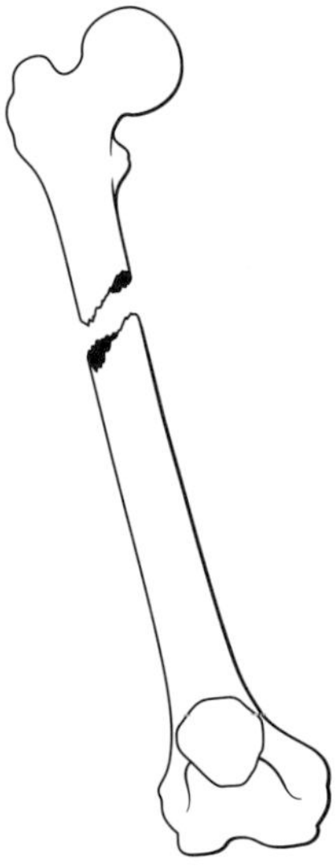

FIGURE 7–12. Spiral fracture.

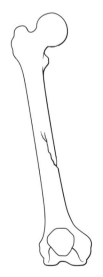

FIGURE 7–11. Greenstick fracture.

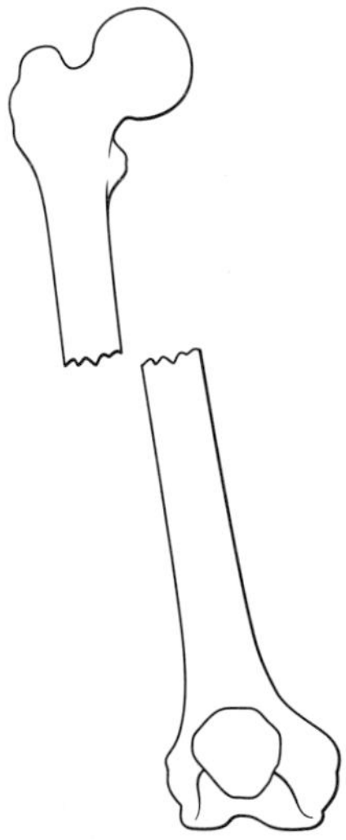

FIGURE 7–13. Transverse fracture with displacement.

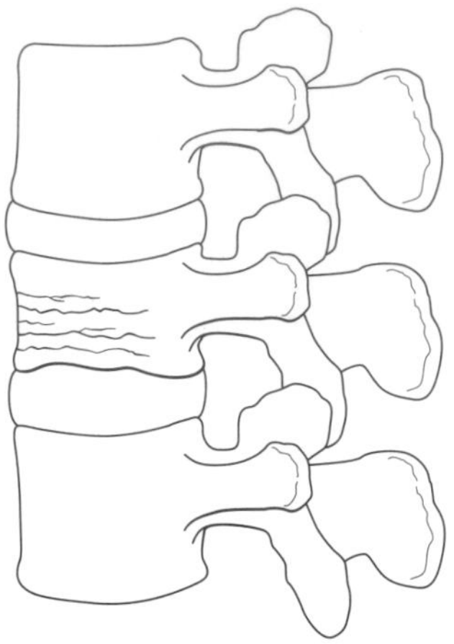

FIGURE 7–14. Compression fracture.

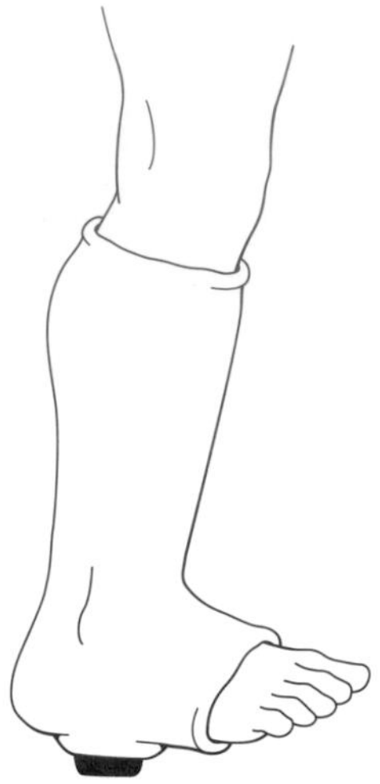

FIGURE 7–15. Cast immobilization of a fracture.

COMPRESSION FRACTURE. This type of fracture occurs when a mass of bone is compressed. It is most commonly seen in the spine (Fig. 7–14).

STRESS (FATIGUE) FRACTURE. Usually no more than a hairline fracture, this is caused by a repetitive stress to the bone. It also may take the form of many microscopic fractures that cannot be seen on X-ray. Rest is the primary treatment for these fractures, and no immobilization is necessary.

Treatment of Fractures

With the exception of stress and compression fractures, the treatment of fractures involves holding the bone fragments together so that healing can occur. The following four methods are those most commonly used to achieve this goal.

CAST. The classic means of immobilizing a fracture is a cast. Because the cast remains on for at least 6 weeks, a significant amount of stiffness may develop. No aquatic therapy can be initiated until the cast has been removed (Fig. 7–15).

SPLINT. Splints are used for fractures not severe enough to warrant a cast. The benefit of this form of immobilization is that it can be removed to begin rehabilitation. A therapeutic pool is probably the most comfortable environment for early mobilization of these minor fractures.

INTERNAL FIXATION. The use of internal hardware to hold the bone fragments together is called internal fixation. The most common forms of internal fixation are screw and plate, intramedullary rod, transfixion screws, and wire. Figure 7–16 shows examples of the screw and plate method and the intramedullary rod method. Because all of the hardware lies under the skin, aquatic therapy can begin as soon as the skin incisions heal. Patients with this type of fixation may have weight-bearing restrictions while the fracture is healing.

EXTERNAL FIXATION. External fixation, as depicted in Figure 7–17, uses a frame external to the body, with pins entering the bone through the skin. Its primary purpose is to hold pieces of a broken bone apart. If this type of fixation is used, it is necessary to wait until the hardware has been removed before aquatic therapy can begin.

POSTURE

Observation of a patient's posture can provide clues to many orthopedic problems. Poor posture can be caused by muscle imbalance, bony deformity, pain, muscle contractures, or general weakness. It may also simply be the result of poor postural habits. In any case, it is often beneficial to try to correct the problem through education and exercise.

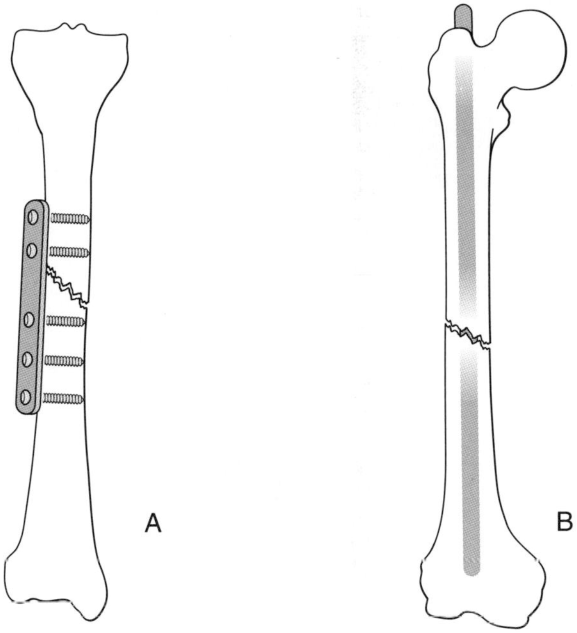

FIGURE 7–16. Internal fixation with *(A)* screw and plate method and *(B)* intramedullary rod method.

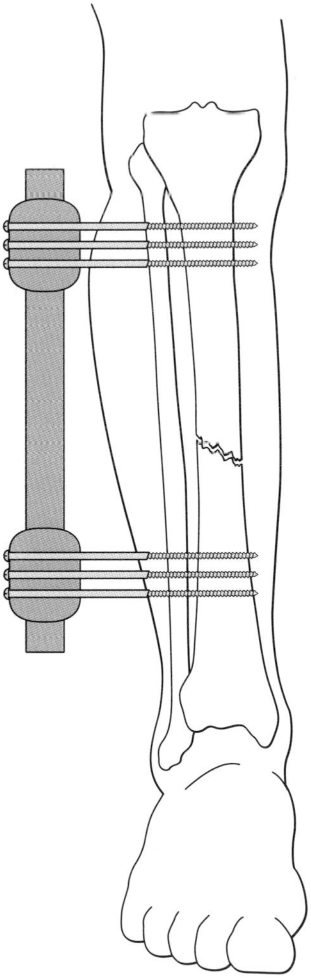

FIGURE 7–17. External fixation.

Common Postural Problems

FEET. Look for excessive pronation or supination. These problems predispose a person to ankle sprains. Flat feet can cause knee, hip, and low back problems.

KNEE. Look for valgus (knock-knee) or varus (bowleg) deformities, which commonly lead to arthritis and, short of surgery, cannot be corrected. Patellar alignment problems (kneecaps that sit too high or too far to the outside of the knee) may be improved with exercises that strengthen the inner quadriceps muscle. Lack of full extension after a knee injury can become a permanent deformity if the tissues are not stretched out early in rehabilitation.

HIP. Hip flexion contractures can lead to knee or back problems. A contracture occurs when the muscles or other tissues that cross a joint shorten, and it results in a limitation of joint motion. A contracture can also prevent normal gait. Even if the contracture has been present for a long period of time, it is important to try to stretch it out to improve the patient's gait.

LUMBAR SPINE. The most common postural problem in the low back is excessive lordosis (swayback), as seen in Figure 7–18. This condition may be caused by tight hip flexors or tight back extensors and weak abdominals. The tight muscles must be stretched, and the abdominals must be strengthened. Practicing the pelvic tilt in various body positions is important because it educates the abdominal muscles to work at a low level all the time. This helps to reduce the lordosis.

FIGURE 7–18. Increased lordosis.

THORACIC SPINE. Thoracic spine postural problems include scoliosis (a lateral "S" curve) and kyphosis (a flexed, slouched posture). Scoliosis deformities may be rigid or mobile. General range of motion exercises can help, and the patient must be encouraged to maintain an axial extension (upright) posture. Figure 7–19 depicts a kyphotic posture. People with a thoracic spine that is more kyphotic than normal need to work on thoracic extension exercises. These patients must concentrate on the axial extension posture as well.

CERVICAL SPINE. The most common postural problem in the neck is an increased cervical lordosis or "poking chin" (Fig. 7–20). The neck extensors must be stretched, and the axial extension posture must be reinforced. This is most simply done by telling the patient to tuck the chin in and pretend that it is being lifted from the crown of the head. Ideally, the ear and the tip of the shoulder should be in the same vertical plane.

SHOULDER. Many shoulder tendonitis and bursitis conditions are caused by a posture that includes shoulders that are protracted (rounded forward). This is often associated with a "poking chin" and thoracic kyphosis, as is shown in Figure 7–21. Protraction of the shoulders results in tightening of the muscles in the front of the shoulder and alters the

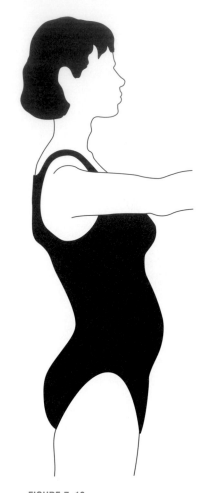

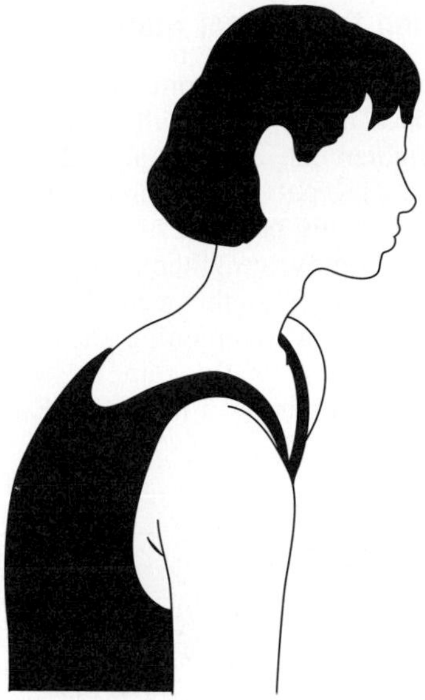

FIGURE 7–19. Thoracic kyphosis.

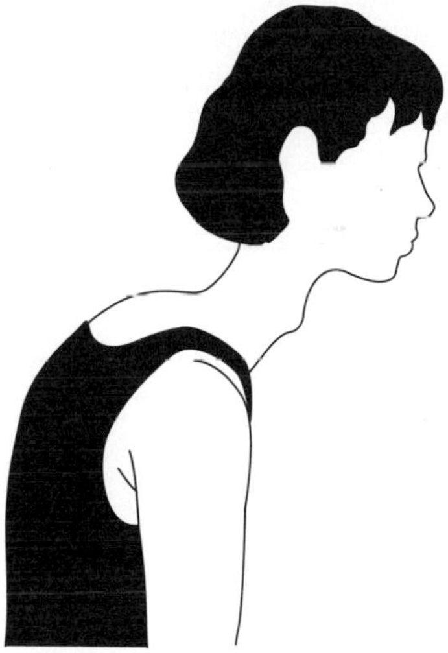

FIGURE 7–20. Cervical lordosis.

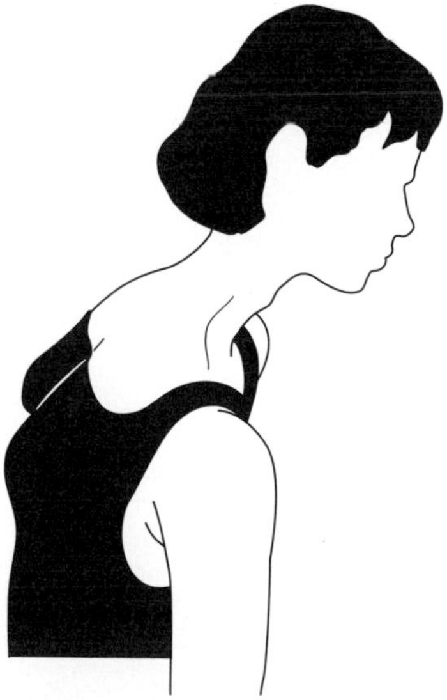

FIGURE 7–21. Protracted shoulders.

mechanics of the rotator cuff muscles. Tight muscles must be stretched, spinal postural problems must be addressed, and the patient must learn to hold the shoulders in a relaxed, retracted position.

Correct Vertical Alignment

In order to achieve a correct vertical alignment posture, the overall posture, rather than just one specific part of the body, must be assessed. Some typical alignment landmarks are depicted in Figure 7–22. The ears should be centered over the shoulders and the shoulders over the hips. Correct alignment does not involve sustained forward head (protraction) or forward body (leaning forward from the waist or hips). There should be no hyperextension of the cervical (neck) or lumbar (low back) sections of the spine and no fully extended joints.

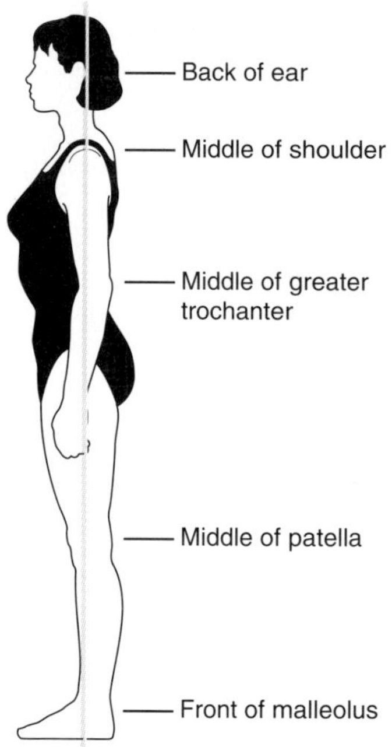

FIGURE 7–22. Typical vertical alignment landmarks.

How to Find the Correct Standing Position

Stand one foot away from the wall. Gently sit with the back against the wall, bending the knees slightly. Tighten the abdominal and buttock muscles; this tilts the pelvis back and flattens the lower spine. Holding this position, inch up the wall to a standing position by straightening the legs and moving the heels closer to the wall (Fig. 7–23). Now walk around while maintaining the same posture. Place back against wall again to see if correct standing position has been maintained.

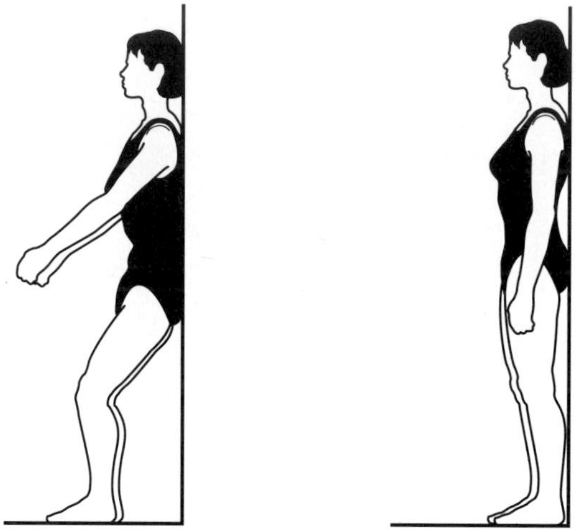

FIGURE 7–23. Inching up the wall to a correct standing posture.

Aquatic Rehabilitation of the Shoulder

Chapter 8

THE STRUCTURE AND FUNCTION OF THE SHOULDER AND SHOULDER GIRDLE
- **The Anatomic Parts**
- **The Muscles and Their Actions**
- **Measuring the Range of Motion of the Shoulder**

SHOULDER STRETCHES
- Pectoral Stretch
- Shoulder Shrugs
- Elbow Touch
- Shoulder Rolls
- Hug Stretch
- Cross-Shoulder Stretch
- Behind Back Pull-back
- Overhead Pullover
- Shoulder Internal Rotation Stretch
- Shoulder Abduction Stretch
- Pectoral Press Stretch
- Shoulder External Rotation Stretch
- Shoulder Extension, Elbows Bent
- Shoulder Extension, Elbows Straight
- Corner Stretch
- Range of Motion Exercises Using a Wand
  - Wand Shoulder Flexion (to 90°)
  - Wand Shoulder Extension
  - Wand Shoulder Abduction
  - Wand Horizontal Abduction and Adduction
  - Wand External Rotation
  - Wand Functional Internal and External Rotation
- Supine Shoulder Stretches
  - Shoulder Overhead Press, Supine
  - Shoulder Abduction, Supine
  - Shoulder External Rotation, Supine

SHOULDER EXERCISES
- Shoulder Press-down
- Resistive Shoulder Adduction and Abduction
- Resistive Shoulder Flexion
- Resistive Shoulder Extension
- Resistive Horizontal Abduction and Adduction
- Resistive Internal and External Rotation
- Rowing
- Side Arm Pull
- Upright Rowing

THE STRUCTURE AND FUNCTION OF THE SHOULDER AND SHOULDER GIRDLE

The Anatomic Parts

THE GLENOHUMERAL JOINT. The glenohumeral joint is the articulation between the head of the humerus and the glenoid fossa of the scapula. It is a synovial, ball-and-socket, multiaxial joint. The capsular laxity allows the joint a wide range of movement but makes it vulnerable to dislocation. The capsular ligaments and several muscles strengthen and support above, behind, and in front of the joint (Fig. 8–1). However, the joint is relatively unsupported below. As a result, a traumatic dislocation of the humeral head can cause chronic shoulder instability.

THE STERNOCLAVICULAR JOINT. The sternoclavicular joint is the articulation between the medial end of the clavicle and the manubrium of the sternum. It is a saddle-shaped synovial joint. There is a cartilaginous disc between the two bone faces that helps the joint move better by reducing the incongruity of the surfaces and that absorbs shock transmitted through the upper limb to the axial skeleton. The ligaments provide significant strength to the joint and allow adequate freedom of movement. Because of the strength of this joint, falls on an outstretched arm are more likely to result in a fracture of the clavicle than in a dislocation of the sternoclavicular joint (see Fig. 8–1).

THE CORACOCLAVICULAR JOINT. The coracoclavicular joint occurs where the undersurface of the clavicle passes in close proximity to the coracoid process of the scapula. The strong union of this fibrous joint guarantees that the scapula and clavicle move as one unit and also helps transmit upper limb shock to the stronger medial end of the clavicle (Fig. 8–2).

THE ACROMIOCLAVICULAR JOINT. The acromioclavicular joint is a small synovial articulation between the lateral end of the clavicle and the acromion process of the scapula. The integrity of the joint is a result of the support of the surrounding ligaments (see Fig. 8–2). Sprains of this joint regardless of severity are commonly referred to as shoulder separations.

The Muscles and Their Actions

A muscle must cross a joint to act directly on that joint. The way in which a muscle crosses a joint affects the action. The shoulder (glenohu-

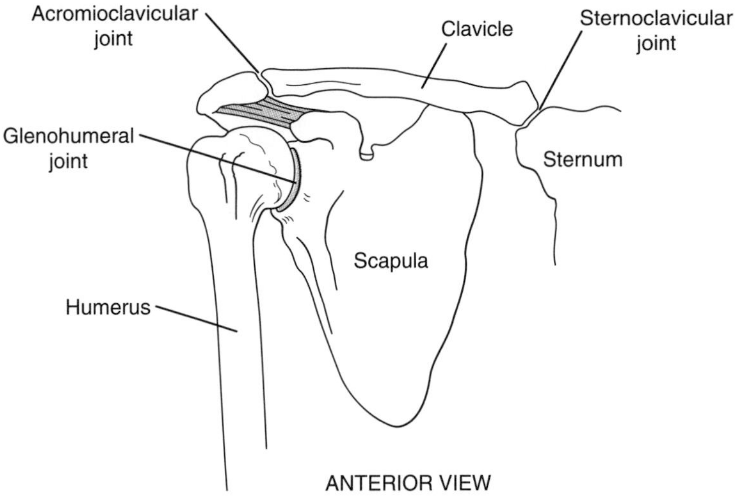

FIGURE 8–1. The bones and joints of the shoulder and shoulder girdle.

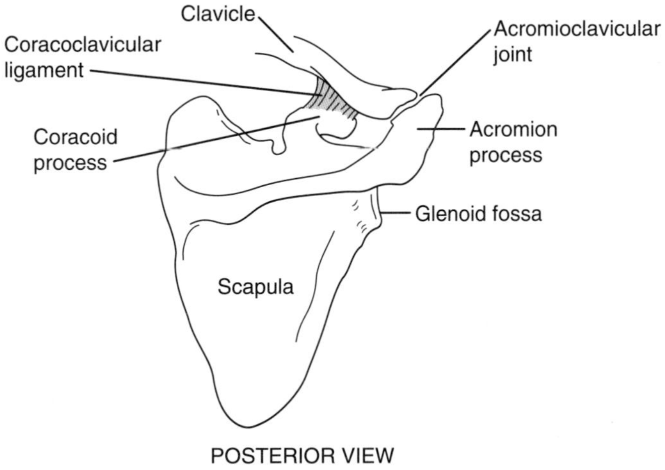

FIGURE 8–2. The coracoclavicular and acromioclavicular joints and associated ligaments.

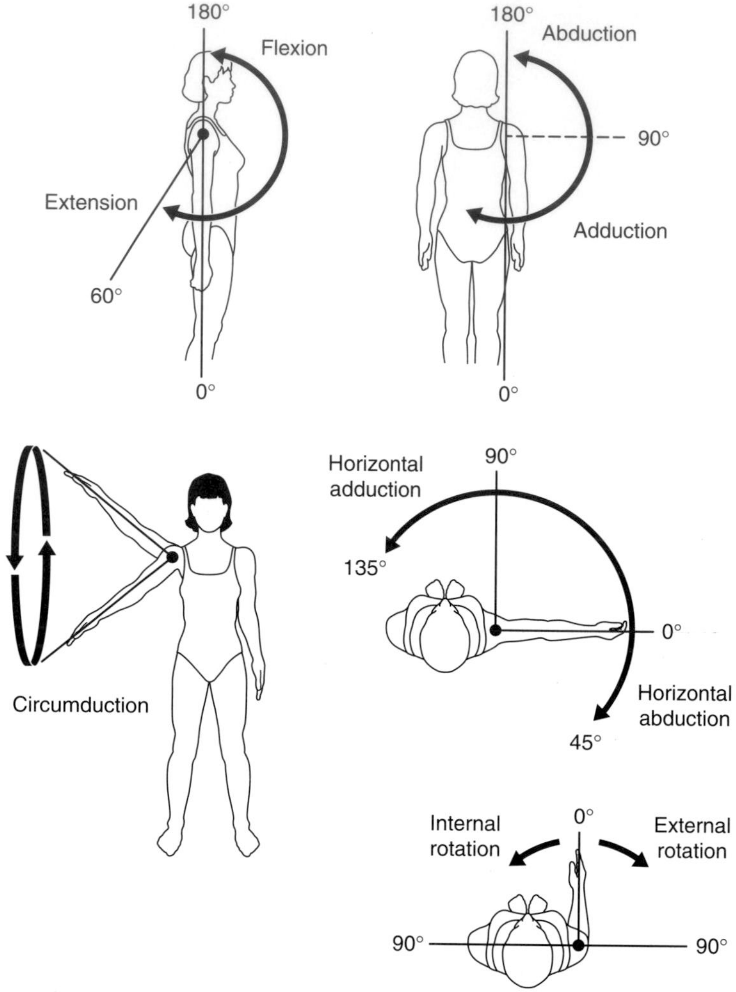

FIGURE 8–3. Movements of the shoulder showing normal ranges of motion. (Modified from Magee D. Orthopedic Physical Assessment. Philadelphia: W.B. Saunders, 1987.)

meral) joint permits the following movements (Fig. 8–3):

- flexion and extension (Table 8–1)
- abduction and adduction (Table 8–2)
- horizontal abduction and adduction (Table 8–3)
- internal and external rotation (Table 8–4)
- circumduction

The shoulder girdle (scapula) permits the following movements (Fig. 8–4; Table 8–5):

- elevation and depression
- upward and downward rotation
- protraction and retraction

Table 8–6 summarizes the muscles involved in the movements of the shoulder and shoulder girdle.

Text continued on page 92

TABLE 8–1. Muscles Involved in Shoulder Flexion and Extension

Muscle	Origin (O)	Insertion (I)	Action
Anterior deltoid 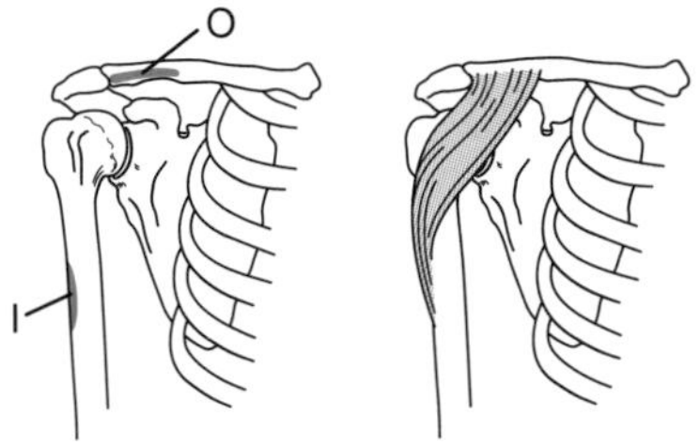	Lateral third of the clavicle	Halfway down the lateral surface of the humerus	Shoulder flexion Accessory movements: Horizontal adduction Medial rotation Abduction of humerus
Coracobrachialis 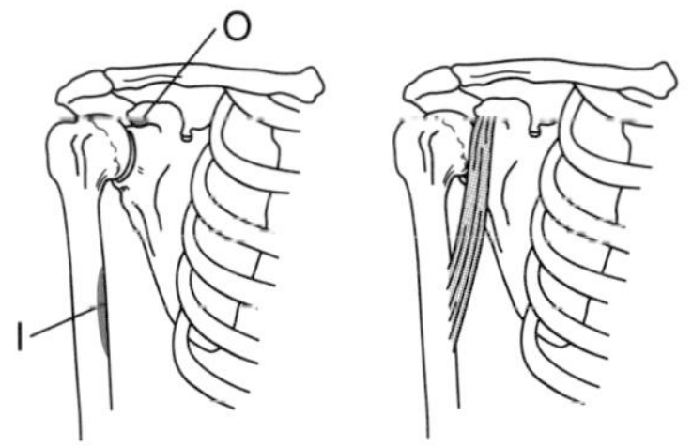	Apex of the coracoid process	Halfway down the medial surface of the humerus (opposite to the insertion of the deltoids)	Shoulder flexion
Latissimus dorsi 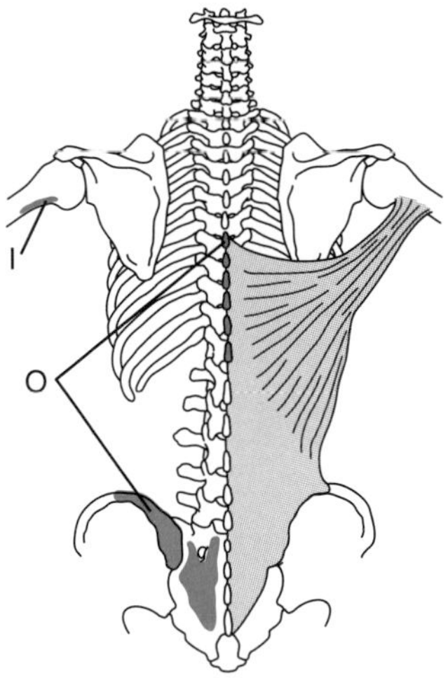	Posterior ilium, sacrum, lumbar fascia, vertebral spines T7 to T12	Floor of the bicipital groove of the humerus, between pectoralis major and teres major	Shoulder extension Accessory movements: Adduction of the humerus Horizontal abduction Medial (internal) rotation

Table continued on following page

TABLE 8–1. Muscles Involved in Shoulder Flexion and Extension *Continued*

Muscle	Origin (O)	Insertion (I)	Action
Teres major 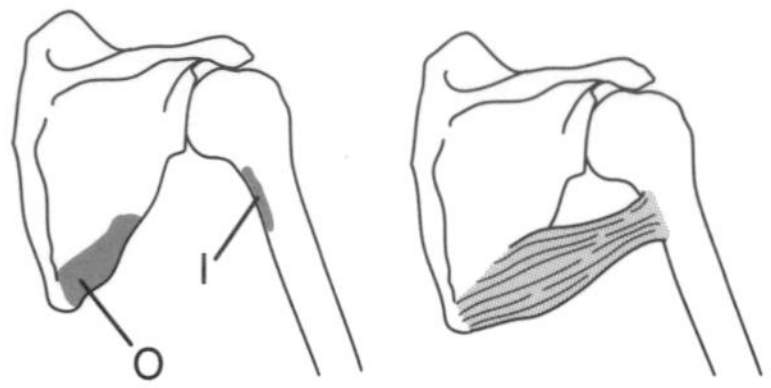	Axillary border of the scapula	Medial lip of the bicipital groove of the humerus	Shoulder extension Accessory movements: Adducts humerus Medial (internal) rotation
Posterior deltoid 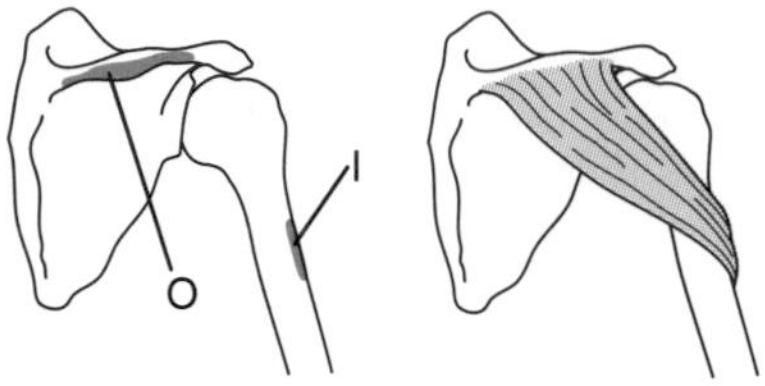	Spine of the scapula	Halfway down the lateral surface of the humerus	Shoulder extension Accessory movements: Horizontal abduction External (lateral) rotation

TABLE 8–2. Muscles Involved in Shoulder Abduction and Adduction

Muscle	Origin (O)	Insertion (I)	Action
Medial deltoid 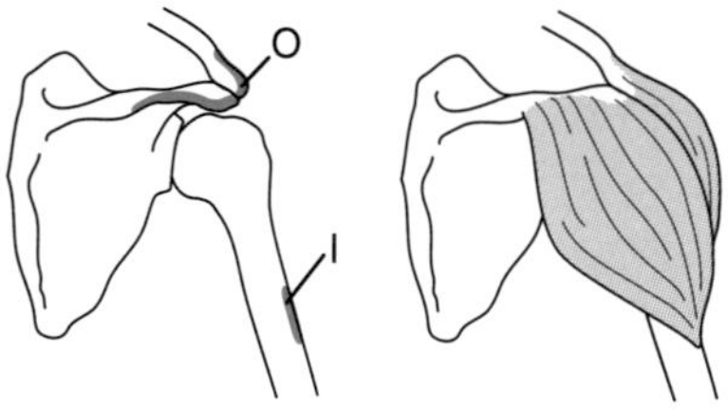	Acromion process of the scapula	Halfway down the lateral surface of the humerus	Shoulder abduction

TABLE 8–2. Muscles Involved in Shoulder Abduction and Adduction *Continued*

Muscle	Origin (O)	Insertion (I)	Action
Supraspinatus 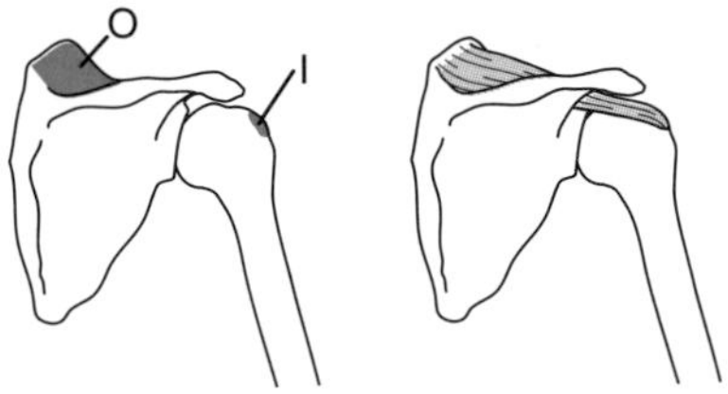	Supraspinous fossa of the scapula	Top of the greater tuberosity of the humerus	Initiates abduction of the humerus
Trapezius (middle fibers) 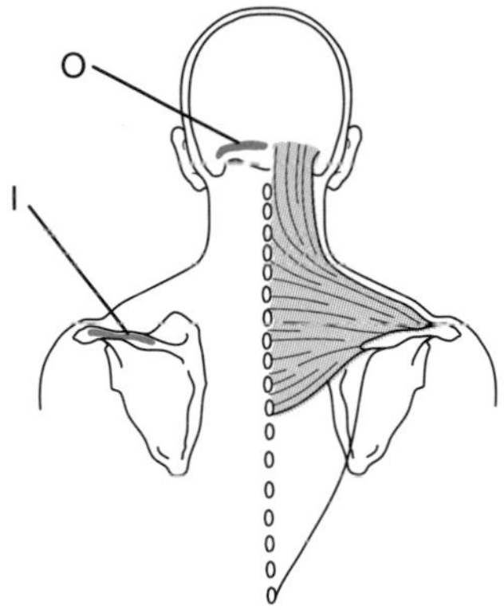	Ligament of the neck Vertebral spines C7 to T12	Acromion process of the scapula (medial margin)	Adduction of the scapula
Rhomboid major and minor 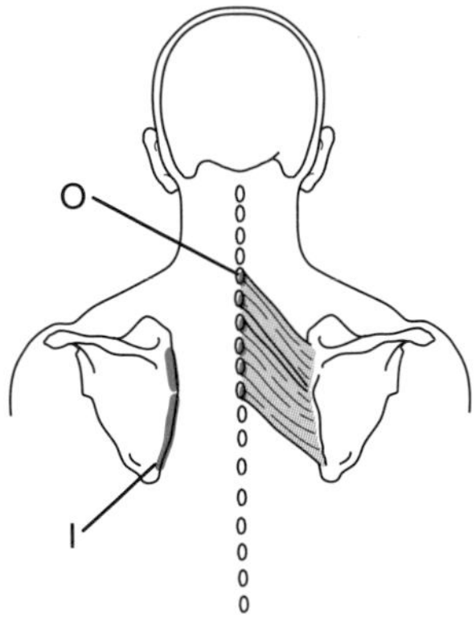	Vertebral spines C7 to T5	Medial border of the scapula	Adduction of the scapula Accessory movements: Downward rotation of the scapula

TABLE 8–3. Muscles Involved in Shoulder Horizontal Abduction and Adduction

Muscle	Origin (O)	Insertion (I)	Action
Posterior deltoid 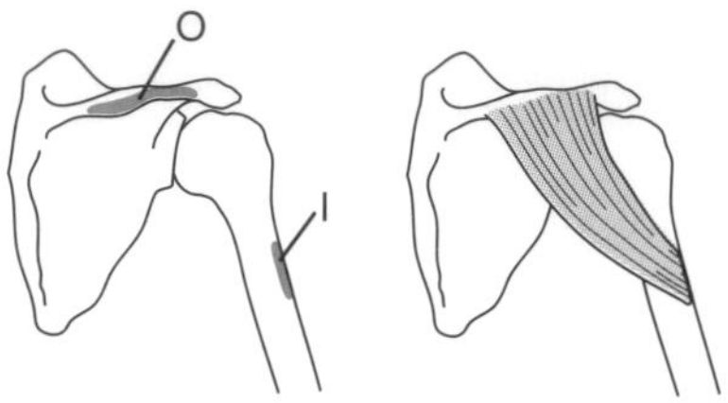	Spine of the scapula	Halfway down the lateral surface of the humerus	Shoulder horizontal abduction
Pectoralis major 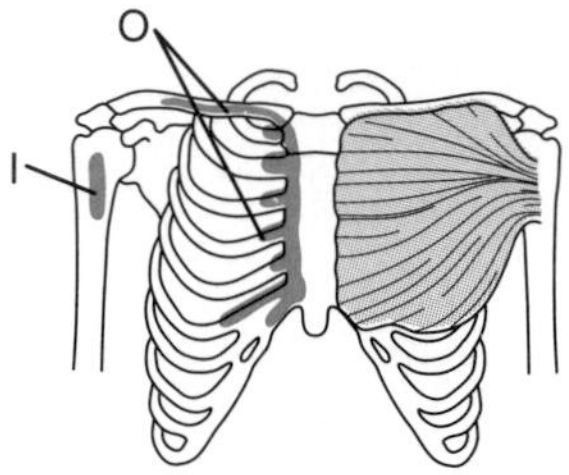	Medial half of the clavicle, sternum, and costal cartilages	Lateral lip of the bicipital groove of the humerus	Shoulder horizontal adduction Accessory movements: Flexes humerus Medial (internal) rotation of the humerus

TABLE 8–4. Muscles Involved in Shoulder Internal (Medial) and External (Lateral) Rotation

Muscle	Origin (O)	Insertion (I)	Action
Subscapularis 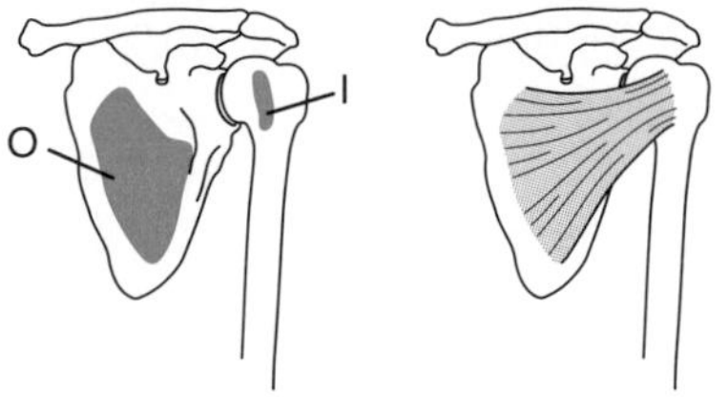	Subscapular fossa	Lesser tuberosity of the humerus	Internal (medial) rotation Accessory movements: Weak adduction of the humerus
Pectoralis major	See Table 8–3		
Latissimus dorsi	See Table 8–1		
Teres major	See Table 8–1		
Infraspinatus 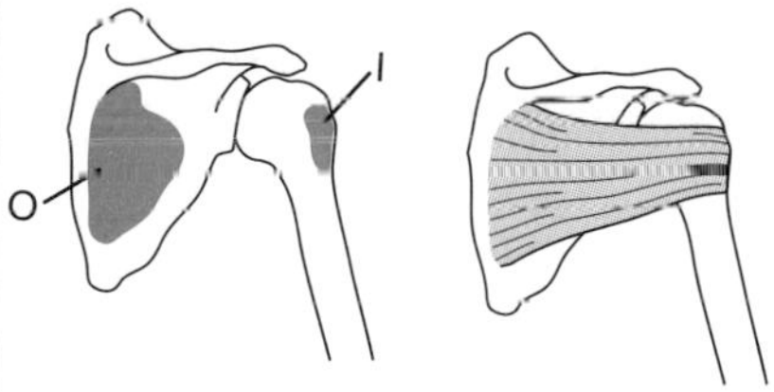	Infraspinous fossa	Posterior greater tuberosity of the humerus	External (lateral) rotation of the humerus Accessory movements: Shoulder extension Horizontal abduction of the humerus
Teres minor 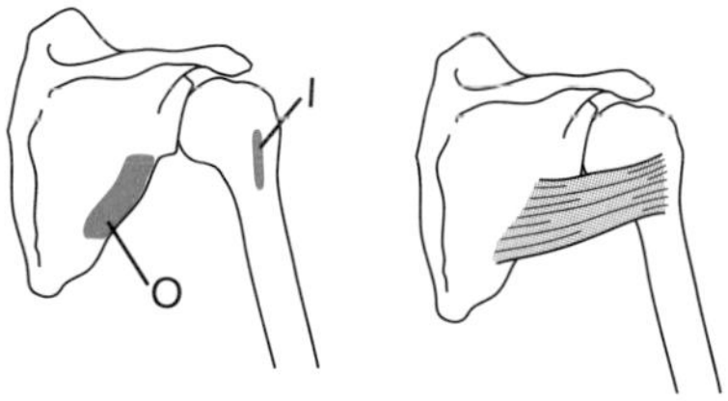	Axillary border of the scapula	Lower posterior greater tuberosity of the humerus	External (lateral) rotation of the humerus Accessory movements: Weak shoulder extension Shoulder adduction

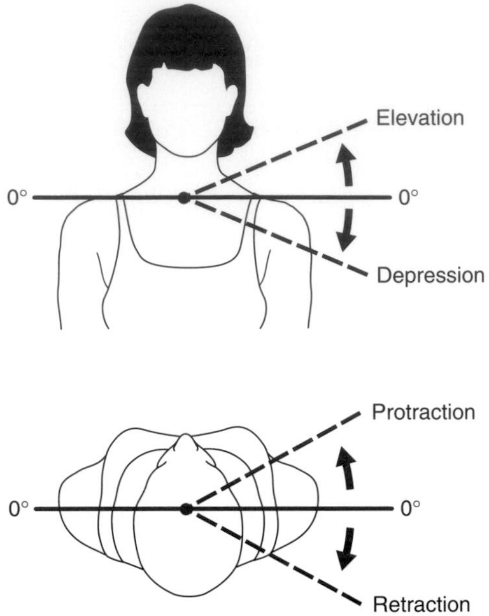

FIGURE 8–4. Scapular movements. (Redrawn from Green W, Heckman J. The Clinical Measurement of Joint Motion. Rosemont, IL: American Academy of Orthopaedic Surgeons, 1994.)

TABLE 8–5. Muscles Involved in the Scapular Movements

Muscle	Origin (O)	Insertion (I)	Action
Trapezius (superior fibers) 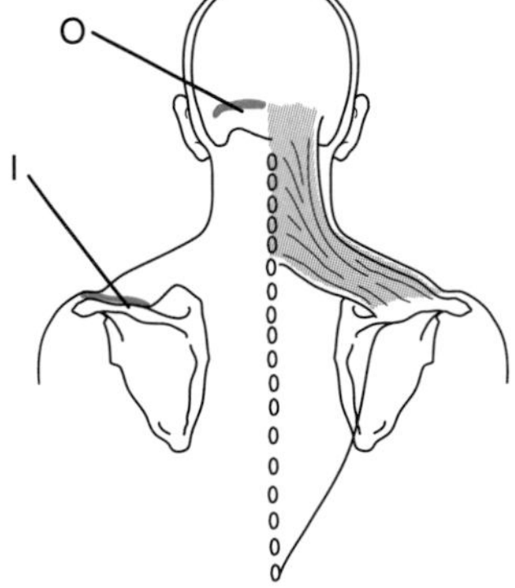	Base of the skull Ligament of the neck	Lateral third of the clavicle (posterior border)	Scapular elevation Accessory movements: Neck extension

TABLE 8–5. Muscles Involved in the Scapular Movements *Continued*

Muscle	Origin (O)	Insertion (I)	Action
Levator scapulae 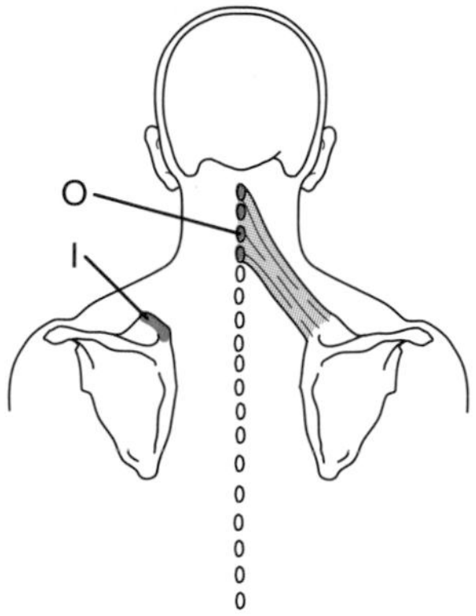	Transverse process of C1 to C4	Upper medial border of the scapula	Scapular elevation
Trapezius (inferior fibers) 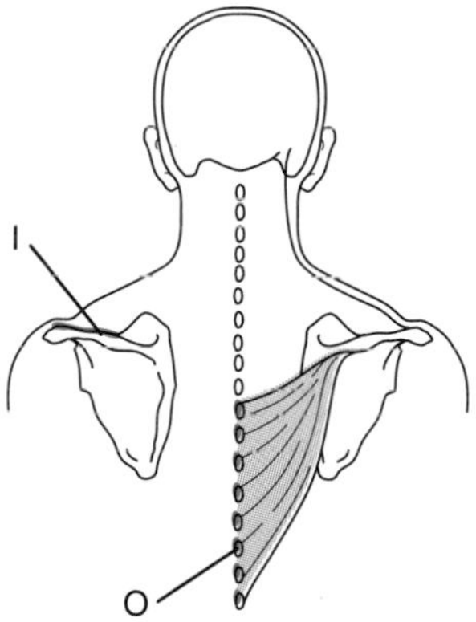	Vertebral spines of the inferior thoracic vertebrae	Scapular spine	Scapular depression Accessory movements: Adduction of the scapula

Table continued on following page

TABLE 8–5. Muscles Involved in the Scapular Movements *Continued*

Muscle	Origin (O)	Insertion (I)	Action
Serratus anterior 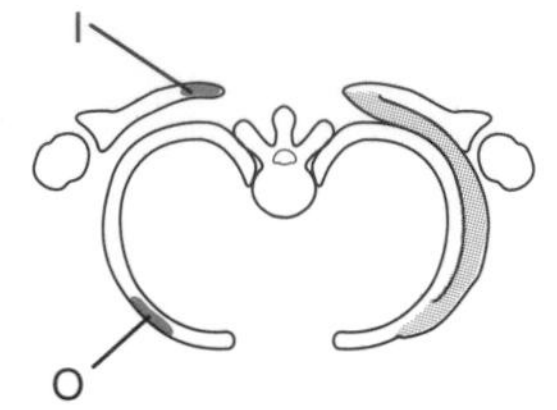	Outer lateral surface of ribs 1 through 9 Aponeuroses covering the intercostal muscles	Costal surface, medial border of the scapula	Abducts scapula Upward rotation of the scapula
Pectoralis minor 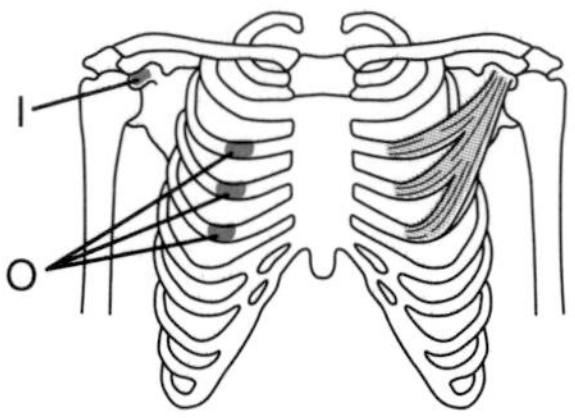	Anterior surface of ribs 3, 4, and 5	Coracoid process of the scapula	Abducts scapula Downward rotation of the scapula

TABLE 8–6. Summary of the Muscles Involved in the Movements of the Shoulder and Shoulder Girdle

Anatomic Movement	Prime Movers	Assistant Movers	Nerve Root Level	Normal Range of Motion
Flexion	Anterior deltoideus Pectoralis minor (clavicular)	Biceps brachii (short head) Coracobrachialis Subscapularis	C5 to T2	0°–180°
Extension	Latissimus dorsi Teres major	Triceps brachii Posterior deltoid	C5 to T2	0°–45°
Abduction	Medial deltoideus Supraspinatus	Pectoralis major (above horizontal) Anterior deltoideus Biceps brachii (long head)	C5 to T1	0°–180°
Adduction	Pectoralis major Latissimus dorsi Teres major	Biceps brachii (short head) Triceps brachii (long head) Coracobrachialis Subscapularis (above horizontal)	C5 to T1	40°–45°
Horizontal adduction	Anterior deltoideus Pectoralis major Coracobrachialis	Biceps brachii	C5 to T1	0°–135° in horizontal plane
Horizontal abduction	Medial deltoideus Posterior deltoideus Infraspinatus Teres minor	Supraspinatus Latissimus dorsi Teres major	C4 to C8	0°–45° in horizontal plane
Internal rotation	Subscapularis Teres major	Anterior deltoideus Pectoralis minor Biceps brachii Latissimus dorsi	C5 to T1	55°
External rotation	Infraspinatus Teres minor	Posterior deltoideus	C4 to C6	40°–45°
Elevation of the scapula	Trapezius Levator scapulae Rhomboids		C1 to C5	
Depression of the scapula	Trapezius Pectoralis minor	Latissimus dorsi	C4 to T1	
Abduction and upward rotation of the scapula	Serratus anterior Trapezius		C2 to C8	
Abduction and downward rotation of the scapula	Rhomboids Pectoralis minor	Levator scapulae	C3 to T1	

Measuring the Range of Motion of the Shoulder

Shoulder range of motion is measured with the goniometer (Fig. 8–5). To measure shoulder flexion and extension, the examiner places the stationary arm of the goniometer along the midaxillary line of the trunk.[1] The moving arm is placed along the midline of the humerus, as viewed from the side.[3]

To measure shoulder abduction, the examiner places the stationary arm of the goniometer parallel to the midline of the body with the axis of the goniometer over the glenohumeral joint.[3] The moving arm is placed along the midline of the humerus, as viewed from behind the subject.[3]

To measure shoulder internal and external rotation, the examiner places the stationary arm of the goniometer parallel to the floor with the shoulder in 90° of abduction and the center of the goniometer at the olecranon process.[4] The moving arm is placed along the dorsal midline of the forearm.

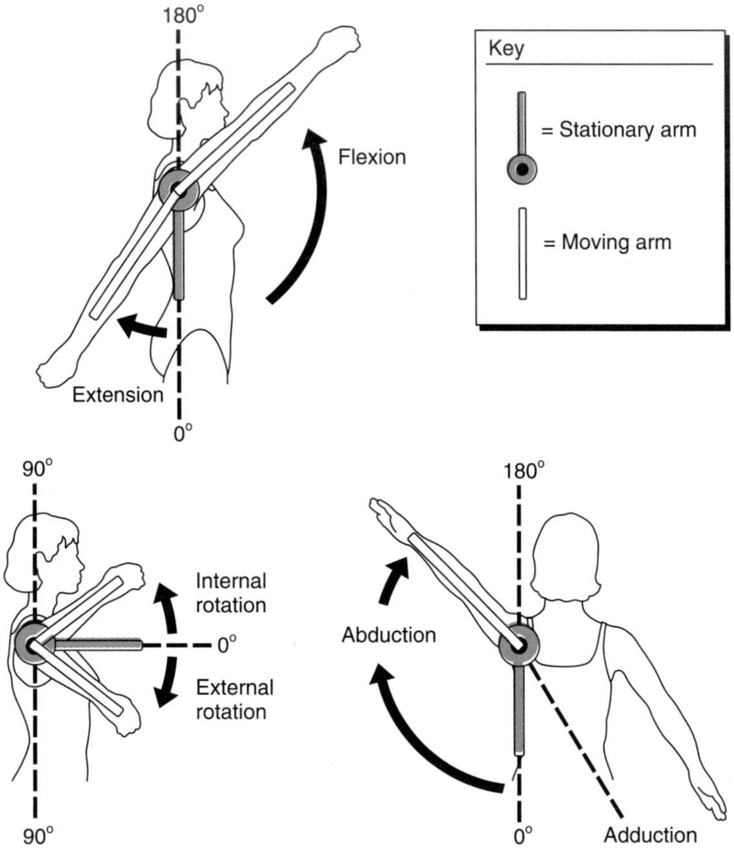

FIGURE 8–5. Measuring the range of motion of the shoulder. (Modified from Green W, Heckman J. The Clinical Measurement of Joint Motion. Rosemont, IL: American Academy of Orthopaedic Surgeons, 1994.)

SHOULDER STRETCHES

Pectoral Stretch (Fig. 8–6)

Prime movers: pectoralis, rhomboids, trapezius, and deltoids.

- Extend the arms in front of the body at shoulder level, with the palms up
- Horizontally abduct the arms, bringing the shoulder blades close to one another
- Keep the palms facing up
- Hold, then relax and return to original position

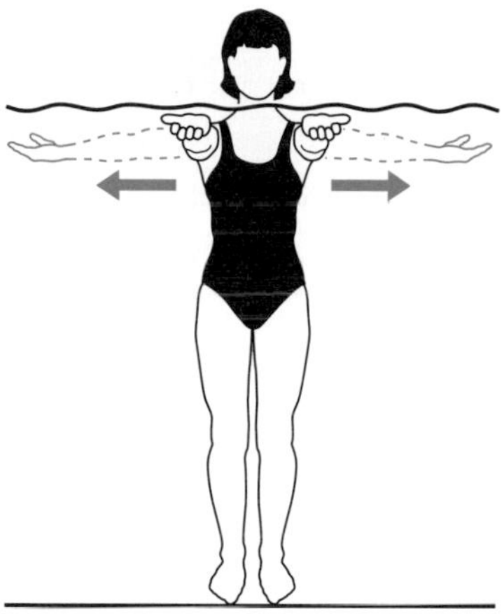

FIGURE 8–6. Pectoral stretch.

Shoulder Shrugs (Fig. 8–7)

Prime movers: trapezius, rhomboids, levator scapulae, and latissimus dorsi.

- Lift both shoulders up toward the ears and hold
- Gently lower the shoulders
- Hold, then relax

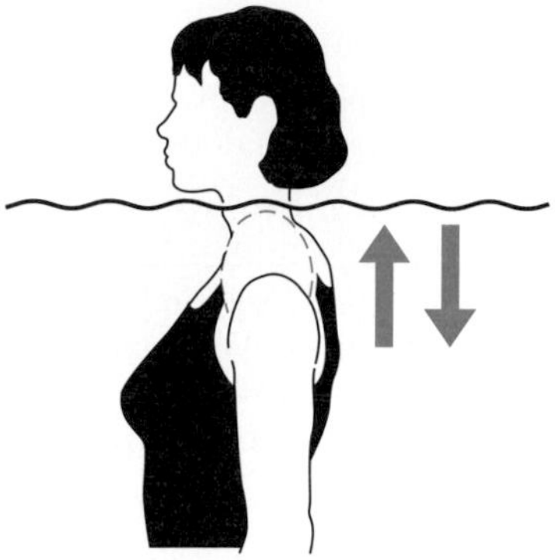

FIGURE 8–7. Shoulder shrugs.

Elbow Touch (Fig. 8–8)

Prime movers: trapezius, rhomboids, posterior deltoids, and pectoralis.

- Place the hands on the shoulders with the elbows out to the sides
- Slowly adduct the elbows until they touch in thc front
- Hold, then relax

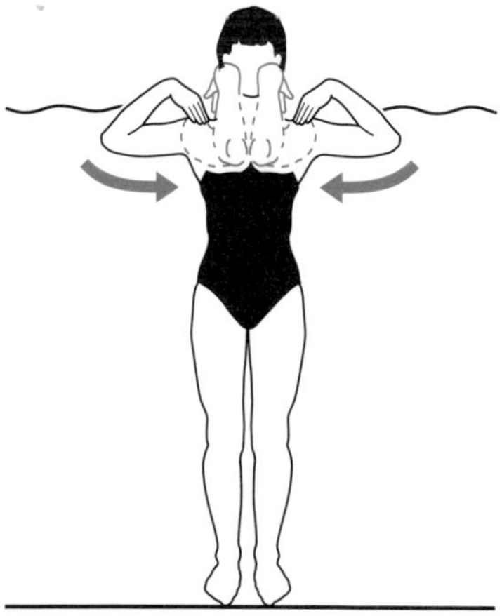

FIGURE 8–8. Elbow touch.

Shoulder Rolls (Fig. 8–9)

Prime movers: trapezius, levator scapulae, rhomboids, pectoralis, latissimus dorsi, and serratus anterior.

- Place the arms at the sides
- Draw an imaginary circle with the shoulders, moving the joints forward, up, back, and down
- Repeat in the opposite direction

NOTE: It is important to emphasize the basic scapular movements: protraction, elevation, retraction, and depression.

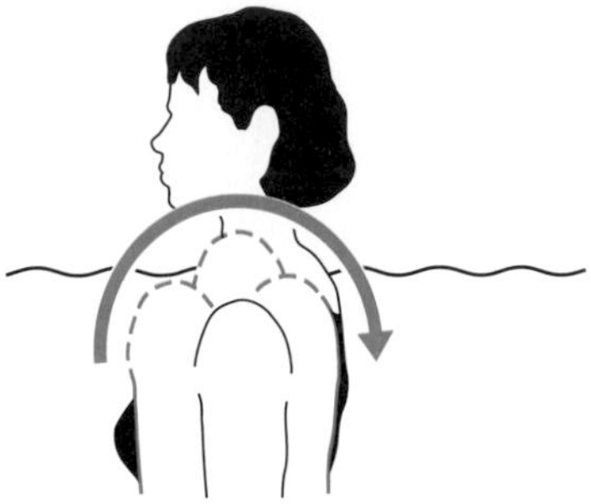

FIGURE 8–9. Shoulder rolls.

Hug Stretch (Fig. 8–10)

Prime movers: trapezius, rhomboids, infraspinatus, teres major, and teres minor.

- Begin with the arms stretched out to the sides
- Place each hand on opposite shoulder
- Flex the chin toward the chest until a gentle stretch is felt at the base of the skull (origin of trapezius)
- Lift the arms slightly and pull forward; the stretch should be felt in the upper and middle portions of the back
- Hold, then relax

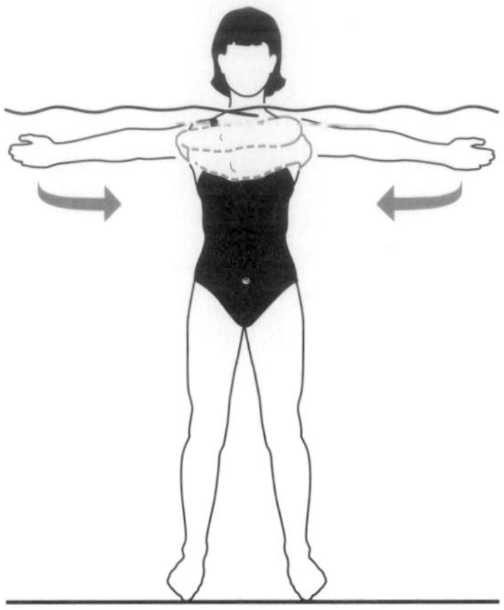

FIGURE 8–10. Hug stretch.

Cross-Shoulder Stretch (Fig. 8–11)

Prime movers: trapezius, rhomboids, infraspinatus, teres major, teres minor, and posterior deltoids.

- Reach across the chest with the (involved) right arm
- Place the left hand above the right elbow and gently pull the arm across the chest
- Hold, then relax
- Repeat with the arms reversed

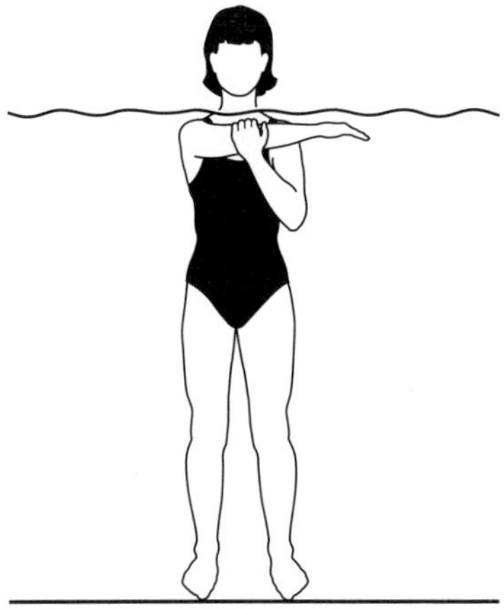

FIGURE 8–11. Cross-shoulder stretch.

Behind Back Pull-back (Fig. 8–12)

Prime movers: pectoralis minor, anterior deltoids, and biceps.

- Grasp the hands behind the back
- Gently lift the clenched hands upward without bending the trunk, hips, or elbows
- Hold, then relax

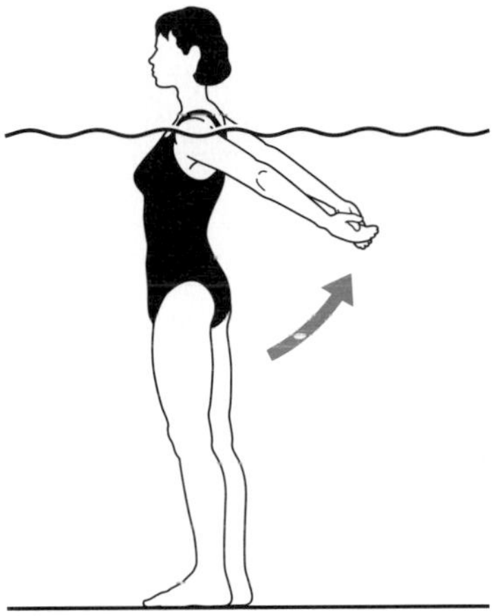

FIGURE 8–12. Behind back pull-back.

Overhead Pullover (Fig. 8–13)

Prime movers: latissimus dorsi, pectoralis, teres major, and triceps.

- Grasp the hands in front of the chest
- Gently reach up as high as possible without arching the back or bending the elbows
- Hold, then lower the arms and relax

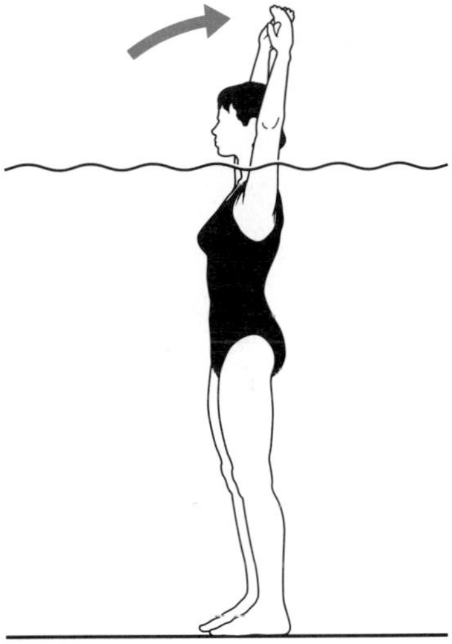

FIGURE 8–13. Overhead pullover.

Shoulder Internal Rotation Stretch (Fig. 8–14)

Prime movers: supraspinatus and long head of biceps.

- Place the arms at the sides with the palms facing back (pronated)
- Flex the elbow on the involved side so that the dorsal surface of the hand is behind the back
- Try to reach the hand up as far as possible; feel a stretch in the anterior shoulder
- Hold, then lower the arm and relax

VARIATION: Perform the movement while holding a flotation device

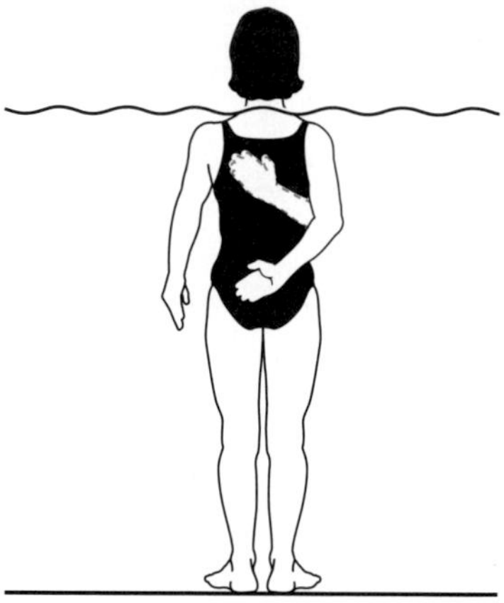

FIGURE 8–14. Shoulder internal rotation stretch.

Shoulder Abduction Stretch (Fig. 8–15)

Prime movers: pectoralis major, latissimus dorsi, and teres major.

- Rest the forearm on the involved side on the edge of the pool with the palm up
- Bring the head down toward the arm while simultaneously moving the trunk away from the pool edge; feel a stretch under the arm
- Hold, then relax

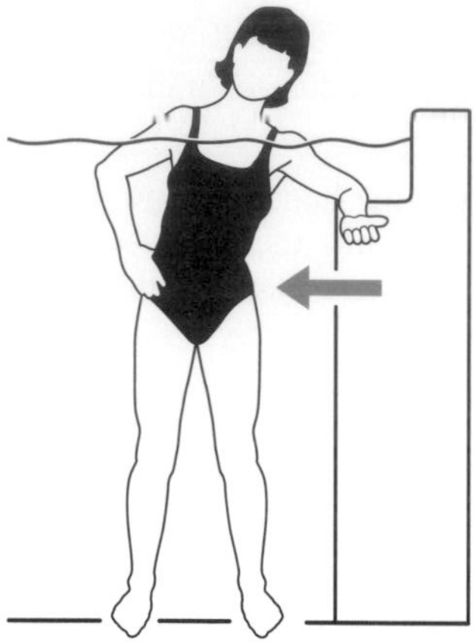

FIGURE 8–15. Shoulder abduction stretch.

Pectoral Press Stretch (Fig. 8–16)

Prime movers: pectoralis and anterior deltoids.

- Stand facing the pool wall with the legs spread slightly and the palms of the hands on the wall; the uninvolved elbow is flexed, the involved comfortably extended
- Keeping the hands stationary, slowly rotate the uninvolved shoulder away from the wall; the involved shoulder moves toward the wall
- Hold, then relax

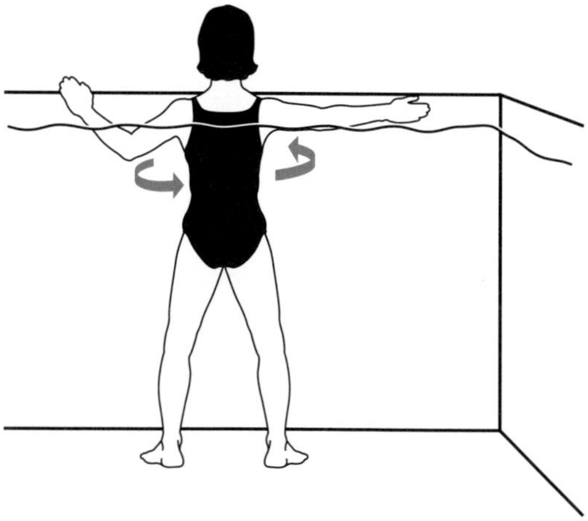

FIGURE 8–16. Pectoral press stretch.

Shoulder External Rotation Stretch (Fig. 8–17)

Prime movers: subscapularis and teres major.

- Place the palm of the involved hand against pool wall with the elbow bent to 90°
- Rotate the trunk on the involved side away from the pool wall, keeping the involved arm fixed and the elbow close to the body
- Turn the body until a stretch is felt across the anterior shoulder
- Hold, then relax

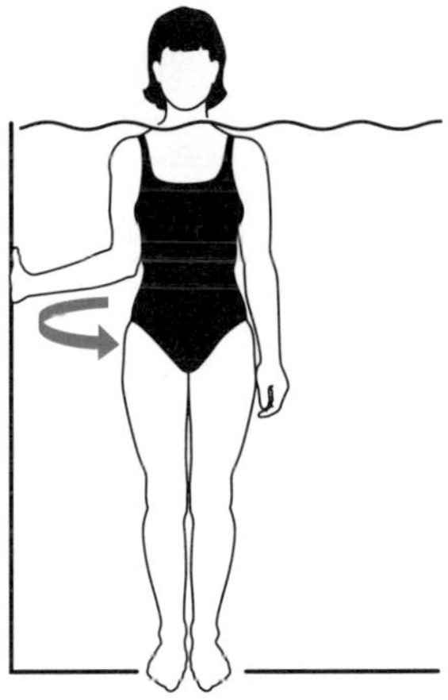

FIGURE 8–17. Shoulder external rotation stretch.

Shoulder Extension, Elbows Bent (Fig. 8–18)

Prime movers: pectoralis, biceps brachii, and anterior deltoid.

- Place the back against a parallel bar
- Hold on to the bar with both hands, palms back
- Keep the feet shoulder-width apart
- Gently lower the body by bending the knees until a stretch is felt in the shoulders
- Hold, then relax

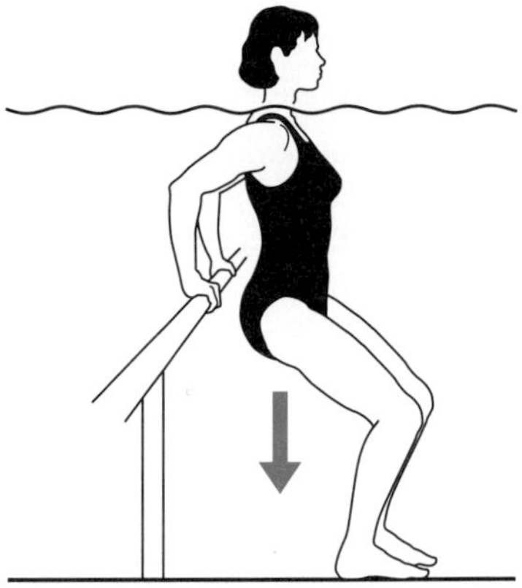

FIGURE 8–18. Shoulder extension, elbows bent.

Shoulder Extension, Elbows Straight (Fig. 8–19)

Prime movers: pectoralis, biceps brachii, and anterior deltoid.

- Hold on to one parallel bar with both hands
- Slowly step forward with one leg, keeping the hands stationary and the back straight, until a stretch is felt in the shoulders
- Hold, then relax

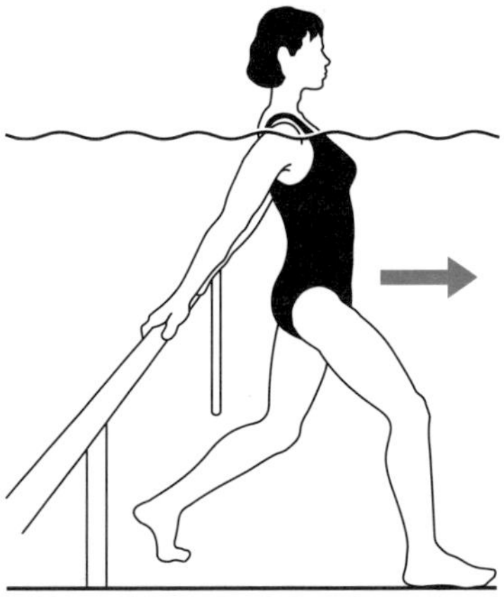

FIGURE 8–19. Shoulder extension, elbows straight.

Corner Stretch (Fig. 8–20)

Prime movers: pectoralis.

- Stand in the corner of the pool with the hands touching the walls at shoulder level, the fingers pointing toward corner, and the feet 2 to 3 feet from the corner
- Bend the elbows and lean forward until a stretch is felt across the chest; do not let the elbows drop
- Hold, then relax

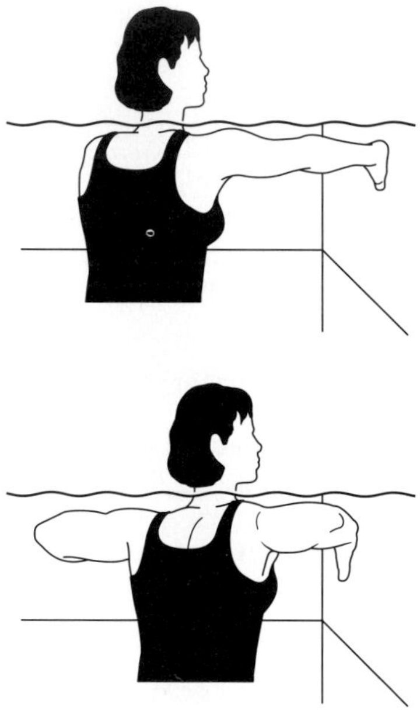

FIGURE 8–20. Corner stretch.

Range of Motion Exercises Using a Wand

In wand exercises, the uninvolved side assists the involved side to obtain maximum range of motion.

Wand Shoulder Flexion (to 90°) (Fig. 8–21)

Prime movers: pectoralis minor, anterior deltoids, biceps brachii, and coracobrachialis.

- Hold the wand in front of the body with both hands, arms straight
- Lift the arms to the surface of the water (90° flexion of shoulders)
- Hold, then lower arms and relax
- Repeat

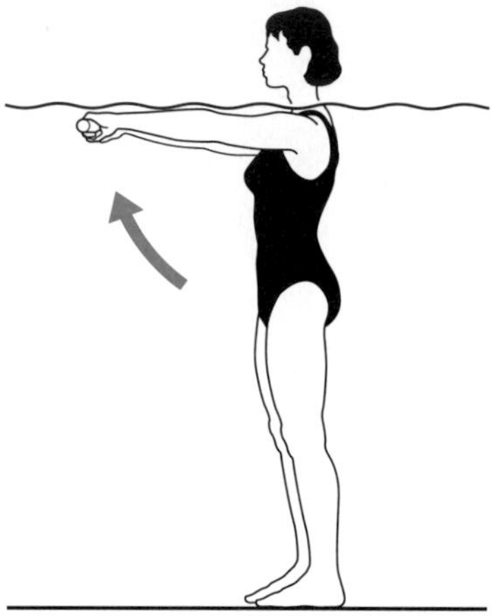

FIGURE 8–21. Wand shoulder flexion (to 90°).

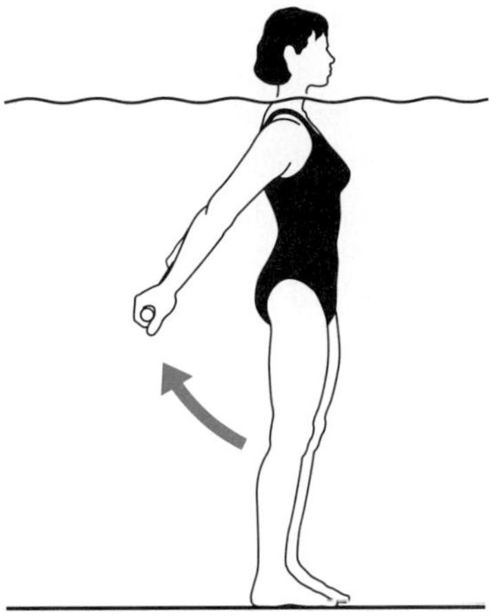

FIGURE 8–22. Wand shoulder extension.

Wand Shoulder Extension (Fig. 8–22)

Prime movers: latissimus dorsi, teres major, triceps, and posterior deltoid.

- Hold the wand with both hands shoulder-width apart behind the back
- Lift the arms upward until a stretch is felt in the involved shoulder
- Hold, then lower arms and relax
- Repeat

VARIATION: Perform movement with floats

Wand Shoulder Abduction (Fig. 8–23)

Prime movers: medial deltoid, supraspinatus, anterior deltoid, and triceps.

- Hold the wand at the ends with both hands, the involved side palm up and the uninvolved side palm down, arms down and straight
- Using the wand, push the involved shoulder into 90° of abduction, with the wand parallel to the floor
- Keep as much of the shoulder in the water as possible
- Hold, then lower the arm and relax

VARIATION: Perform movement in a supine position

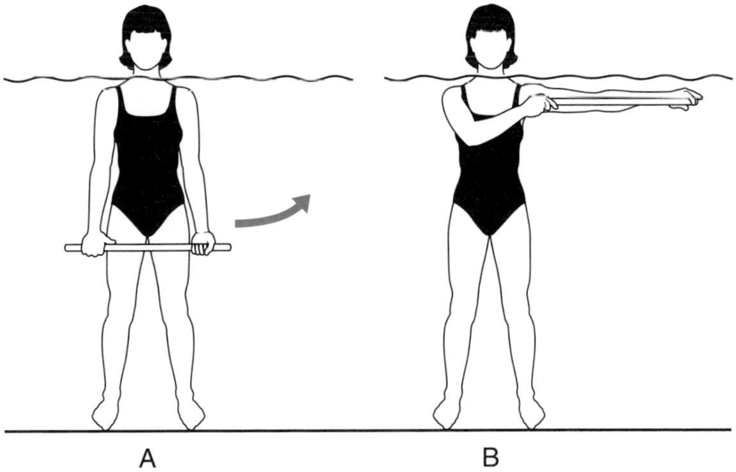

FIGURE 8–23. Wand shoulder abduction.

Wand Horizontal Abduction and Adduction (Fig. 8–24)

Prime movers: deltoids, pectoralis, infraspinatus, teres minor, coracobrachialis, latissimus dorsi, teres major, and biceps brachii.

- Hold the wand at the ends with both hands in front of the body at shoulder level, palms down
- Without allowing the trunk to rotate, push the wand across the body with the uninvolved arm, putting the involved shoulder in a position of horizontal abduction; hold
- Pull the wand back across the body, putting the involved shoulder in a position of horizontal adduction
- Hold, then return to the original position

Wand External Rotation (Fig. 8–25)

Prime movers: latissimus dorsi, subscapularis, pectoralis major, teres major, infraspinatus, teres minor, deltoids, and biceps.

- Stand with the back against the pool wall
- Hold the wand in both hands with the involved side palm up and the uninvolved side palm down
- Keeping the elbow of the involved side bent to 90° and close to the body, use the uninvolved arm to push the involved arm into a position of external rotation
- Hold, then return to the original position

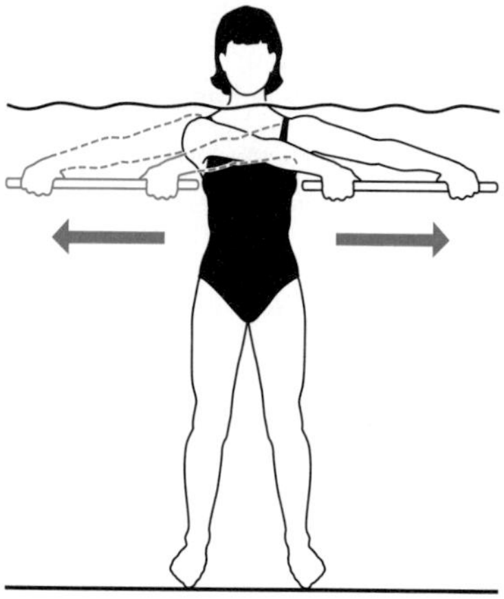

FIGURE 8–24. Wand horizontal abduction and adduction.

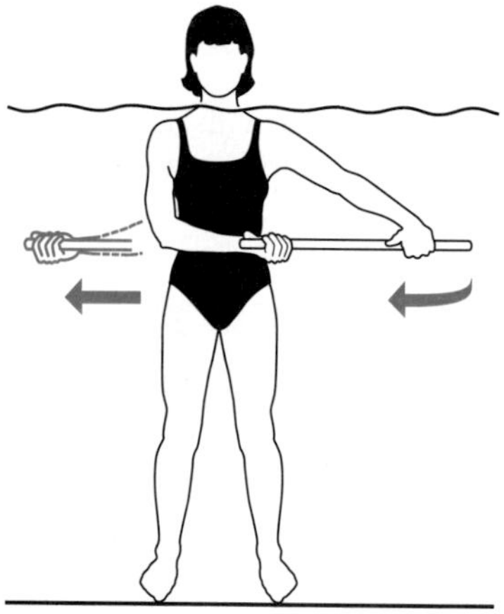

FIGURE 8–25. Wand external rotation.

Wand Functional Internal and External Rotation (Fig. 8–26)

Prime movers: latissimus dorsi, subscapularis, pectoralis major, teres major, infraspinatus, teres minor, deltoids, and long head of biceps.

- Place one arm at the side with the palm facing back; flex the elbow so that the dorsal surface of the hand is behind the back
- Holding the wand, reach up above head with the opposite arm and flex the elbow to place the hand behind the head
- Hold the wand with both hands vertically behind the back
- Pull the wand up to stretch internal rotation of the inferior arm; hold, then relax
- Pull the wand down to stretch external rotation of the superior arm; hold, then relax
- Repeat with arms reversed

VARIATION: This exercise can be performed in a supine position, on the surface of the water, with floats around the neck, waist, and ankles

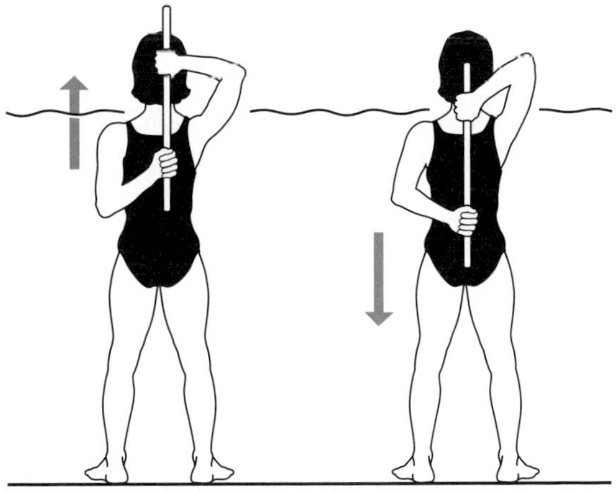

FIGURE 8–26. Wand functional internal and external rotation.

Supine Shoulder Stretches

These exercises are performed with the patient floating supine with floats around the neck and hips. The feet are fixed by resting on the edge of the pool or on a ladder. Each exercise may be performed with a wand (active-assisted movement), float (supportive movement), or paddle (resistive movement).

Shoulder Overhead Press, Supine (Fig. 8–27)

Prime movers: latissimus dorsi, supraspinatus, pectoralis, teres major, and deltoids.

- Join the hands and press upward from the shoulders
- Keep the movement along the surface of the water
- Hold, then relax

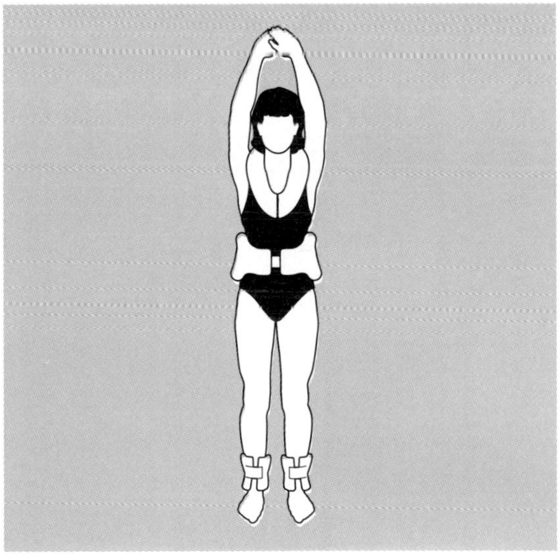

FIGURE 8–27. Shoulder overhead press, supine.

Shoulder Abduction, Supine (Fig. 8–28)

Prime movers: latissimus dorsi, supraspinatus, pectoralis, teres major, and deltoids.

- Start with the arms at the sides
- Abduct the shoulders as far as possible, keeping the arms near the surface of the water
- Hold, then return to the original position

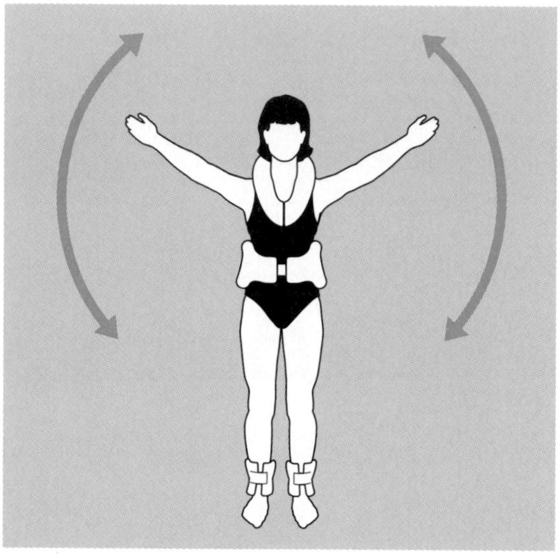

FIGURE 8–28. Shoulder abduction, supine.

Shoulder External Rotation, Supine (Fig. 8–29)

Prime movers: latissimus dorsi, supraspinatus, subscapularis, pectoralis, teres major, and deltoids.

- Hold the wand in the hands above the head, palms up
- Pull the wand down toward the top of the head; try to achieve a position of 90° shoulder abduction and 90° elbow flexion bilaterally
- Hold, then relax

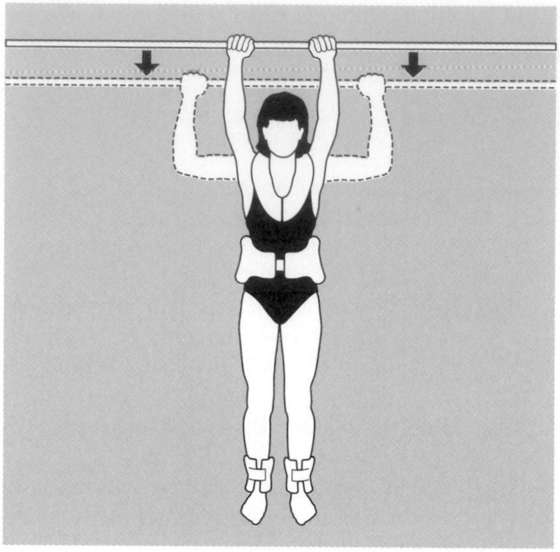

FIGURE 8–29. Shoulder external rotation, supine.

SHOULDER EXERCISES

Shoulder Press-down (Fig. 8–30)

Prime movers: trapezius, pectoralis minor, latissimus dorsi, and deltoids.

- Hold flotation devices slightly in front of the body, at chest level and with the elbows bent
- Press down, extending the elbows
- Return to the original position

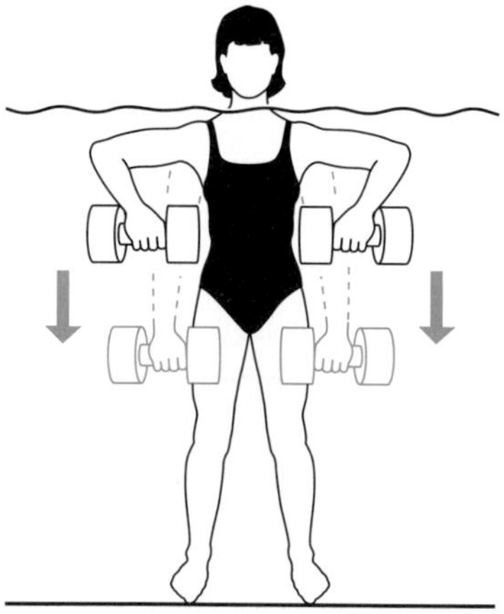

FIGURE 8–30. Shoulder press-down.

Resistive Shoulder Adduction and Abduction (Fig. 8–31)

Prime movers: adduction: pectoralis major, latissimus dorsi, teres major, short head of biceps brachii, and short head of triceps brachii; abduction: medial deltoid, supraspinatus, anterior deltoid, and triceps brachii.

- Hold resistive devices out to the sides slightly below shoulder level
- Pull the arms toward the hips (adduction) maintaining elbow extension throughout the exercise
- Do not twist or rotate the trunk
- Return to the original position (abduction)

VARIATION: During abduction, alter forearm pronation and supination to alter the degree of difficulty of the exercise

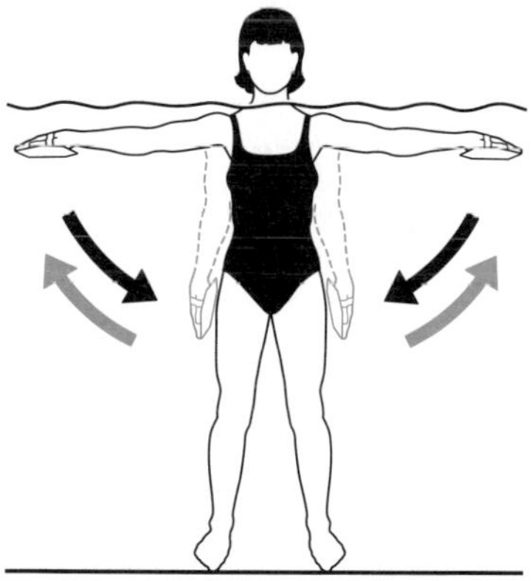

FIGURE 8–31. Resistive shoulder adduction and abduction.

Resistive Shoulder Flexion (Fig. 8–32)

Prime movers: anterior deltoid, pectoralis minor, biceps brachii, and coracobrachialis.

- Hold resistive devices in the hands at the sides, palms forward
- Raise the involved arm in front of the body and lift it toward the surface of the water, keeping the elbow straight but not locked
- Return to the original position

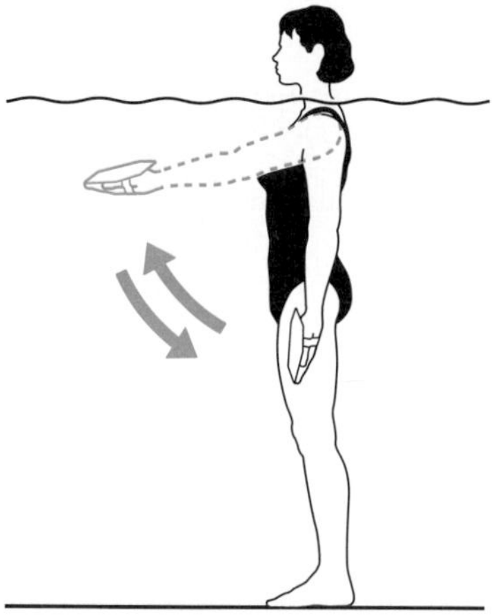

FIGURE 8–32. Resistive shoulder flexion.

Resistive Shoulder Extension (Fig. 8–33)

Prime movers: latissimus dorsi, teres major, triceps brachii, and posterior deltoid.

- Hold resistive devices in the hands at the sides, palms back
- Lift the involved arm posteriorly toward the surface of the water, keeping the elbow straight but not locked
- Return to the original position

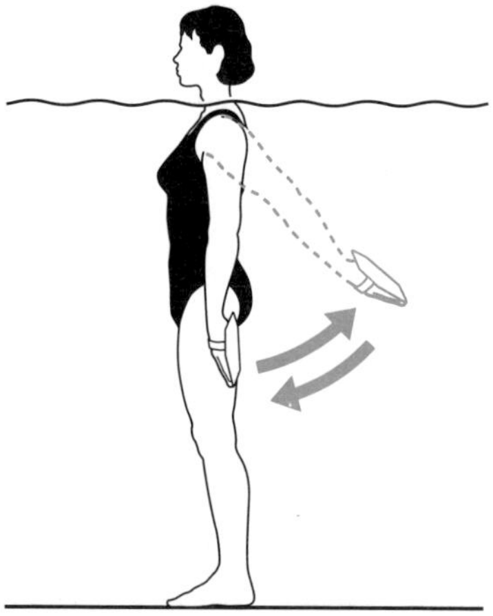

FIGURE 8–33. Resistive shoulder extension.

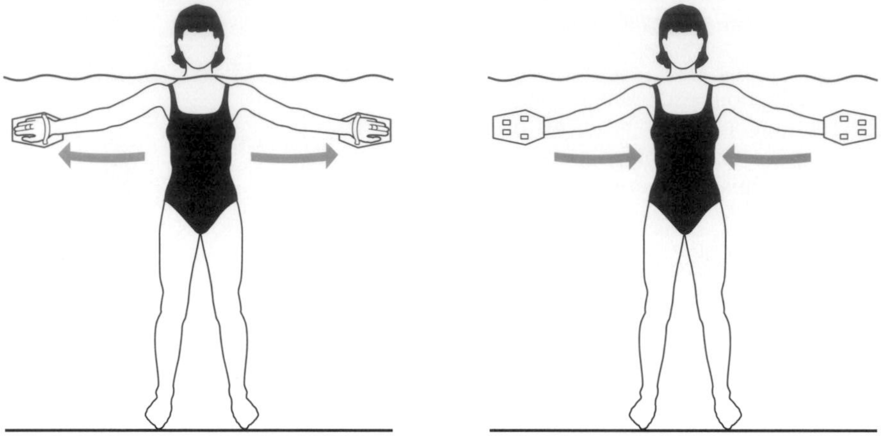

FIGURE 8–34. Resistive horizontal abduction and adduction.

Resistive Horizontal Abduction and Adduction (Fig. 8–34)

Prime movers: horizontal abduction: medial deltoid, posterior deltoid, infraspinatus, teres minor, latissimus dorsi, and teres major; horizontal adduction: anterior deltoid, pectoralis major, pectoralis minor, coracobrachialis, and biceps brachii.

- Hold resistive paddles in front of the body at shoulder level, with the elbows slightly flexed
- With the palms facing posteriorly, move the hands away from the midline of the body (abduction)
- Turn the palms forward and adduct the arms to return to the original position

Resistive Internal and External Rotation (Fig. 8–35)

Prime movers: internal rotation: subscapularis, teres major, anterior deltoid, pectoralis minor, and biceps brachii; external rotation: infraspinatus, teres minor, and posterior deltoid.

- Hold a resistive device in the hand of the involved arm with the elbow held against the side and bent to 90°
- Gently externally rotate the shoulder, keeping the forearm parallel to the floor and the elbow close to the side.
- Then rotate shoulder internally, crossing the hand in front of the body past the midline.

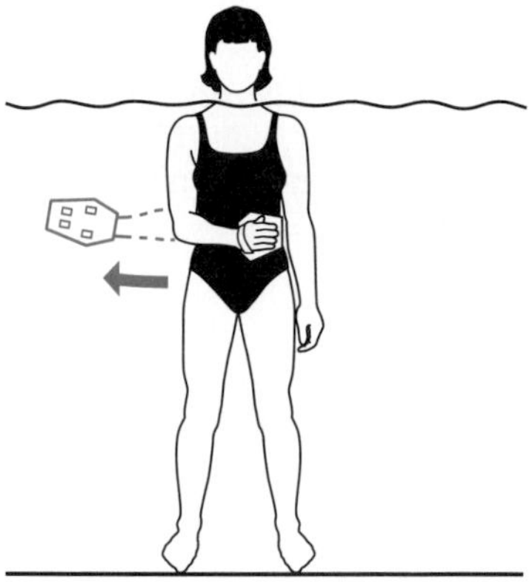

FIGURE 8–35. Resistivc internal and external rotation.

Rowing (Fig. 8–36)

Prime movers: latissimus dorsi, rhomboids, trapezius, and posterior deltoids.

- Secure stretch bands (bungee cords) to the ladder or any other fixed object in the pool, and face the ladder, holding the handles in both hands
- Place one foot on the ladder for support
- Gently pull the hands back at chest level, leading with the elbows and adducting the scapulae
- Return to the original position

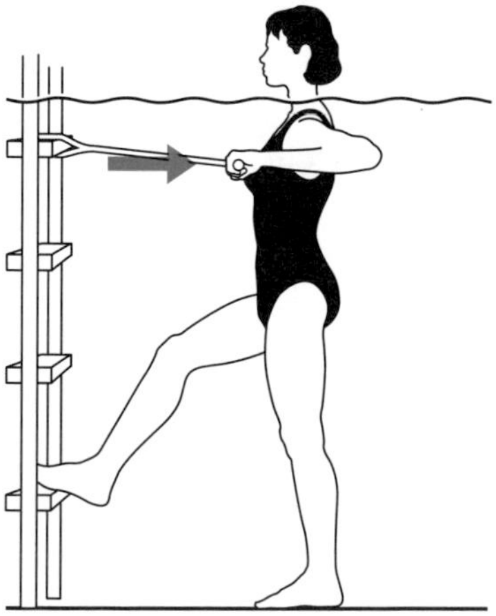

FIGURE 8–36. Rowing.

Side Arm Pull (Fig. 8–37)

Prime movers: medial deltoid, supraspinatus, anterior deltoid, and triceps.

- Secure a stretch band (bungee cord) to the ladder or any other fixed object in the pool, and stand with the uninvolved side of the body facing the ladder
- Place the uninvolved hand on the ladder for support
- Reach across the body with the other hand, grasp the handle of the stretch band, and gently abduct the arm, keeping the elbow straight
- Return to the original position

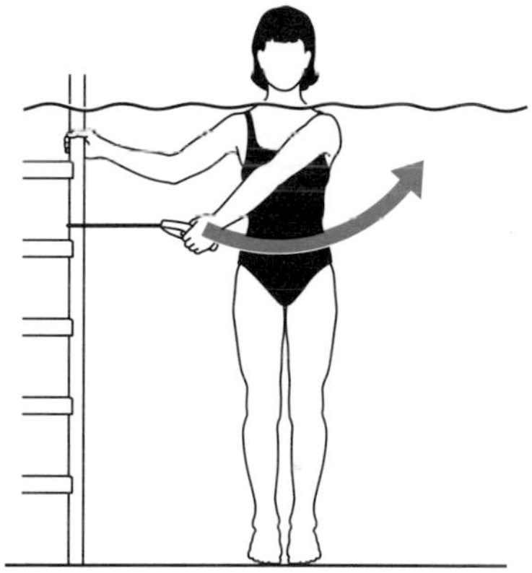

FIGURE 8–37. Side arm pull.

Upright Rowing (Fig. 8–38)

Prime movers: trapezius, anterior deltoid, and biceps.

- Stand on one end of a stretch band (bungee cord) and hold the handle with both hands
- Leading with the elbow (abduction), pull the hands toward the surface of the water; keep the hands close to the body
- Return to the original position

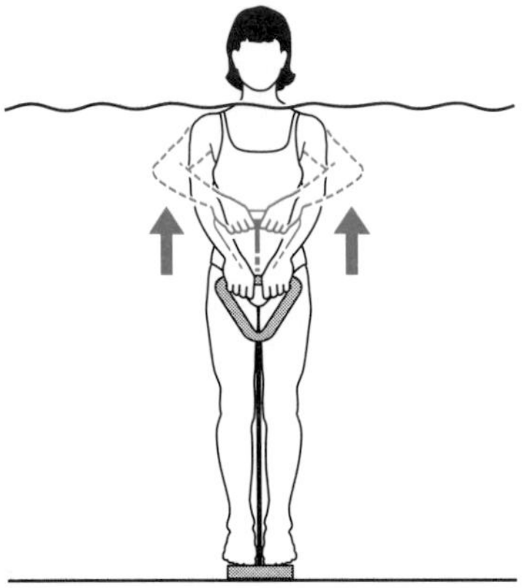

FIGURE 8–38. Upright rowing.

COMMON CONDITIONS OF THE SHOULDER

Shoulder Arthritis

Shoulder arthritis is a general term used for any arthritic condition when it is located in the shoulder.

Origin

The shoulder is affected by osteoarthritis less than the joints of the lower extremities are because it does not bear weight. Shoulder arthritis is usually caused by a specific predisposing factor, such as a previous injury, disease, or systemic rheumatoid arthritis.

Pathology

Arthritis can affect either the glenohumeral joint or the acromioclavicular joint (Fig. 8–39). The various pathologic processes that may be involved are described in Chapter 7.

Signs and Symptoms

Pain, decreased range of motion, and decreased strength are common with this condition. The decreased range of motion may be caused by damage to the joint itself or by soft tissue shortening. The symptoms may be intensified if arthritis is combined with an acute injury.

Body Parts Affected

- Bones (scapula, humerus, clavicle)
- Joint surfaces (articular cartilage)
- Soft tissues (joint capsule, muscles, tendons, ligaments)

Exercise Priorities

- Establish a controlled exercise program (be careful that the patient does not overdo it)
- Maximize shoulder range of motion
- Strengthen all shoulder muscles

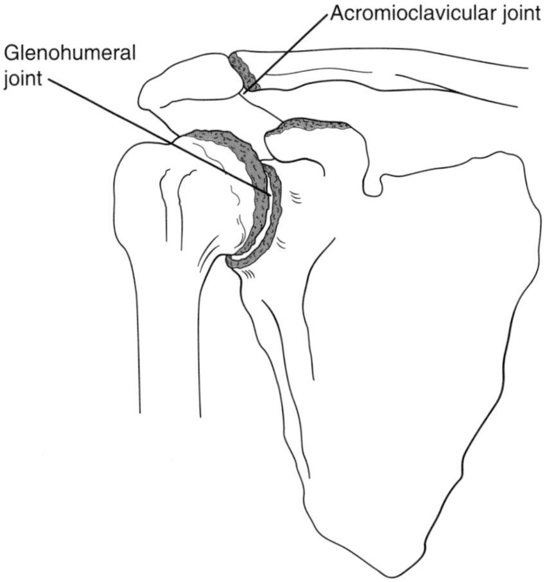

FIGURE 8–39. Shoulder arthritis.

Shoulder (Acromioclavicular) Sprain

Also known as a shoulder separation, this injury involves the acromioclavicular ligament and possibly the coracoclavicular ligament.

Origin

The most common mechanism of injury is a blow to the superior-posterior aspect of the shoulder. This can occur with a fall on the shoulder or on an outstretched hand. It can also occur with a traction injury whereby the arm is pulled away from the body.

Pathology

A first-degree sprain is a partial tear of the acromioclavicular ligament (Fig. 8–40). A second-degree sprain involves a complete tear of the acromioclavicular ligament and a partial tear of the coracoclavicular ligament. A third-degree sprain involves a complete tear of both ligaments. Full recovery from this injury is very slow, often taking a year or more.

Signs and Symptoms

A "tent pole" deformity is common with moderate to severe sprains. This occurs because the end of the clavicle rises, lifting the skin like a tent pole. It is very painful if palpated and if the arm is horizontally adducted.

Body Parts Affected

- Ligaments (acromioclavicular and coracoclavicular)
- Bones (humerus, clavicle, scapula)
- Soft tissues (shoulder muscles, tendons, shoulder joint capsule)

Exercise Priorities

- Restore full range of motion
- Strengthen all shoulder muscles (start with pain-free movements and add exercises as tolerated)

Shoulder Fracture

Common shoulder fractures include those of the acromion, humerus, scapula, and clavicle (Fig. 8–41).

Origin

Fractures to this part of the body are usually caused by a fall or some sort of direct blow, such as would occur in a car accident.

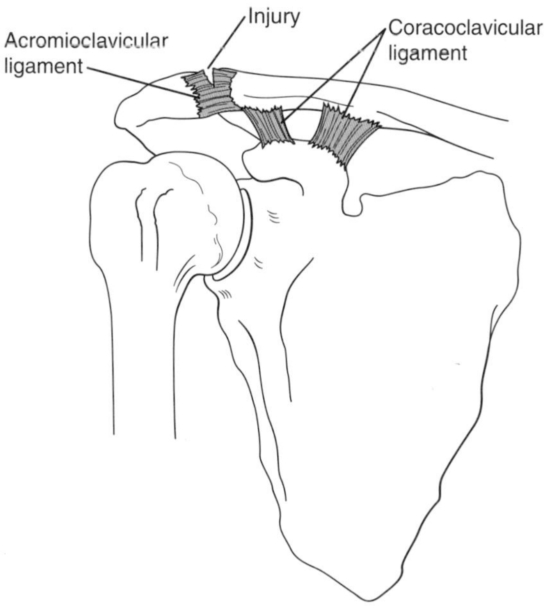

FIGURE 8–40. Shoulder sprain.

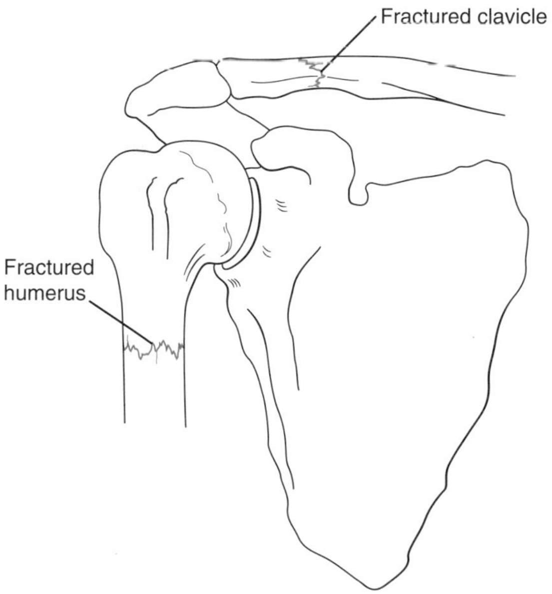

FIGURE 8–41. Common shoulder fractures.

Pathology

The various types of fractures are outlined in Chapter 7. Undisplaced fractures are usually treated conservatively by having the patient rest the arm in a sling for 4 to 6 weeks. Some doctors may want to begin rehabilitation within this period. More severe fractures may require open reduction and internal fixation, which also allows an early start to mobilization. It must be conveyed to the patient that any fracture that involves a joint is usually more difficult to rehabilitate and results in a significant risk of osteoarthritis in that joint.

Signs and Symptoms

After the acute pain resolves, the patient has pain only with movement. The degree of weakness and loss of range of motion can vary greatly.

Body Parts Affected

- Bones (scapula, clavicle, humerus)
- Glenohumeral and acromioclavicular joints
- Soft tissues (shoulder muscles, ligaments, joint capsule)

Exercise Priorities

- Restore range of motion as soon as possible (the longer this is postponed, the harder it is to achieve)
- Maintain range of motion in adjacent areas (neck, elbow, wrist)
- Strengthen all shoulder muscles

Shoulder Tendonitis

This common injury involves inflammation of one or more tendons of the shoulder. Usually, the rotator cuff tendons are involved, most commonly the supraspinatus tendon (Fig. 8–42).

Origin

This injury can be caused by a direct blow, but it is usually a repetitive strain injury. Overhead activities cause an impingement of the rotator cuff tendons between the humerus and the coracoacromial ligament. If the cuff tendons become inflamed, they swell. This in turn causes more impingement and sets up a cycle of impingement and inflammation.

Pathology

The pathology of tendonitis is described in Chapter 7. This particular injury is relatively slow to heal because the blood supply to the rotator cuff is generally poor and because many activities of daily living involve overhead activities.

Signs and Symptoms

The "painful arc," shown in Figure 8–43, is the most common sign of shoulder tendonitis. Increased pain also occurs with overhead activities and with reaching behind the back (ie, stretching of the supraspinatus). Pain is often referred to the deltoid region.

Body Parts Affected

- Rotator cuff muscles and tendons
- Coracoacromial ligament
- Large shoulder muscles (pectoralis major, latissimus dorsi, deltoid, long head of biceps)

Exercise Priorities

- Gently stretch the injured tendon
- Strengthen all rotator cuff muscles within a range that does not impinge the tendons (less than 90° of shoulder flexion and abduction)
- Start with strengthening exercises that are pain free and gradually add other exercises as tolerated

Shoulder Bursitis

This injury has a presentation similar to that of shoulder tendonitis. The treatment routine is also very similar.

Origin

Bursitis is almost always an overuse injury. As with shoulder tendonitis, it is most often caused by excessive amounts of overhead activities. It may become a chronic problem, depending on the patient's occupation or athletic activity.

Pathology

The subacromial bursa and the subdeltoid bursa (Fig. 8–44) are the ones most commonly involved. The pathology of bursitis is discussed in Chapter 7.

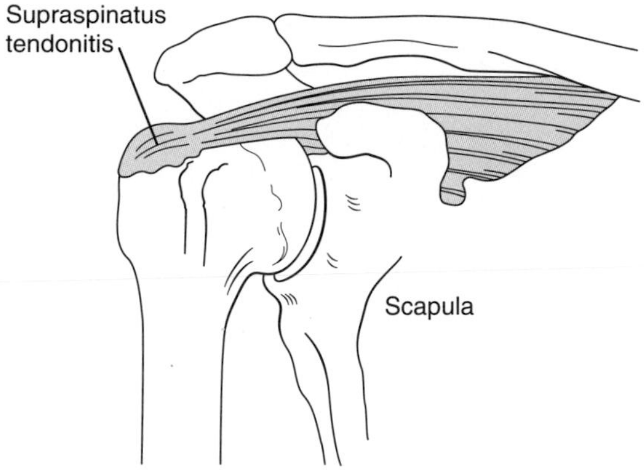

FIGURE 8–42. Shoulder tendonitis.

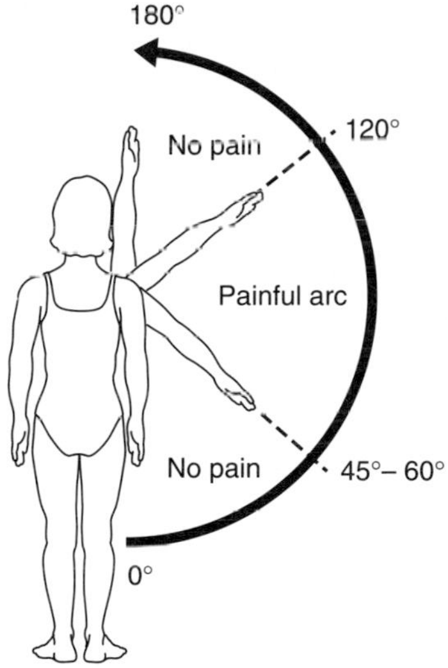

FIGURE 8–43. Painful arc syndrome.

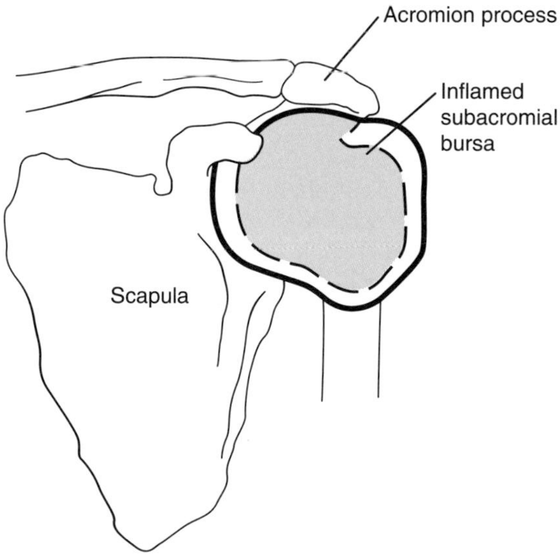

FIGURE 8–44. Shoulder bursitis.

Signs and Symptoms

A "painful arc" (see Fig. 8–43) is a common sign of shoulder bursitis. However, true bursitis may be painful even without impingement of the bursa. The pain may subside and then recur without warning.

Body Parts Affected

- Bursa (subacromial, subdeltoid)
- Coracoacromial ligament
- Muscles of the shoulder

Exercise Priorities

- Restore range of motion as soon as possible
- Gradually institute a strengthening program of all shoulder muscles, staying within the pain-free range

Rotator Cuff Damage

The surgical repair of a torn rotator cuff is a very common procedure.

Origin

The tear may have occurred from a single traumatic incident, such as a fall on the shoulder. It may also be the result of a repetitive strain injury (the tendon becomes chronically inflamed, weakens, and then ruptures).

Pathology

The surgery is done to repair third-degree strains, usually of the supraspinatus or subscapularis muscles. The various procedures used in the repair involve stitching the torn structures together or stapling the torn tendon to the bone (Fig. 8–45).

Signs and Symptoms

Before the surgical repair, the shoulder is very weak. Some movements may not be possible at all. After the operation, active movement is weak and painful. The rate at which the pain subsides varies from person to person.

Body Parts Affected

- Rotator cuff muscles and tendons
- Larger shoulder muscles (pectoralis muscles, deltoid, latissimus dorsi)

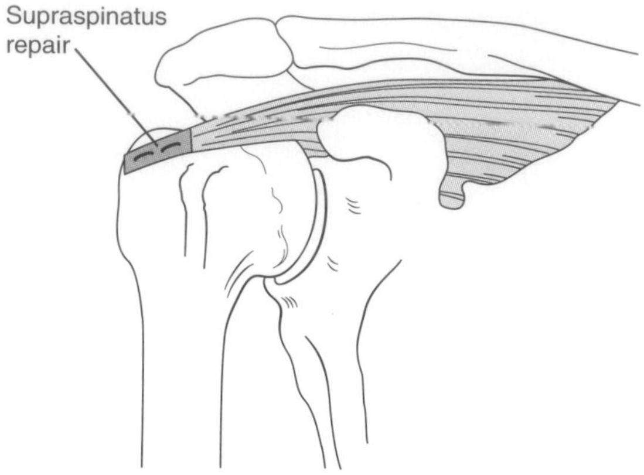

FIGURE 8–45. Rotator cuff reconstruction.

Exercise Priorities

- Check with the surgeon to determine whether there are any restrictions on movement
- Start with assistive exercise in the early phases to increase range of motion
- Start a strengthening program with the uninvolved muscles first; gradually add exercises for all shoulder muscles

Frozen Shoulder (Adhesive Capsulitis)

This syndrome is characterized by increasing shoulder pain and stiffness.

Origin

Although the exact cause of adhesive capsulitis is not known, it is often secondary to an acute problem. It may occur after a period of immobilization (eg, after a fracture), after a repetitive strain injury, or for no apparent reason.

Pathology

In this condition, intra-articular lesions develop within the joint capsule. Thickening and stiffening of the joint capsule then occur (Fig. 8–46). There is usually a gradual spontaneous recovery, but without treatment this recovery can take 2 years or longer.

Signs and Symptoms

Pain and stiffness are the chief complaints, with the most limited movements being external rotation, abduction, and internal rotation. There is often a reversed scapulohumeral rhythm (by which the scapula moves more than the glenohumeral joint during abduction) and referred pain down the arm. As the condition progresses, pain decreases, but the stiffness may start to involve adjacent muscles, such as those of the neck.

Body Parts Affected

- Joint capsule
- Shoulder muscles and tendons

Exercise Priorities

- Restore range of motion (pain may not be a useful guideline)
- Begin strengthening exercises as tolerated

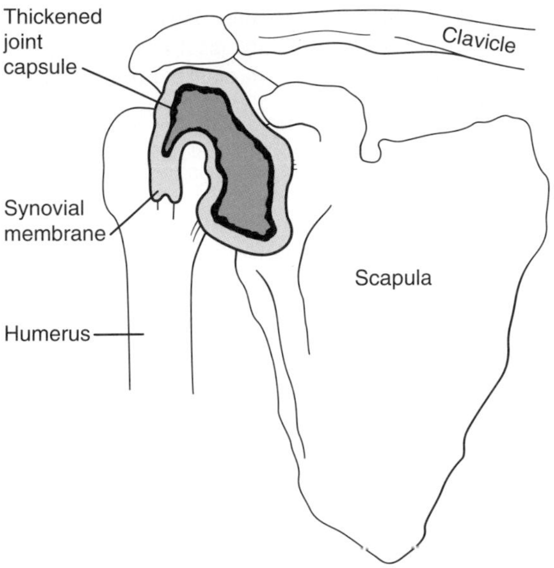

FIGURE 8–46. Adhesive capsulitis.

Shoulder Dislocation

This injury involves the subluxation of the glenohumeral joint.

Origin

The most common cause of shoulder dislocation is an abduction and external rotation force on the humerus. This produces an anterior dislocation. If the dislocation results from a fall on an outstretched hand, the humeral head dislocates posteriorly (Fig. 8–47).

Pathology

During a dislocation, the joint capsule may be torn or stretched. There may also be some damage to the rotator cuff muscles. Recurrent dislocations occur if there is a laxity in the joint. This may require corrective surgery, which involves tightening of the anterior or posterior rotator cuff tendons. Rehabilitation takes essentially the same course regardless of whether surgery is performed.

Signs and Symptoms

Before the dislocation has been reduced, the acromion is very prominent, and there is a marked "step defect." It is visually obvious that the shoulder has been dislocated. After reduction, the shoulder looks normal, but it is still quite painful. After the pain subsides, the patient may be left with some joint laxity and a feeling of apprehension when the arm is

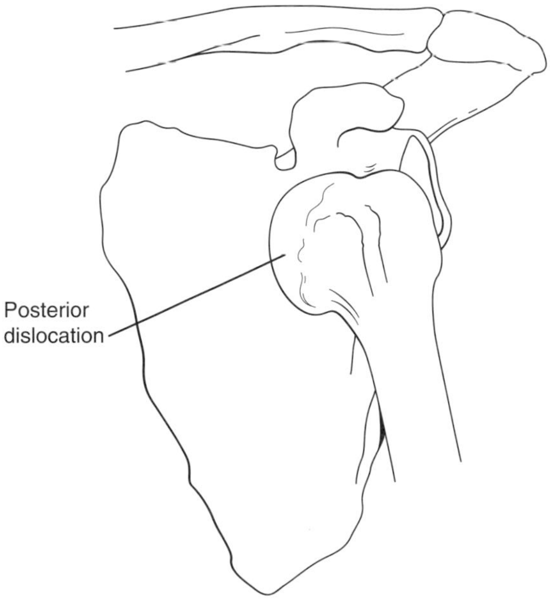

FIGURE 8–47. Shoulder dislocation.

abducted and externally rotated. This fearful feeling probably occurs because subconsciously the patient is aware that abduction with external rotation is an unstable position.

Body Parts Affected

- Joint capsule
- Rotator cuff muscles and tendons
- Large shoulder muscles (pectoralis muscles, deltoid, latissimus dorsi)
- Nerves of the brachial plexus

Exercise Priorities

- Gradually restore range of motion as tolerated (do not push for full flexion or full external rotation)
- Strengthen weak rotator cuff muscles (try to achieve equal strength between internal rotators and external rotators)
- Strengthen all large shoulder muscles

Reflex Sympathetic Dystrophy

Reflex sympathetic dystrophy involving the shoulder results from malfunction of the sympathetic nervous system after an injury. The whole arm becomes hypersensitive, and a vicious cycle of pain and stiffness is established.

Origin

The precipitating incident is usually a fracture or severe soft tissue injury somewhere in the upper extremity. There is no way to predict at the time of injury whether reflex sympathetic dystrophy will develop.

Pathology

Although the exact mechanism of this syndrome is not known, it is clear that the autonomic nervous system, the vascular system, and the sensory nerves are affected. The hypersensitivity and severe pain lead to guarded movement. The long-term changes that result from the decreased movement include the formation of fibrous tissue in associated soft tissue, osteoporosis, muscle atrophy, and degenerative changes within the joint.

Signs and Symptoms

As previously mentioned, pain and stiffness are always severe problems. The malfunctioning autonomic nervous system may also lead to changes in the skin, such as increased sweating, shiny skin, and cyanosis.

Body Parts Affected

- Nervous system
- Circulatory system
- Muscles, bones, and joints of the entire limb
- Brain (coping strategies for dealing with the severe pain may be necessary)

Exercise Priorities

- Increase range of motion
- Try not to cause excessive pain (various pain-relieving methods may be tried before exercise to allow more movement, including physical therapy modalities, nerve blocks, pain medications, and psychologic coping methods)

Shoulder Hemiarthroplasty

A shoulder hemiarthroplasty involves the replacement of the humeral head only. The glenoid fossa is not replaced.

Origin

This operation is usually performed because there is a significant amount of damage to the glenohumeral joint. Such a condition may occur with advanced arthritis or after a severe injury.

Pathology

This surgery involves the excision of the humeral head. A prosthetic head is then put in its place, and the muscles are reattached to the bones (Fig. 8–48).

Signs and Symptoms

Most patients find that the postoperative pain quickly subsides to a level lower than that of their preoperative pain. The degree of limitation of range of motion varies from person to person.

Body Parts Affected

- Check with the surgeon for any range of motion restrictions
- Increase range of motion (full range may not be attainable)
- Increase strength of all shoulder muscles

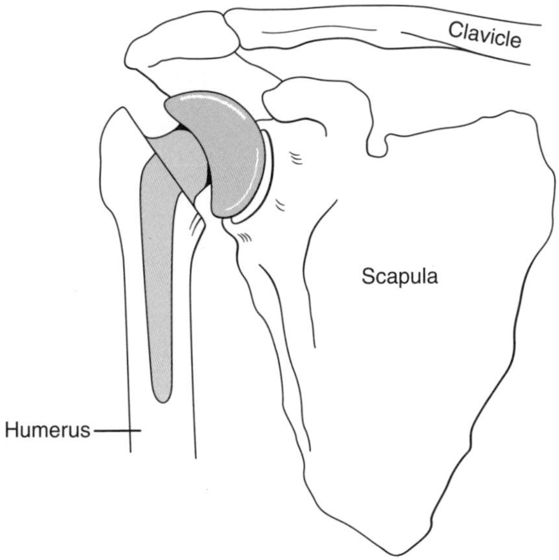

FIGURE 8–48. Shoulder hemiarthroplasty.

Exercise Priorities

- Maximize range of motion

THE AQUATIC EXERCISE THERAPY PROTOCOL FOR CONDITIONS OF THE SHOULDER

Phase One

Patients with shoulder dislocations and those who have had rotator cuff repairs should stay in Phase One for 4 to 8 weeks to allow the injured structures time to heal. For all other conditions, patients should be able to perform all the indicated exercises before progressing to the next level. The patient may not progress at all strengthening exercises at exactly the same rate.

Warm-up

Perform each exercise for 2 minutes.

- Bent Arm Pull (see Fig. 5–12)
- Breast Stroke (see Fig. 5–14)
- Pendulum Exercises: Pendulum Pulls and Pendulum Crisscross (see Figs. 5–18, 5–19)

Stretch

Perform six repetitions of each exercise, holding for 10 seconds. For wand exercises, use the uninvolved arm to maximize shoulder range of motion.

- Pectoral Stretch (see Fig. 8–6)
- Shoulder Shrugs (see Fig. 8–7)
- Shoulder Rolls (see Fig. 8–9)
- Hug Stretch (see Fig. 8–10)
- Cross-Shoulder Stretch (see Fig. 8–11)
- Wand Shoulder Flexion (to 90°) (see Fig. 8–21)
- Wand Shoulder Extension (see Fig. 8–22)
- Wand Shoulder Abduction (see Fig. 8–23)
- Wand Horizontal Abduction and Adduction (see Fig. 8–24)
- Wand External Rotation (see Fig. 8–25)

Strengthen

Perform one set of 8 to 12 repetitions. Use resistance of the water only.

- Resistive Shoulder Flexion (see Fig. 8–32)
- Resistive Shoulder Extension (see Fig. 8–33)
- Resistive Shoulder Adduction and Abduction (see Fig. 8–31)
- Resistive Horizontal Abduction and Adduction (see Fig. 8–34)
- Resistive Internal and External Rotation (see Fig. 8–35)

Phase Two

Patients with shoulder dislocation and those who have had rotator cuff repairs should stay in Phase Two for 4 weeks after progressing from Phase One. Patients with all other conditions can progress when able.

Warm-up

Perform each exercise for 2 minutes.

- Straight Arm Pull (see Fig. 5–13)
- Breast Stroke (see Fig. 5–14)
- Pendulum Exercises: all (see Figs. 5–16, 5–17, 5–18, 5–19)

Stretch

Perform five repetitions of each exercise, holding for 20 seconds.

- Elbow Touch (see Fig. 8–8)
- Behind Back Pull-back (see Fig. 8–12)

- Shoulder Internal Rotation Stretch (see Fig. 8–14)
- Shoulder Abduction Stretch (see Fig. 8–15)
- Pectoral Press Stretch (see Fig. 8–16)
- Shoulder Extension, Elbows Bent (see Fig. 8–18)
- Corner Stretch (see Fig. 8–20)

Strengthen

Perform two sets of 8 to 12 repetitions. Use small resistive paddles.

- Resistive Shoulder Flexion (see Fig. 8–32)
- Resistive Shoulder Extension (see Fig. 8–33)
- Resistive Shoulder Adduction and Abduction (see Fig. 8–31)
- Resistive Horizontal Abduction and Adduction (see Fig. 8–34)
- Resistive Internal and External Rotation (see Fig. 8–35)

Phase Three

Warm-up

Perform each exercise for 2 minutes.

- Straight Arm Pull (see Fig. 5–13)
- Cross-Body Pull (see Fig. 5–15)
- Pendulum Exercises: all (see Figs. 5–16, 5–17, 5–18, 5–19)

Stretch

Perform five repetitions of each exercise, holding 30 seconds. Continue with any stretches from Phase One and Phase Two that are still limited in range. Add the following stretches:

- Shoulder Overhead Press, Supine (see Fig. 8–27)
- Shoulder External Rotation Stretch (see Fig. 8–17)
- Shoulder Extension, Elbows Straight (see Fig. 8–19)
- Wand Functional Internal and External Rotation (see Fig. 8–26)

Strengthen

Perform three sets of 8 to 12 repetitions. Use larger resistive paddles.

- Resistive Shoulder Flexion (see Fig. 8–32)
- Resistive Shoulder Extension (see Fig. 8–33)
- Resistive Shoulder Adduction and Abduction (see Fig. 8–31)
- Resistive Horizontal Abduction and Adduction (see Fig. 8–34)
- Resistive Internal and External Rotation (see Fig. 8–35)
- Shoulder Press-down (see Fig. 8–30)
- Rowing (see Fig. 8–36)
- Side Arm Pull (see Fig. 8–37)
- Upright Rowing (see Fig. 8–38)

Phase Four

Warm-up

Perform each exercise for 2 minutes.

- Straight Arm Pull (see Fig. 5–13)
- Cross-Body Pull (see Fig. 5–15)
- Pendulum Exercises: all (see Figs. 5–16, 5–17, 5–18, 5–19)
- Combination Arm Movements (see Fig. 5–20)

Stretch

Perform five repetitions of each exercise, holding 30 seconds. Continue with any stretches from Phase Two and Phase Three that are still limited in range.

- Overhead Pullover (see Fig. 8–13)
- Shoulder Abduction, Supine (see Fig. 8–28)
- Shoulder External Rotation, Supine (see Fig. 8–29)

Strengthen

Perform four sets of 15 to 20 repetitions. Progress to the following upper extremity exercises in deep water:

- Deep Water Bent Arm Pull (see Fig. 6–4)
- Deep Water Straight Arm Pull (see Fig. 6–5)
- Deep Water Shoulder Circles (see Fig. 6–6)
- Deep Water Breast Stroke (see Fig. 6–7)
- Deep Water Shoulder Press (see Fig. 6–8)
- Deep Water Elbow Press (see Fig. 6–9)
- Deep Water Wave (see Fig. 6–10)
- Deep Water Wrist Side Press (see Fig. 6–11)

REFERENCES

1. Magee D. Orthopedic Physical Assessment. Philadelphia: W.B. Saunders, 1987.
2. Green W, Heckman J. The Clinical Measurement of Joint Motion. Rosemont, IL: American Academy of Orthopaedic Surgeons, 1994.
3. Arnheim D. Modern Principles of Athletic Training. St. Louis: Times Mirror/Mosby College Publishing, 1985.

Aquatic Rehabilitation of the Elbow and Forearm

CHAPTER 9

THE STRUCTURE AND FUNCTION OF THE ELBOW AND FOREARM

The Anatomic Parts

The elbow is a uniaxial, synovial hinge joint that is made up of three articulations: the ulnohumeral joint, the radiohumeral joint, and the proximal radioulnar joint (Fig. 9–1).

THE ULNOHUMERAL JOINT. The ulnohumeral joint is located between the trochlear notch of the ulna and the trochlea (or medial surface) of the humerus. When the elbow is kept close to the side of the body and the arm is extended into the anatomic position (palms facing forward), the medial edge of the hand lies a few inches from the thigh (because of the shape of the bones). In this

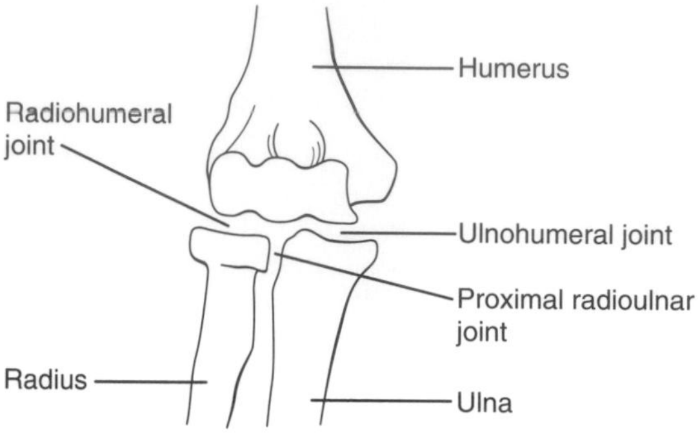

FIGURE 9–1. The joints of the elbow.

position, the elbow is flexed to 70°, and the forearm supinated 10°.[1] This position is called the carrying angle of the elbow. Normally, handheld loads can be carried most effectively at this angle (Fig. 9–2).

THE RADIOHUMERAL JOINT. The radiohumeral joint lies between the proximal surface of the radial head and the capitulum (or lateral surface) of the humerus.

THE RADIOULNAR JOINT. In the forearm, there are two articulations between the radius and the ulna, one proximal and one distal, that together form the radioulnar joint. The proximal joint lies between the head of the radius and a notch on the lateral surface of the proximal end of the ulna. The distal joint lies between the circular head of the ulna and a notch in the radius.

SUPPORTING STRUCTURES. The supporting structures of the elbow include the fibrous capsule, the ligaments, the interosseous membrane, and the muscles that cross the joint. The fibrous capsule is attached to the bones just above and below the joint and encompasses the proximal radioulnar joint. The collateral ligaments of the elbow strengthen the capsule, both medially, by means of the fan-shaped ulnar collateral ligament, which provides most of the elbow's stability, and laterally, by means of the cord-like radial collateral ligament. Both of these ligaments run from the humeral condyles to the ulna, leaving the radius free to pivot on the capitulum during pronation and supination (Fig. 9–3).

The head of the radius is held in position against the ulna by a ring of connective tissue called the annular ligament.

The interosseous membrane joins the middle portions of the radius and the ulna. Although it is not a true joint, it provides a broader surface of origin for the many muscles of the forearm, and if injured, it can affect the mechanics of the elbow joint.

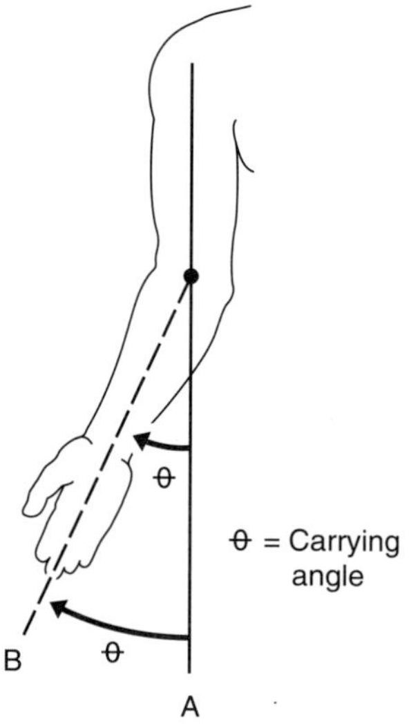

FIGURE 9–2. The carrying angle of the elbow.

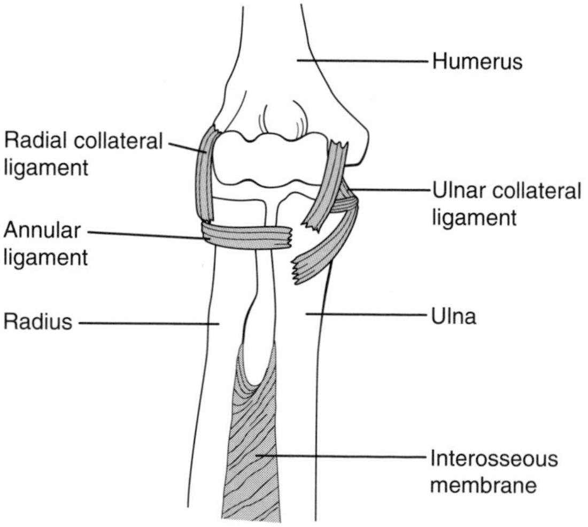

FIGURE 9–3. The elbow joint and supporting ligaments.

The Muscles and Their Actions

A muscle must cross a joint to act directly on that joint. The way in which a muscle crosses a joint affects the action. The muscles discussed in this section are involved at three joints: the shoulder, the elbow, and the radioulnar joint of the forearm. The biceps and triceps cross both the shoulder and the elbow but work more powerfully at the elbow. The elbow and forearm permit the following movements (Fig. 9–4):[2]

- Flexion and extension (Table 9–1)
- Hyperextension
- Pronation and supination (Table 9–2)

Table 9–3 summarizes the muscles involved in the movements of the elbow and forearm.

Measuring the Range of Motion of the Elbow and Forearm

To measure elbow flexion and extension[3] (Fig. 9–5), the examiner places the stationary arm of the goniometer along the lateral midline of the humerus (pointing toward the acromion process). The moving arm is placed along the lateral midline of the radius (pointing toward the styloid process).

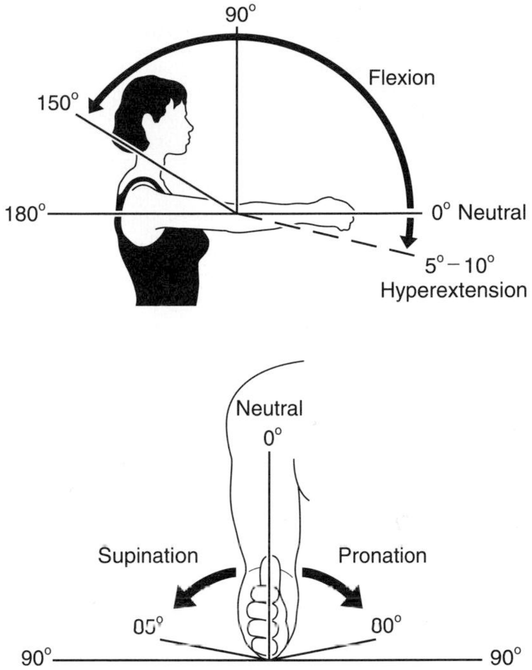

FIGURE 9–4. Movements of the elbow and the forearm, showing normal ranges of motion. (Adapted from Green W, Heckman J. The Clinical Measurement of Joint Motion. Rosemont, IL: American Academy of Orthopaedic Surgeons, 1994.)

TABLE 9–1. Muscles Involved in Elbow Flexion and Extension

Muscle	Origin (O)	Insertion (I)	Action
Biceps brachii 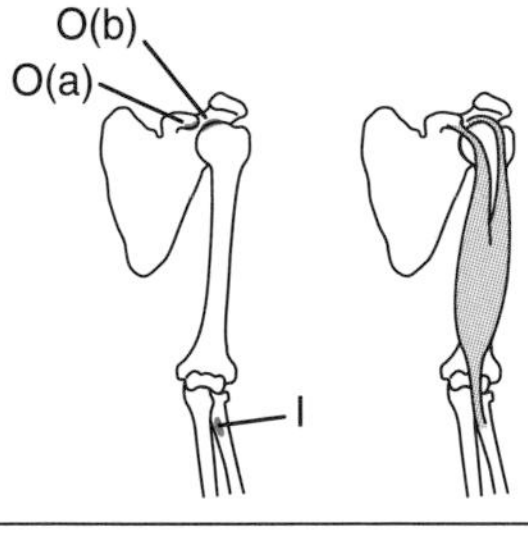	a. Coracoid process b. Top of the glenoid fossa of the scapula	Tuberosity of the radius	Elbow flexion Accessory movements: Flexion of the humerus at the shoulder Supinates hand
Brachialis 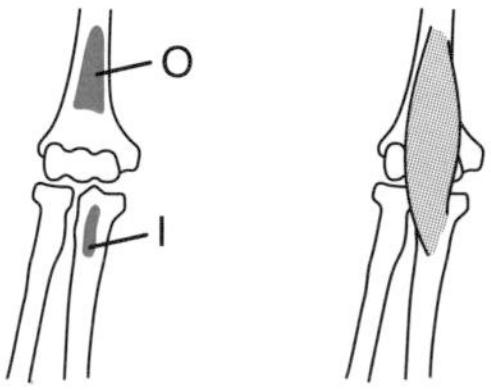	Lower two-thirds of the anterior humerus	Coronoid process of the ulna	Elbow flexion

Table continued on following page

TABLE 9–1. Muscles Involved in Elbow Flexion and Extension *Continued*

Muscle	Origin (O)	Insertion (I)	Action
Brachioradialis 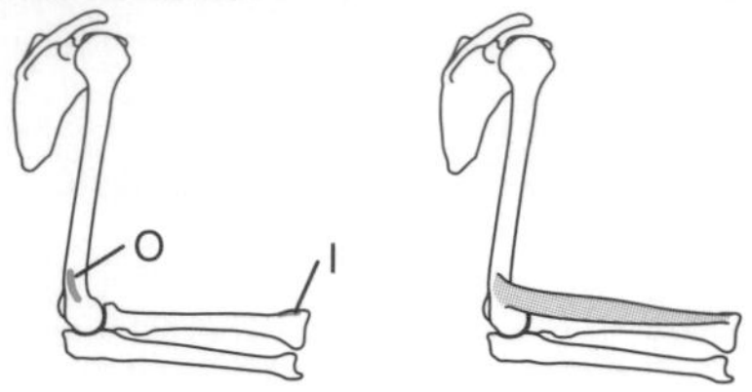	Lateral supracondylar ridge of the humerus	Styloid process of the radius	Elbow flexion Acccessory movement: Semisupinates
Triceps brachii 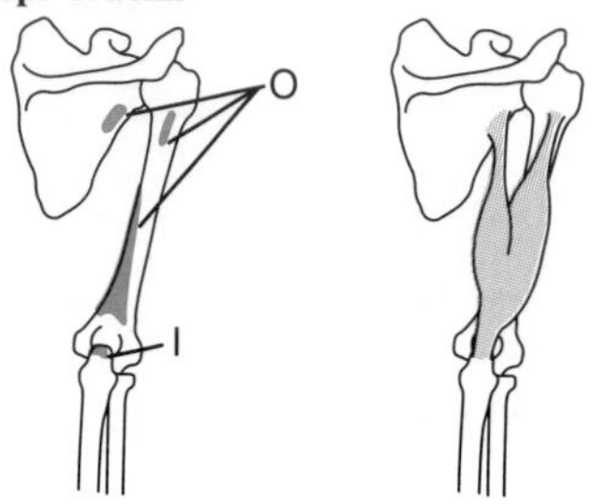	Just under the glenoid fossa Upper posterior humerus Lower posterior humerus	Olecranon process of the ulna	Elbow extension Accessory movement: Weak extension of the humerus at the shoulder
Anconeus 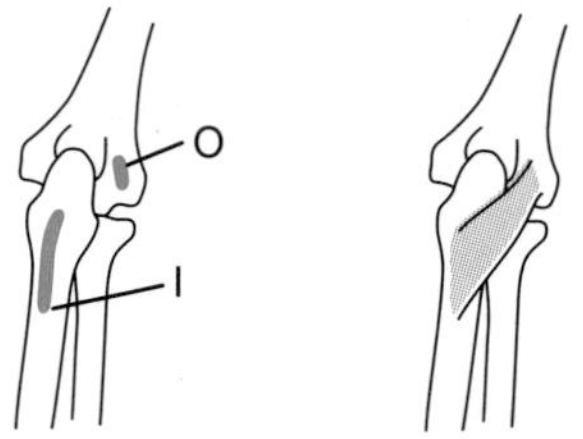	Back of the lateral epicondyle of the humerus	Olecranon process and upper posterior ulna	Helps to extend the elbow Maintains the health of the elbow joint by putting tension on the synovium to prevent pinching

TABLE 9–2. Muscles Involved in Forearm Pronation and Supination

Muscle	Origin (O)	Insertion (I)	Action
Pronator teres 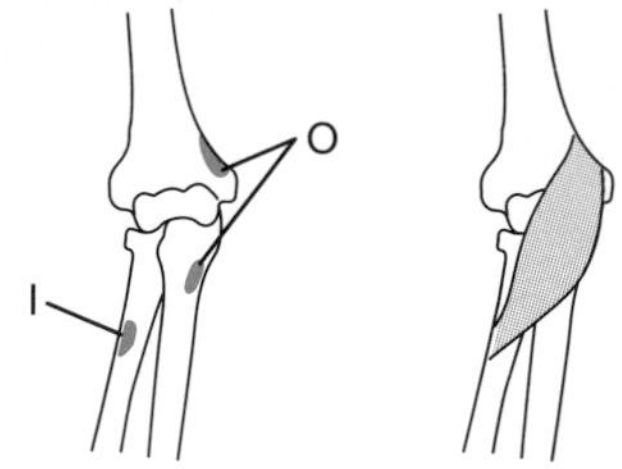	Medial epicondyle of the humerus Coronoid of the ulna	Outer surface of the middle radius	Forearm pronation Accessory movement: Flexes the forearm at the elbow
Pronator quadratus 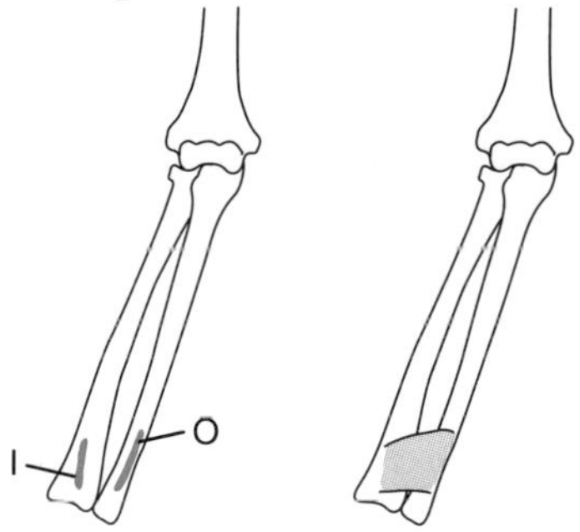	Lower front of the ulna	Lower front of the radius	Pronates the forearm (especially during extension of the elbow)
Supinator 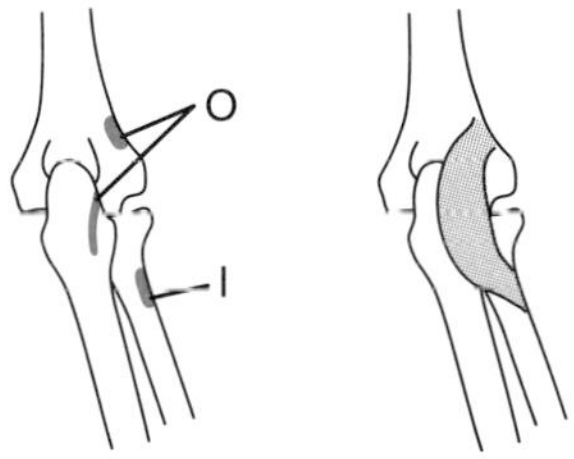	Lateral supracondylar ridge of the humerus and the ulna	Outer surface of the upper radius	Supinates the forearm

TABLE 9–3. Summary of the Muscles Involved in the Movements of the Elbow and Forearm

Anatomic Movement	Prime Movers	Assistant Movers	Nerve Root Level	Normal Range of Motion
Flexion	Biceps brachii Brachialis Brachioradialis	Flexor carpi radialis Flexor carpi ulnaris	C5 to T1	140°–150°
Extension	Triceps brachii	Anconeus Extensor carpi radialis longus Extensor carpi radialis brevis Extensor carpi ulnaris	C6 to T1	
Pronation	Pronator quadratus	Flexor carpi radialis Pronator teres	C6 to T1	80°
Supination	Supinator	Extensor carpi radialis Extensor pollicis longus Adductor pollicis longus Biceps brachii	C5 to T1	85°

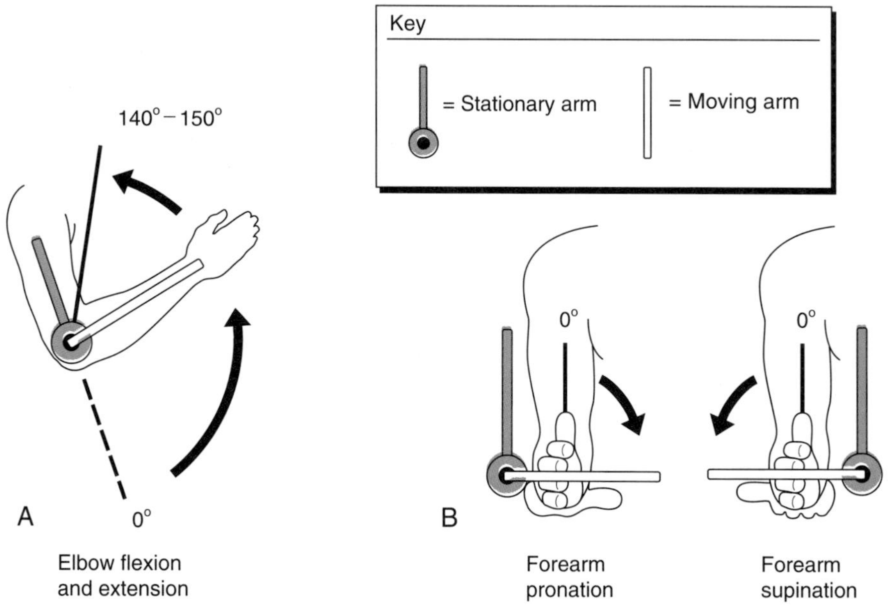

FIGURE 9–5. Measuring the range of motion of the elbow and forearm.

To measure forearm pronation, the examiner places the stationary arm of the goniometer on the dorsal surface of the wrist parallel to the long axis of the humerus, with the thumb pointing up. The moving arm is placed on the back of the hand *after* the movement has been performed.

To measure forearm supination, the examiner places the stationary arm of the goniometer on the palm side of the hand parallel to the humerus. The moving arm is placed on the hand *after* the movement has been performed.

ELBOW AND FOREARM STRETCHES

Biceps Stretch (Fig. 9–6)

Prime movers: biceps brachii, brachialis, brachioradialis, flexor carpi radialis, flexor carpi ulnaris, and deltoids.

- Hold the hands at the sides and flex the wrists so that palms are facing the bottom of the pool
- Straighten the elbow and press the arms back with elbows straight; feel the stretch along the front of the arms
- Hold, then relax

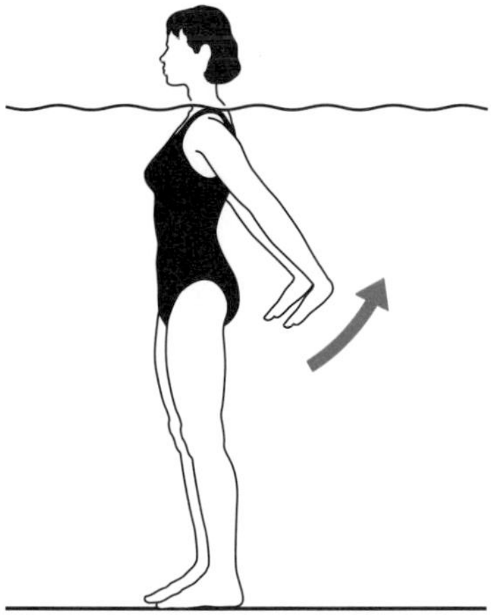

FIGURE 9–6. Biceps stretch.

Triceps Stretch (Fig. 9–7)

- Place the hand on the involved side behind the head with the palm touching the back of the neck
- Reach down the spine as far as possible
- Assist the stretch by placing the opposite hand on the elbow and pulling gently
- Hold, then relax

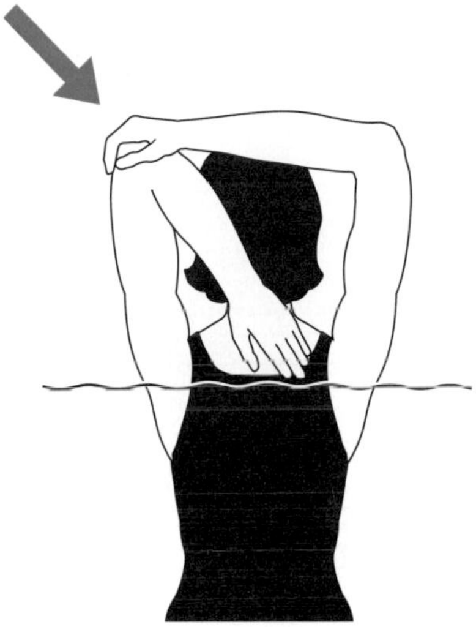

FIGURE 9–7. Triceps stretch.

Mild Triceps Stretch (Fig. 9–8)

- Flex the elbow of the involved hand, placing the palm on the shoulder
- Raise the elbow to shoulder level
- Use the uninvolved hand to push the elbow up, keeping the involved hand on the shoulder
- Hold, then relax

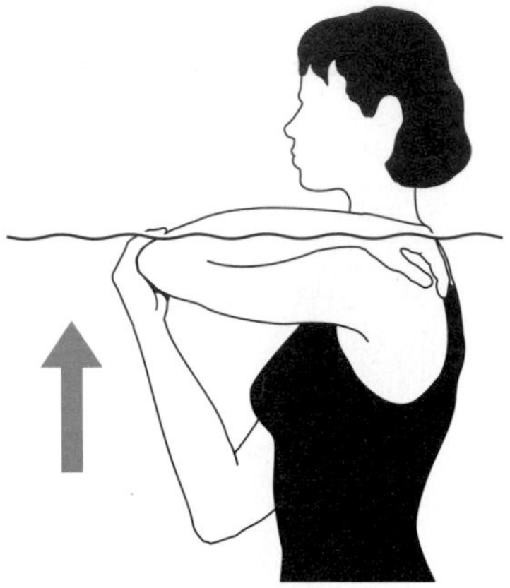

FIGURE 9–8. Mild triceps stretch.

Forearm Stretch (Fig. 9–9)

Prime movers: flexor carpi radialis, flexor carpi ulnaris, extensor carpi radialis longus, extensor carpi radialis brevis, and extensor carpi ulnaris.

- Stand with the arms in front of the body, with hands joined, the palms facing down, and the arms straight
- Flex the wrists until a stretch is felt in the forearm
- Hold, then relax

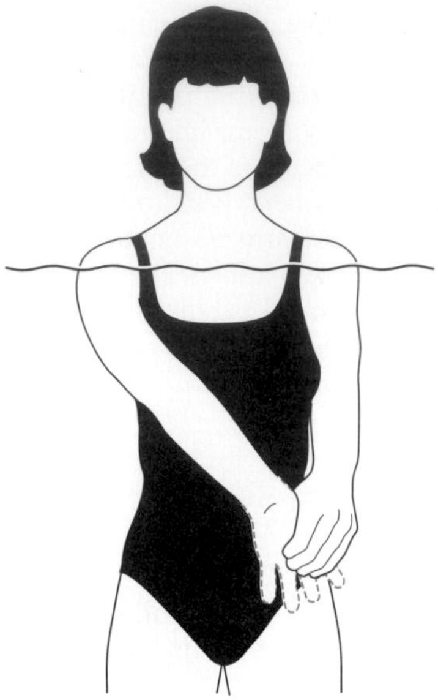

FIGURE 9–9. Forearm stretch.

ELBOW AND FOREARM EXERCISES

Elbow Bend (Fig. 9–10)

Prime movers: biceps brachii, brachialis, brachioradialis, flexor carpi radialis, flexor carpi ulnaris, triceps, and deltoids.

- Hold resistive devices in both hands, with the arms straight at the sides
- Flex the elbows and abduct the shoulders, moving the hands toward the surface of the water
- Return to the original position
- Repeat

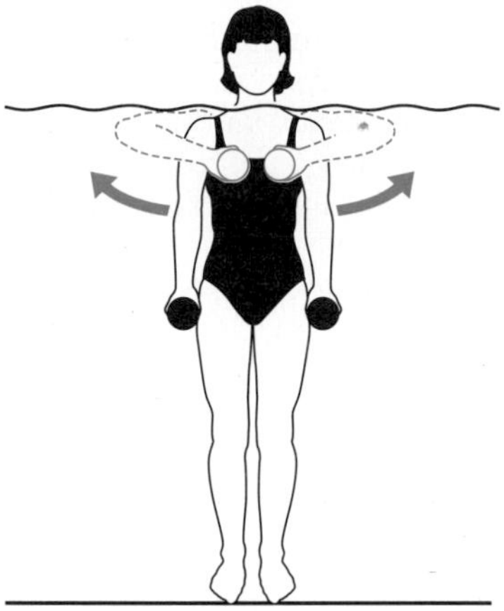

FIGURE 9–10. Elbow bend.

Biceps Curl (Fig. 9–11)

Prime movers: biceps brachii, brachialis, brachioradialis, and triceps.

- Secure stretch bands (bungee cords) to the ladder or any other fixed object in the pool, and stand with your back to the ladder, holding the handles with the arms at the sides
- Keeping the elbows as close to the sides as possible, flex the elbows through full range
- Lower to the original position

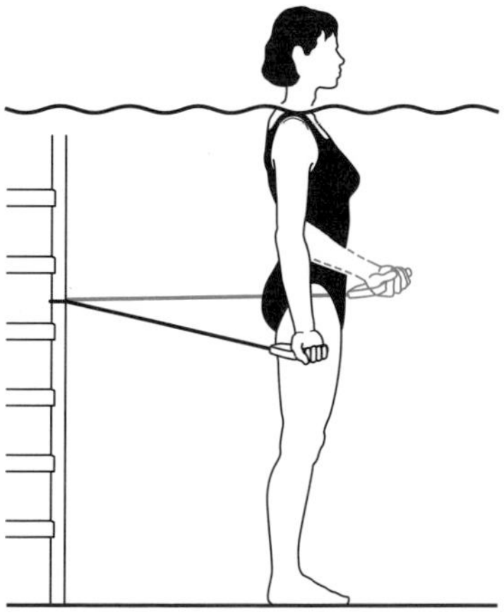

FIGURE 9–11. Biceps curl.

Resistive Pronation and Supination
(Fig. 9–12)

Prime movers: pronator teres, pronator quadratus, supinator, and biceps brachii.

- Stand with the elbows pressed against the sides of the body and flexed to 90°
- Hold the hands palms up, then gently turn the hands so the palms are facing down
- Progress by holding resistive device in hand

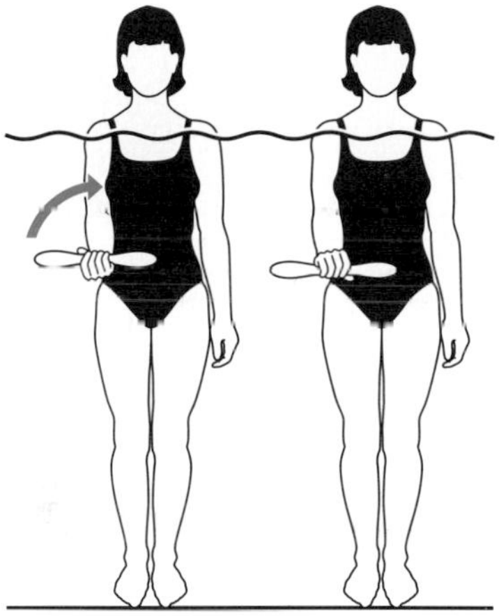

FIGURE 9–12. Resistive pronation and supination.

Combined Elbow Bend (Fig. 9–13)

Prime movers: biceps brachii, brachialis, brachioradialis, flexor carpi radialis, flexor carpi ulnaris, triceps, pronator teres, pronator quadratus, and supinator.

- Stand with the hands at the sides and the palms facing forward (anatomic position)
- Flex the elbows until the hands touch the shoulders
- Turn the hands until the palms are facing down
- Extend the elbows, keeping them close to the body

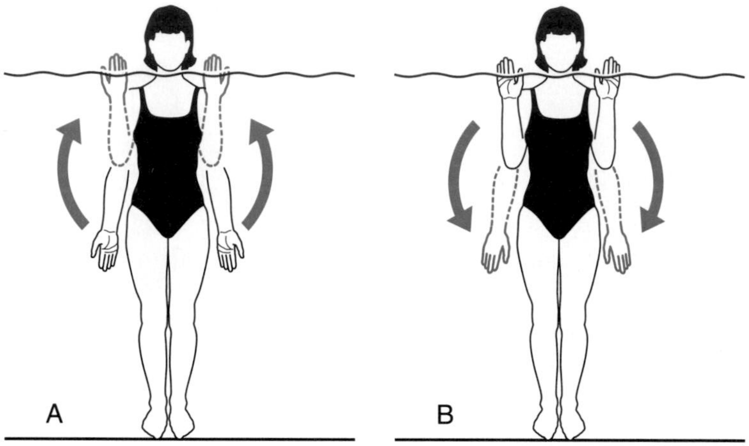

FIGURE 9–13. Combined elbow bend.

Triceps Extension (Fig. 9–14)

Prime mover: triceps.

- Stand upright with the elbow on the involved side flexed, holding a flotation device in the hand with the palm down
- Hold onto the edge of the pool with the opposite hand
- Keeping the elbow close to the side of the body, extend the forearm at the elbow
- Return to the original position

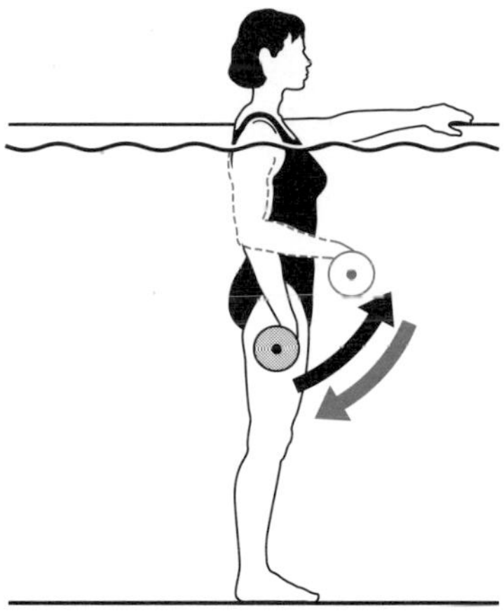

FIGURE 9–14. Triceps extension.

Triceps Dip (Fig. 9–15)

Prime movers: triceps, flexor carpi radialis, flexor carpi ulnaris, deltoids, and latissimus dorsi.

- Grasp the parallel bars with both hands and hold the body above the bars, with the elbows extended and knees flexed
- Slowly flex the elbows and lower the body as far as possible into the water
- Extend the elbows, returning to the original position

NOTE: The deeper the water, the less the resistance

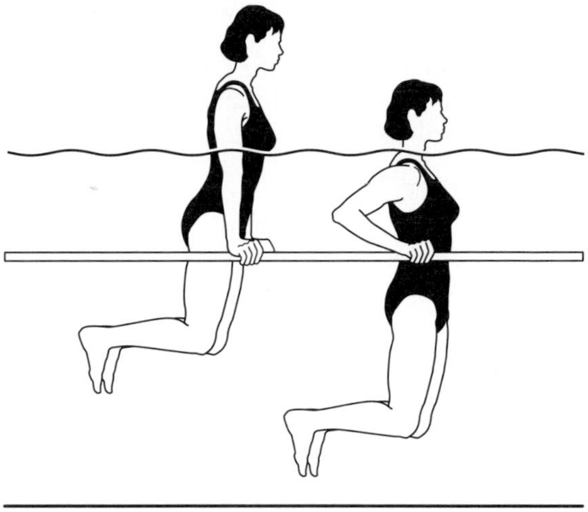

FIGURE 9–15. Triceps dip.

COMMON CONDITIONS OF THE ELBOW AND FOREARM

Elbow Arthritis

Elbow arthritis is a general term used to describe any of the arthritic conditions of the elbow (Fig. 9–16).

Origin

As with other upper extremity joints, arthritis of the elbow is usually caused by a pre-existing condition.

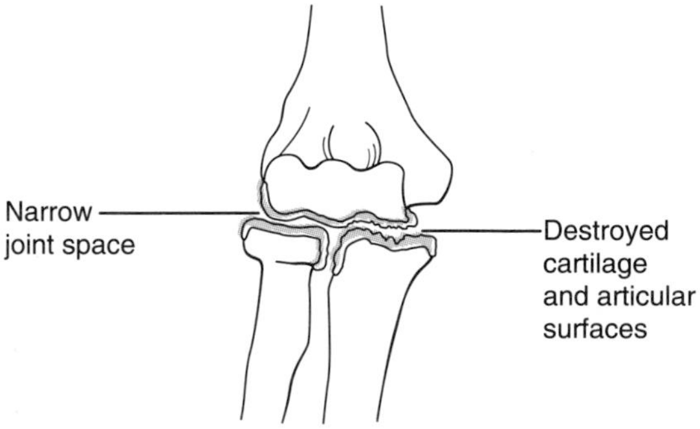

FIGURE 9–16. Elbow arthritis.

Pathology

The ulnohumeral and the superior radioulnar joints are commonly involved. See Chapter 7 for detailed pathology.

Signs and Symptoms

As with other joints, arthritis of the elbow is characterized by pain, stiffness, and decreased strength. Decreased range of motion may impair activities of daily living.

Body Parts Affected

- Bones (humerus, radius, ulna)
- Joint surfaces (articular cartilage)
- Soft tissue (joint capsule, muscles, tendons, ligaments)

Exercise Priorities

- Establish a controlled exercise program (be careful that the patient does not overdo it)
- Maximize range of motion
- Strengthen all elbow muscles

Elbow Fracture

In the elbow region, fractures may involve the humerus, radius, or ulna (Fig. 9–17).

Origin

Elbow fractures are usually caused by a fall on the elbow or a direct blow.

Pathology

The various types of fractures are outlined in Chapter 7. The fractures into this joint are most often repaired with some form of internal fixation. In spite of this, rehabilitation is a slow process, and full range of motion often is not achieved.

Signs and Symptoms

After the initial pain settles, stiffness is a major problem. Full range of motion is not always attainable.

Body Parts Affected

- Bones (humerus, radius, ulna)
- Soft tissue (joint capsule, muscles, ligaments)
- Nerves (damage may have occurred during the injury)

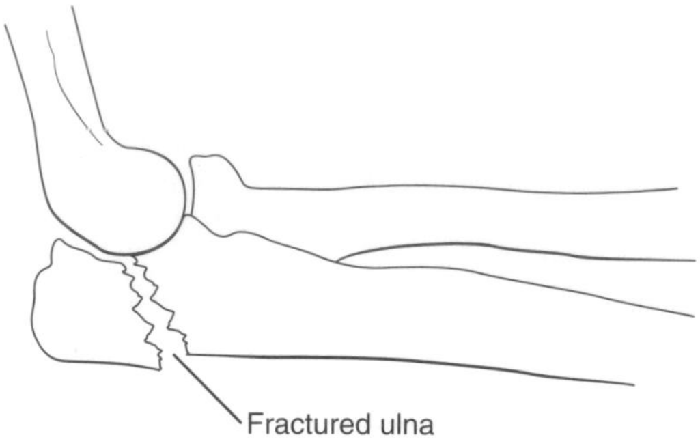

FIGURE 9–17. Elbow fracture.

Exercise Priorities

- Maximize range of motion (including pronation and supination)
- Strengthen all elbow muscles

Elbow Tendonitis

This common injury involves an inflammation of the tendons at the elbow that flex or extend the wrist and fingers.

Origin

As described in Chapter 7, this injury is often caused by overuse. The precipitating incident is usually an activity that demands more strength and endurance than the muscle–tendon mechanism possesses.

Pathology

"Tennis elbow" is the common term for lateral epicondylitis. It involves the muscles that extend the wrist and fingers. Medial epicondylitis is usually referred to as "golfer's elbow." It involves the muscles that flex the wrist and fingers (Fig. 9–18).

Signs and Symptoms

Tennis elbow is characterized by point tenderness on the lateral epicondyle and pain with resisted wrist extension. Lifting and gripping activities may also elicit pain. Golfer's elbow involves point tenderness on the medial epicondyle and pain with wrist flexion. For both kinds of elbow tendonitis, range of motion is usually full, but stretching of the involved muscles causes pain.

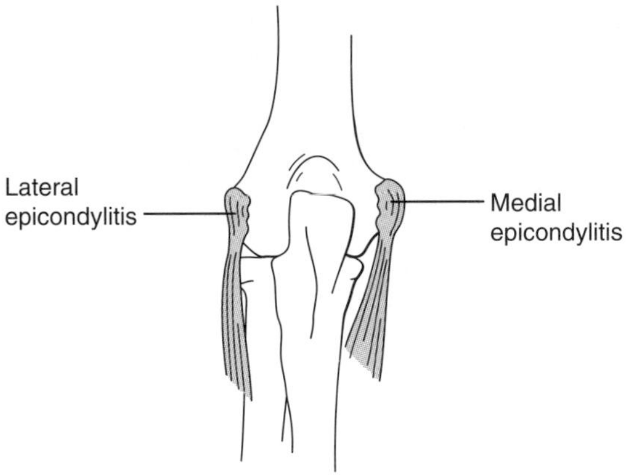

FIGURE 9–18. Elbow tendonitis.

Body Parts Affected

- Muscles and tendons (wrist flexors and extensors)

Exercise Priorities

- Stretch involved muscles
- Strengthen involved muscles
- Eccentric exercise, which involves the lengthening of a muscle, is important (eg, slowly allowing a flotation device to rise toward the surface during a given exercise)

Elbow Dislocation

Elbow dislocation is a dislocation of either the radius or the ulna from its normal position (Fig. 9–19).

Origin

Dislocation of the ulna usually occurs in conjunction with a fracture. Radial dislocation, however, need not involve a fracture. It can occur by itself from a forced pronation stress. It is also a common childhood injury, occurring when a child falls while being held by the hand.

Pathology

Joint dislocations always result in stretching or tearing of the joint capsule and ligaments. Because damage to the nerves and vessels in the area may also occur, these injuries should be checked by a doctor as soon as possible. Arthritis often develops because of damage to the articular cartilage.

Signs and Symptoms

At the time of injury, the bony abnormality is obvious. After the dislocation has been reduced, pain and reduced range of motion are the primary characteristics. If muscle spasm and guarding persist, muscle contractures may develop.

Body Parts Affected

- Bones (humerus, radius, ulna)
- Joint capsule and ligaments
- Muscles of the elbow
- Adjacent nerves and vessels

Exercise Priorities

- Restore range of motion as soon as possible (the longer the elbow remains stiff, the poorer the prognosis)
- Strengthen all elbow muscles

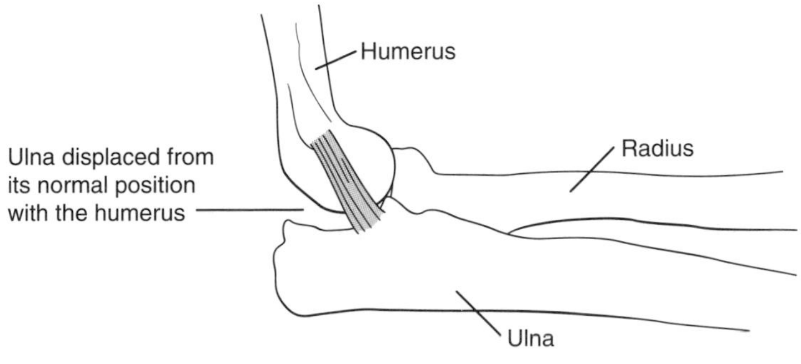

FIGURE 9–19. Elbow dislocation.

THE AQUATIC EXERCISE THERAPY PROTOCOL FOR CONDITIONS OF THE ELBOW AND FOREARM

Phase One

Warm-up

Perform each exercise for 2 to 3 minutes.

- Bent Arm Pull (see Fig. 5–12)
- Breast Stroke (see Fig. 5–14)

Stretch

Perform six repetitions of each exercise, holding for 10 seconds. The wrist exercises are found in Chapter 10.

- Biceps Stretch (see Fig. 9–6)
- Praying Hands (see Fig. 10–9)
- Forearm Stretch (see Fig. 9–9)
- Closed Wave (see Fig. 10–5)
- Palm Stretch (see Fig. 10–8)
- Reverse Praying Hands (see Fig. 10–10)

Strengthen

Perform one set of 8 to 12 repetitions.

- Elbow Bend (use water resistance only) (see Fig. 9–10)
- Biceps Curl (cupped hands) (see Fig. 9–11)
- Wrist Rotation (see Fig. 10–19)

Phase Two

Warm-up

- Bent Arm Pull (see Fig. 5–12)
- Breast Stroke (see Fig. 5–14)

Stretch

Perform five repetitions, holding for 20 seconds.

- Mild Triceps Stretch (see Fig. 9–8)
- Wrist Circles (see Fig. 10–14)
- Biceps Stretch (see Fig. 9–6)
- Praying Hands (see Fig. 10–9)
- Forearm Stretch (see Fig. 9–9)

Strengthen

Perform two sets of 8 to 12 repetitions. Perform the exercises from Phase One with hand paddles or webbed gloves. Then add the following:

- Wrist Flexion (use resistive paddles) (see Fig. 10–17)
- Wrist Extension (see Fig. 10–16)
- Resistive Pronation and Supination (see Fig. 9–12)
- Elbow bend (see Fig. 9–10)
- Biceps curl (use resistive paddles) (see Fig. 9–11)

Phase Three

Warm-up

- Bent Arm Pull (see Fig. 5–12)
- Breast Stroke (see Fig. 5–14)

Stretch

Perform five repetitions, holding for 30 seconds.

- Supinator Stretch (see Fig. 10–11)
- Pronator Stretch (see Fig. 10–12)
- Triceps Stretch (see Fig. 9–7)
- Biceps Stretch (see Fig. 9–6)
- Praying Hands (see Fig. 10–9)
- Forearm Stretch (see Fig. 9–9)

Strengthen

Perform three sets of 8 to 12 repetitions. Perform the exercises of Phase Two with resistive paddles. Then add the following:

- Resistive Pronation and Supination (see Fig. 9–12)
- Triceps Stretch (see Fig. 9–7)
- Wrist Flexion (extend by using flotation bells, which provide eccentric exercise as the bells are allowed to rise) (see Fig. 10–17)
- Combined Elbow Bend (see Fig. 9–13)

Phase Four

Warm-up

- Bent Arm Pull (see Fig. 5–12)
- Breast Stroke (see Fig. 5–14)

Stretch

Perform five repetitions, holding for 30 seconds.

- Supinator Stretch (see Fig. 10–11)
- Pronator Stretch (see Fig. 10–12)
- Triceps Stretch (see Fig. 9–7)
- Biceps Stretch (see Fig. 9–6)
- Praying Hands (see Fig. 10–9)

Strengthen

Perform four sets of 8 to 12 repetitions. Use larger resistive paddles when able.

- Triceps Dip (see Fig. 9–15)
- Wrist Radial and Ulnar Deviation (see Fig. 10–18)
- Resistive Pronation and Supination (see Fig. 9–12)
- Wrist Flexion (use flotation bells to provide eccentric exercise as the bells are allowed to rise) (see Fig. 10–17)
- Wrist Extension (use flotation bells to provide eccentric exercise as the bells are allowed to rise) (see Fig. 10–16)
- Combined Elbow Bend (see Fig. 9–13)

REFERENCES

1. Magee D. Orthopedic Physical Assessment. Philadelphia: W.B. Saunders, 1987.
2. Green W, Heckman J. The Clinical Measurement of Joint Motion. Rosemont, IL: American Academy of Orthopaedic Surgeons, 1994.
3. Arnheim D. Modern Principles of Athletic Training. St. Louis: Times Mirror/Mosby College Publishing, 1985.

CHAPTER 10

AQUATIC REHABILITATION OF THE WRIST AND HAND

THE STRUCTURE AND FUNCTION OF THE WRIST AND HAND

The Anatomic Parts

THE DISTAL RADIOULNAR JOINT. The distal radioulnar joint is the articulation between the circular head of the ulna and a notch in the radius. The joint is supported by ligaments anteriorly and posteriorly. The small capsule of this uniaxial pivot joint allows the radius to roll around the ulna during pronation and supination (Fig. 10–1).

THE RADIOCARPAL JOINT. The radiocarpal

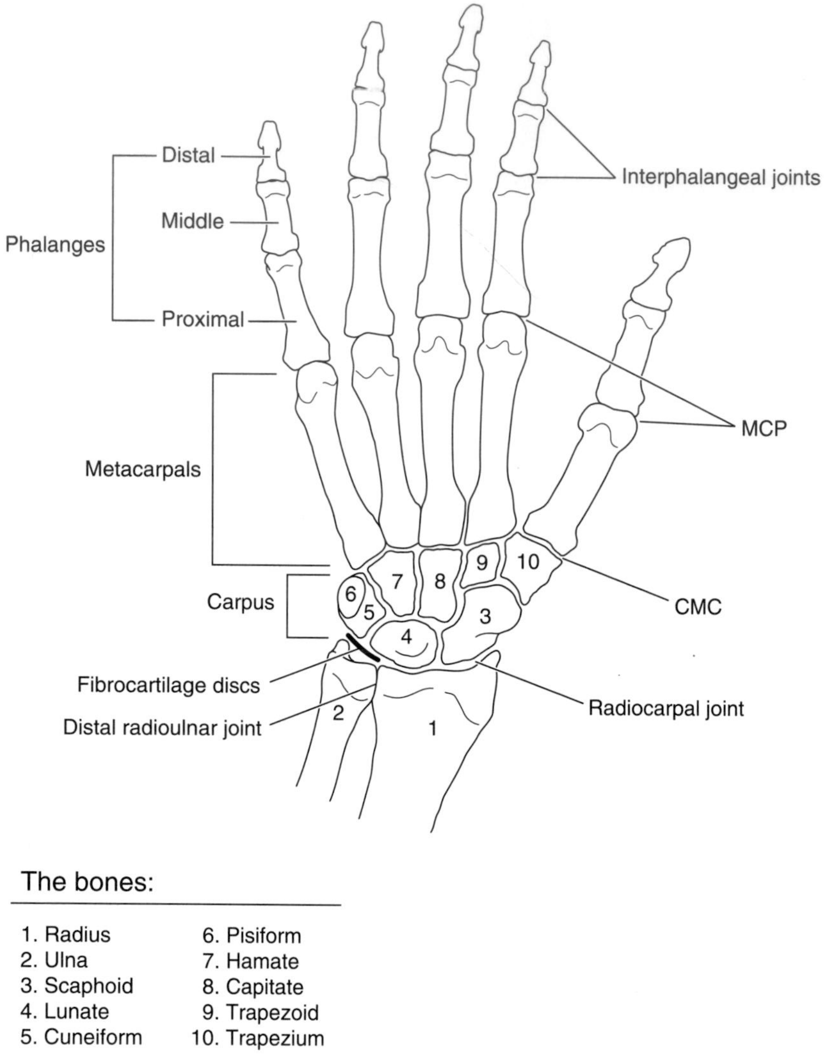

FIGURE 10–1. The bones and joints of the wrist, hand, and fingers (palmar view). CMC = Carpometacarpal joint; MCP = metacarpophalangeal joint.

(wrist) joint is formed by the articulation of the radius with the scaphoid and lunate bones of the carpus. The ulna articulates with the fibrocartilage discs and the cuneiform bone of the carpus at the medial portion of the joint (see Fig. 10–1).

THE INTERCARPAL JOINTS. The intercarpal joints comprise the articulations between the rows of proximal and distal carpal bones (see Fig. 10–1). The joint capsule is secured on all sides (dorsal and palmar surfaces) by the short intercarpal ligaments and the interosseous ligaments (Fig. 10–2). The intercarpal joints allow a slight gliding movement between the bones. These joints become "close-packed" during extension and increase in stability during hyperextension of the wrist.[1]

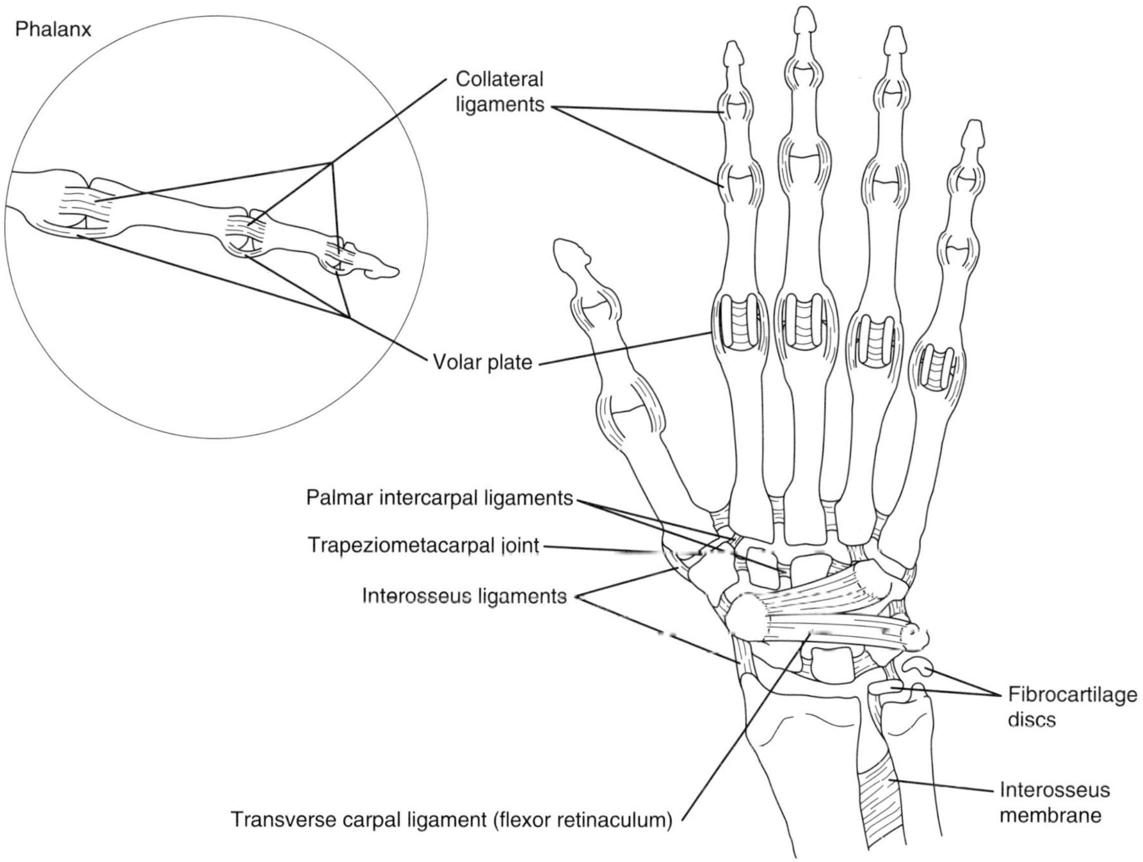

FIGURE 10–2. The ligaments of the wrist and hand joint cavity (palmar view). (Insets modified from Arnheim D. Modern Principles of Athletic Training, 8th ed. St. Louis: Times Mirror/Mosby College Publishing, 1993.)

THE CARPOMETACARPAL JOINTS. The only carpometacarpal joint with any significant movement is that of the thumb. Also known as the trapeziometacarpal joint, this saddle-shaped joint provides the articulation between the trapezium of the carpus and the base of the metacarpal bone of the thumb (see Fig. 10–1). The range of movement of this joint is almost as extensive as that of a ball-and-socket joint. The most useful movement of the thumb is opposition (the ability to touch the pads of each finger with the thumb).

THE METACARPOPHALANGEAL JOINTS. The metacarpophalangeal (knuckle) joints are the articulations between the metacarpal bones and the most proximal phalanges (see Fig. 10–1). These joints are condyloid except for the thumb knuckle, which is a hinge joint. The joint capsules are reinforced by the palmar and collateral ligaments (see

Fig. 10–2). The knuckle joints permit flexion, extension, adduction, and abduction.

THE INTERPHALANGEAL JOINTS. The interphalangeal (finger) joints are hinged joints that provide the articulations between adjacent phalanges. The joint capsules are reinforced by the palmar and collateral ligaments. At the finger joints, only flexion and extension can occur (see Fig. 10–2).

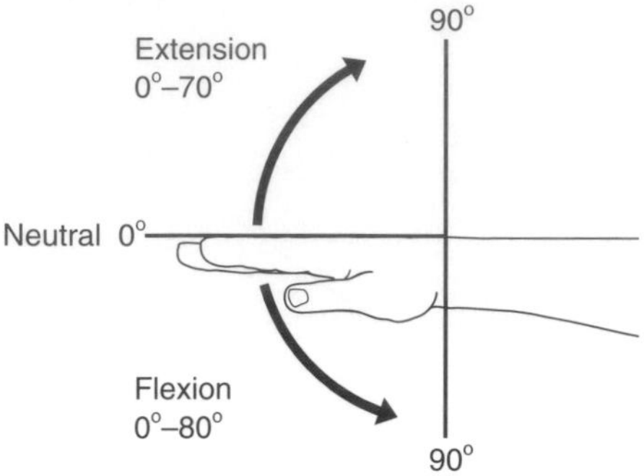

Muscles and Their Actions

A muscle must cross a joint to act directly on that joint. The way in which a muscle crosses a joint affects the action. Some of the muscles discussed in this section are involved at four joints: the elbow, the wrist complex, the hand, and the fingers. The wrist permits the following movements[2] (Fig. 10–3):

- flexion and extension (Tables 10–1 and 10–2)
- radial and ulnar deviation

The muscles acting on the thumb are shown in Table 10–3, and those acting on the hand and fingers are shown in Table 10–4. Table 10–5 summarizes the muscles involved in the movements of the wrist.

Text continued on page 142

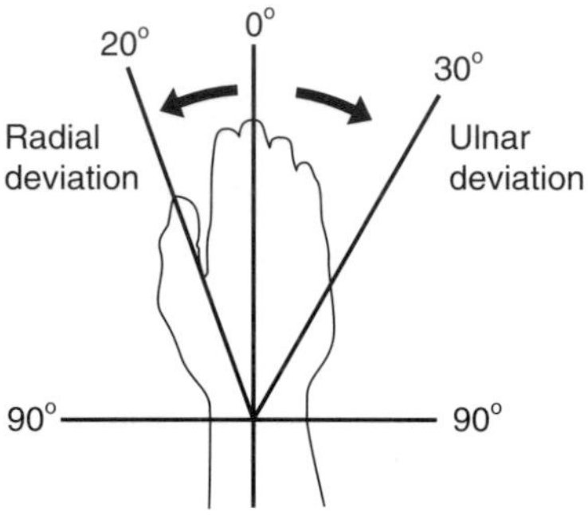

FIGURE 10–3. Movements of the wrist and hand, showing normal ranges of motion. (Adapted from Green W, Heckman J. The Clinical Measurement of Joint Motion. Rosemont, IL: American Academy of Orthopaedic Surgeons, 1994.)

TABLE 10–1. The Muscles Involved in Wrist Flexion

Muscle	Origin (O)	Insertion (I)	Action
Flexor carpi radialis 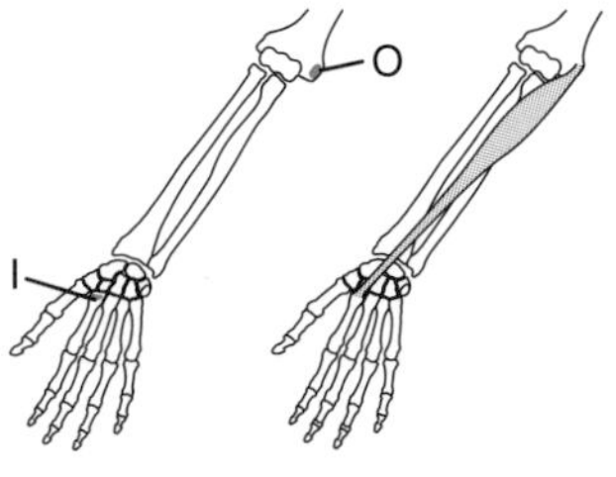 ANTERIOR VIEW	Medial epicondyle of the humerus (common tendon)	Base of the palmar surface of the second metacarpal bone	Wrist flexion Accessory movements: Forearm flexion Wrist abduction

TABLE 10–1. The Muscles Involved in Wrist Flexion *Continued*

Muscle	Origin (O)	Insertion (I)	Action
Flexor carpi ulnaris 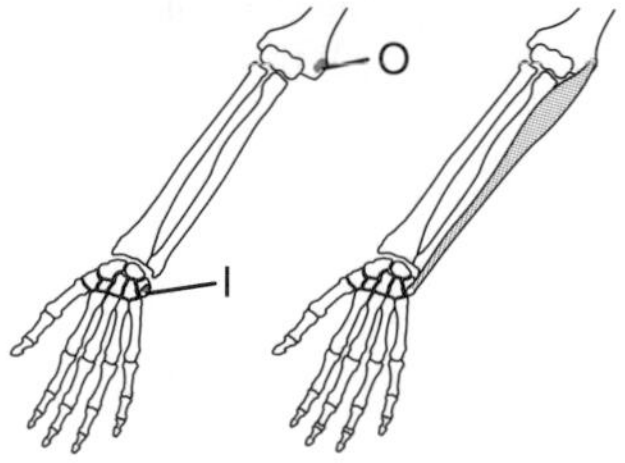 ANTERIOR VIEW	Medial epicondyle of the humerus (common tendon humeral head)	Base of the palmar surface of the metacarpals (pisiform bone, hamate, and base of the fifth metacarpal)	Wrist flexion Accessory movements: Forearm flexion Wrist adduction
Palmaris longus 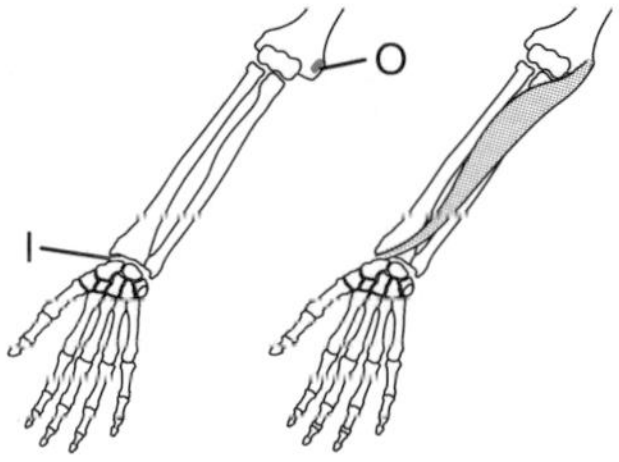 ANTERIOR VIEW	Medial epicondyle of the humerus	Annular ligament of the wrist and the palmar aponeurosis	Tightens the fascia of the palm (weak wrist flexion)

TABLE 10–2. The Muscles Involved in Wrist Extension

Muscle	Origin (O)	Insertion (I)	Action
Extensor carpi ulnaris 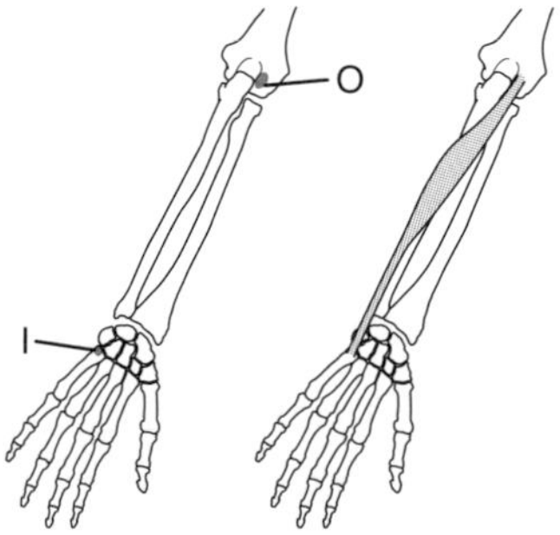 POSTERIOR VIEW	Lateral epicondyle of the humerus	Base of the dorsal surface of the fifth metacarpal	Wrist extension Accessory movements: Forearm extension Wrist adduction

Table continued on following page

TABLE 10–2. The Muscles Involved in Wrist Extension *Continued*

Muscle	Origin (O)	Insertion (I)	Action
Extensor carpi radialis longus 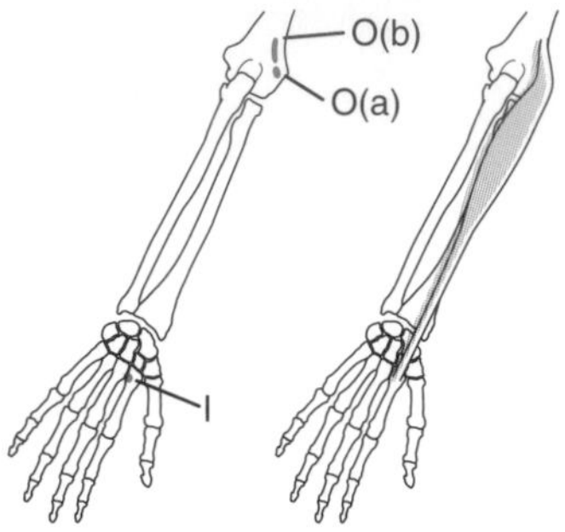 POSTERIOR VIEW	a. Lateral epicondyle of the humerus b. Distal third of the lateral supracondylar ridge of the humerus	Base of the dorsal surface of the second metacarpal	Wrist extension Accessory movement: Wrist abduction
Extensor carpi radialis brevis 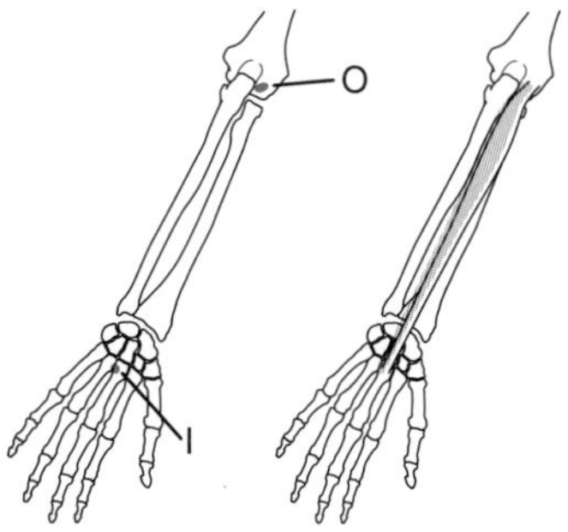 POSTERIOR VIEW	Lateral epicondyle of the humerus	Base of the dorsal surface of the third metacarpal	Wrist extension Accessory movement: Wrist abduction

TABLE 10–3. The Muscles Acting on the Thumb

Muscle	Origin (O)	Insertion (I)	Action
Extensor pollicis longus 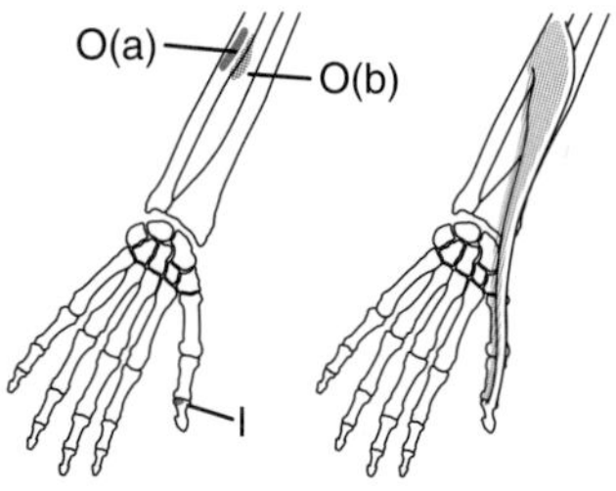 POSTERIOR VIEW	a. Posterior ulna (middle third) b. Interosseous membrane	Base of the dorsal surface of the distal phalanx of the thumb	Thumb extension Accessory movement: Assists wrist extension

TABLE 10–3. The Muscles Acting on the Thumb *Continued*

Muscle	Origin (O)	Insertion (I)	Action
Extensor pollicis brevis 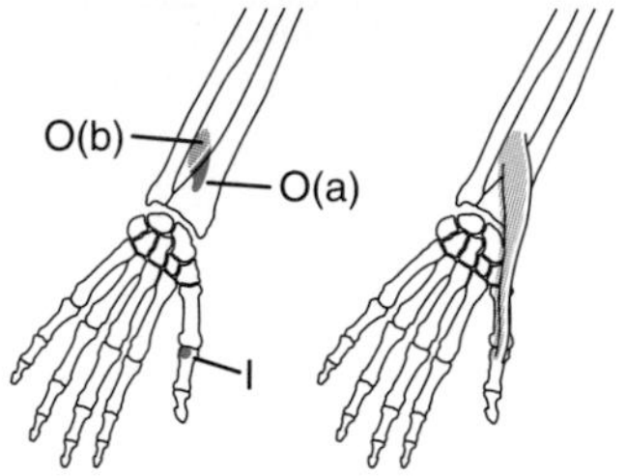 POSTERIOR VIEW	a. Dorsal surface of the radius and ulna b. Interosseous membrane	Base of the dorsal surface of the proximal phalanx of the thumb	Thumb extension Accessory movements: Abducts first metacarpal Abducts wrist
Abductor pollicis longus 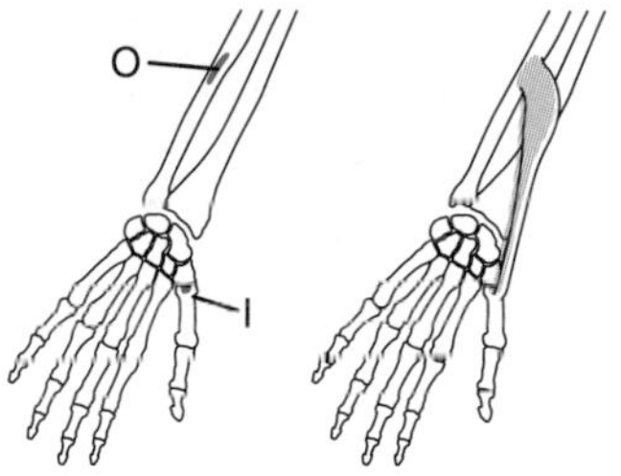 POSTERIOR VIEW	Middle of the ulnar side of the radius below the insertion of the anconeus muscle	Radial side of the base of the first metacarpal	Thumb abduction Accessory movement: Wrist abduction
Abductor pollicis brevis 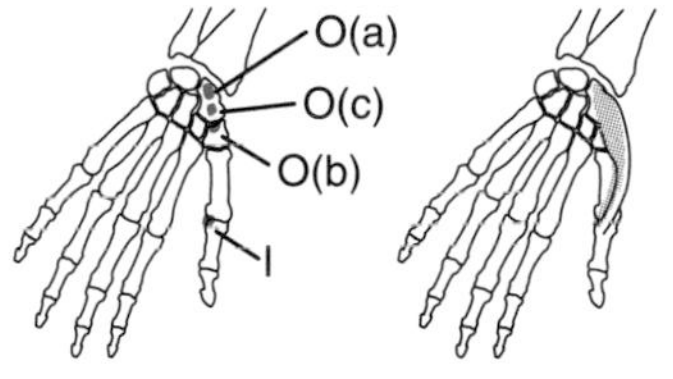 POSTERIOR VIEW	a. Tuberosity of the scaphoid bone b. Ridge of the trapezium c. Transverse carpal ligament	Base of the palmar surface of the proximal phalanx of the thumb	Thumb flexion Accessory movement: Medial rotation of the metacarpal of the thumb
Flexor pollicis longus 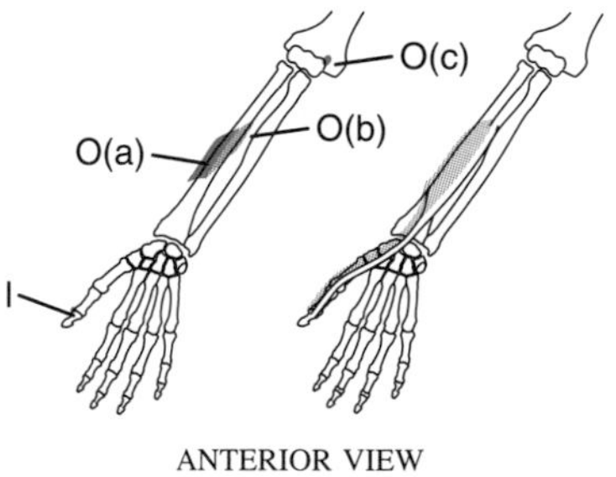 ANTERIOR VIEW	a. Volar surface of the radius b. Interosseous membrane c. Medial epicondyle of the humerus	Base of the palmar surface of the distal phalanx of the thumb	Thumb flexion Accessory movements: Wrist flexion Adducts the metacarpal and wrist

Table continued on following page

TABLE 10–3. The Muscles Acting on the Thumb *Continued*

Muscle	Origin (O)	Insertion (I)	Action
Flexor pollicis brevis 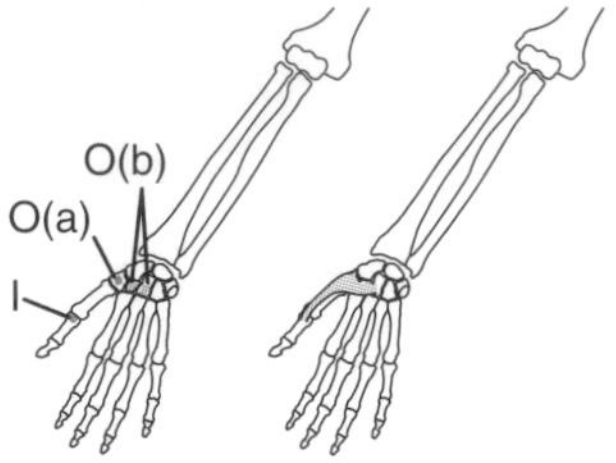 ANTERIOR VIEW	a. Crest of the trapezium (superficial) b. Trapezoid and capitate bones, and palmar ligaments of the distal carpal bones	Base of the palmar surface of the proximal phalanx of the thumb	Thumb flexion Accessory movement: Adduction of the metacarpal of the thumb
Adductor pollicis 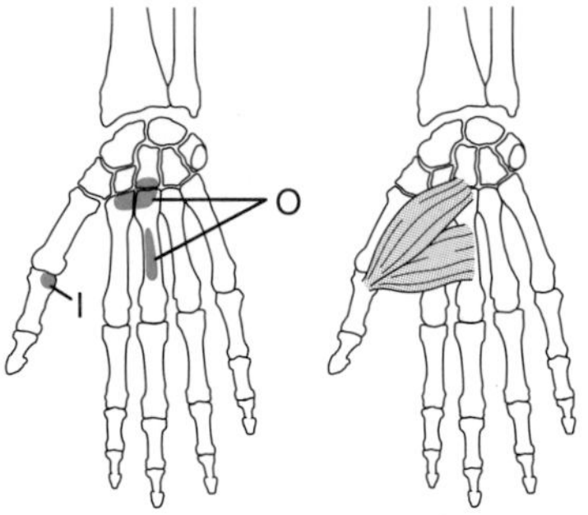 ANTERIOR VIEW	Oblique head (caput obliquus): Capitate bone Base of the second and third metacarpal bones on the palmar surface Transverse head (caput transversus): Distal two-thirds of the palmar surface of the third metacarpal bone (not shown)	Base of the medial surface of the proximal phalanx of the thumb	Thumb adduction Accessory movement: Hyperadduction of the metacarpal of the thumb (touching thumb to palm of hand)
Opponens pollicis 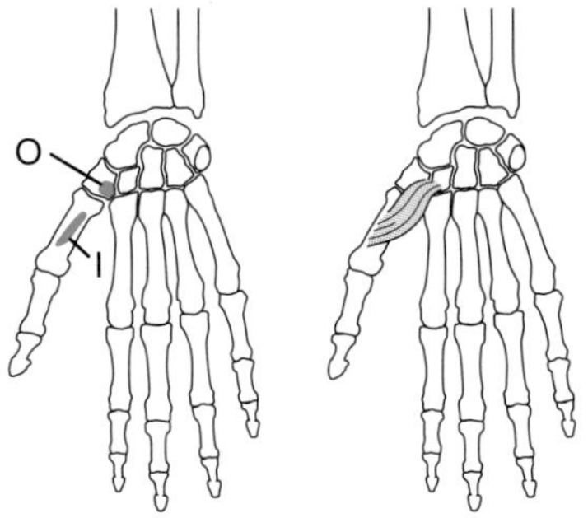 ANTERIOR VIEW	Trapezium bone and transverse ligament	Entire length of the first metacarpal bone on the radial side	Thumb opposition (partial circumduction)

TABLE 10–4. The Muscles Involved in the Movements of the Hand and Fingers

Muscle	Origin (O)	Insertion (I)	Action
Flexor digitorum superficialis 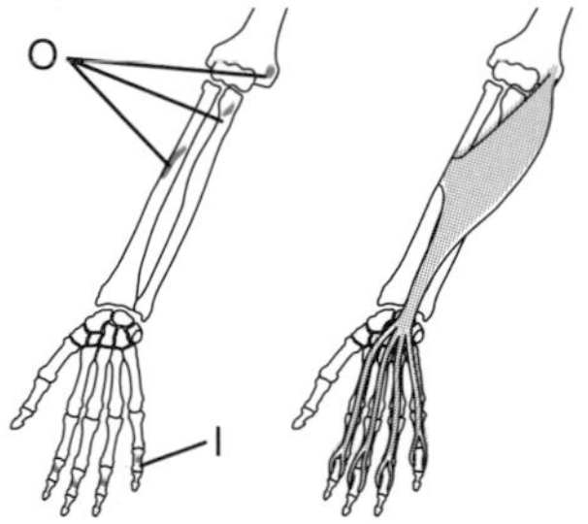 ANTERIOR VIEW	Medial epicondyle of the humerus Anterior upper radius and ulna	Sides of the middle phalanges of the fingers (the tendons are split)	Flexes the fingers (middle and proximal phalanges) Accessory movements: Assists wrist flexion Flexes forearm at the elbow
Flexor digitorum profundus 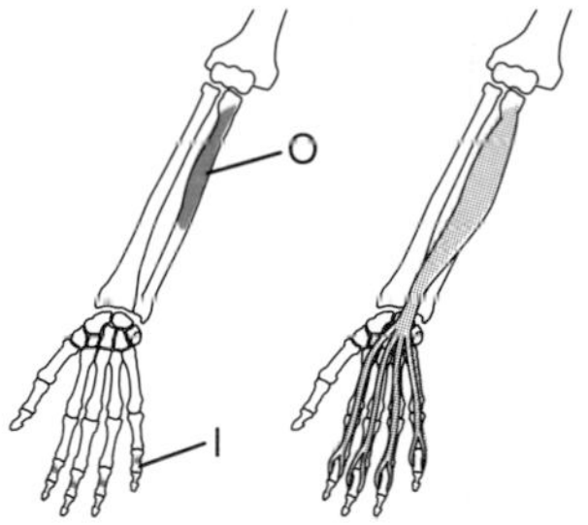 ANTERIOR VIEW	Upper anterior ulna	Dorsal bases of the distal phalanges (the tendon splits)	Flexes the fingers (all phalanges) Accessory movement: Assists wrist flexion
Extensor digitorum 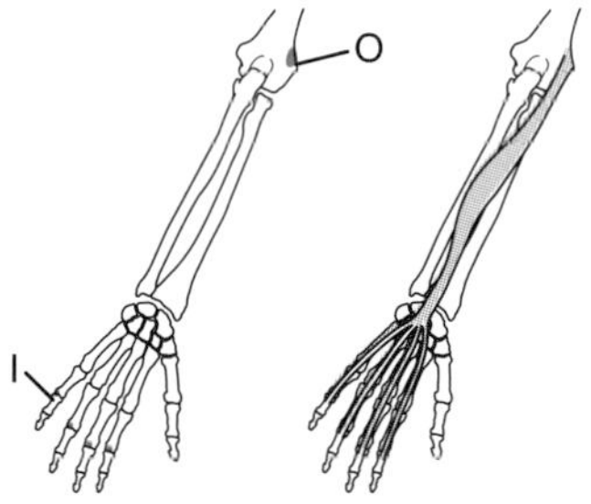 POSTERIOR VIEW	Lateral epicondyle of the humerus (common tendon)	Bases of the middle and distal phalanges of the fingers	Extends the proximal phalanges and wrist Accessory movement: Extends the forearm at the elbow

Table continued on following page

TABLE 10–4. The Muscles Involved in the Movements of the Hand and Fingers *Continued*

Muscle	Origin (O)	Insertion (I)	Action
Lumbricales 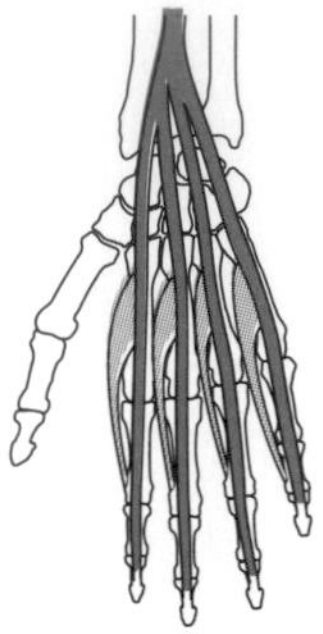 DORSAL VIEW	Tendons of flexor digitorum profundus	Pass to the radial side of the metacarpal bone, to the dorsal expansion of the finger extensor tendons	Flexion of the metacarpophalangeal joints of the fingers
Abductor digiti minimi 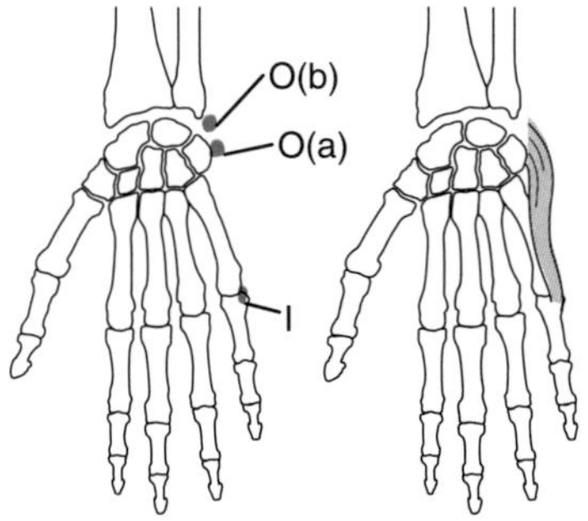 DORSAL VIEW	a. Pisiform bone b. Tendon of flexor carpi ulnaris	Tendon divides: Ulnar side—base of the proximal phalanx (little finger) Ulnar border of the aponeurosis of extensor digiti minimi brevis	Finger abduction (little finger)
Interossei dorsales 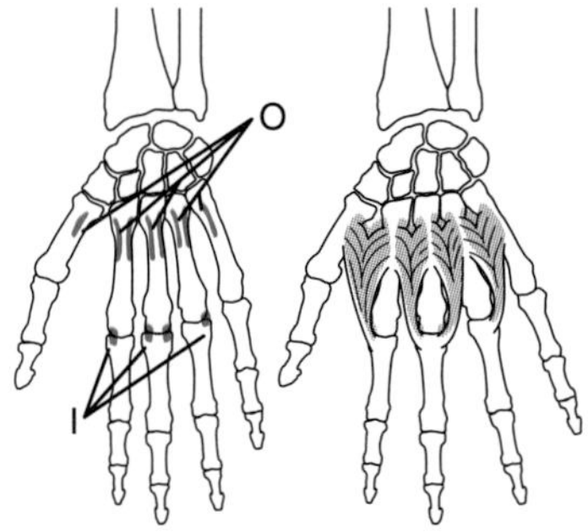 DORSAL VIEW	Each by two heads from adjacent sides of metacarpal bones	Base of proximal phalanges of the second, third, and fourth digits Dorsal expansion of the finger extensor tendons	Finger abduction Accessory movements: Assists flexion of the proximal phalanges Assists extension of the middle and distal phalanges

TABLE 10–4. The Muscles Involved in the Movements of the Hand and Fingers *Continued*

Muscle	Origin (O)	Insertion (I)	Action
Opponens digiti minimi 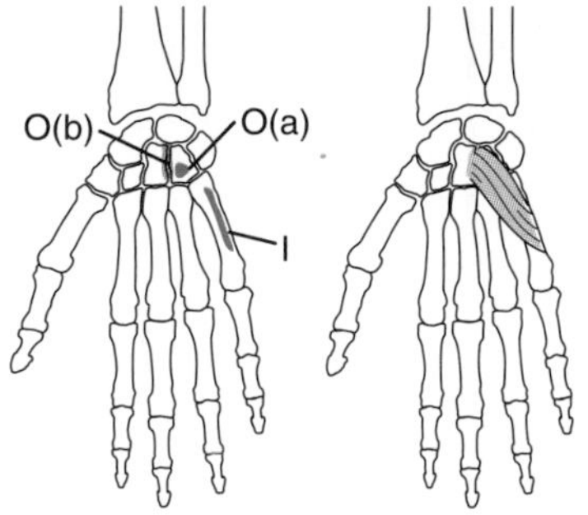 DORSAL VIEW	a. Convex surface of hamate bone b. Flexor retinaculum	Entire length of the fifth metacarpal bone	Opposition of the fifth metacarpal bone
Interossei palmares 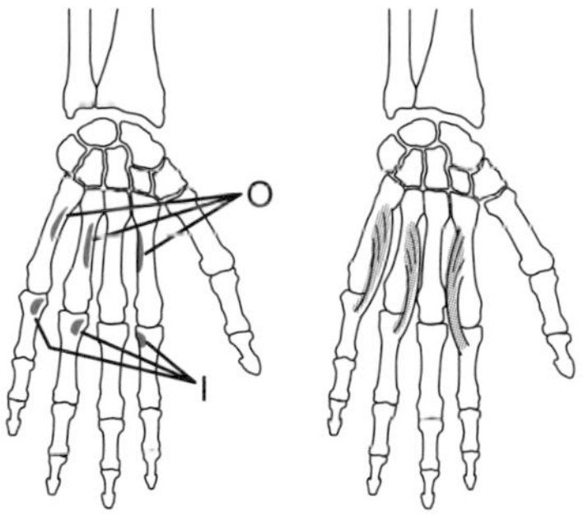 DORSAL VIEW	Entire length of the second, fourth, and fifth metacarpal bones on the palmar surface	Bases of the proximal phalanges of the second, fourth, and fifth metacarpal bones	Finger adduction Accessory movements: Assists flexion of the proximal phalanges Assists extension of the middle and distal phalanges

TABLE 10–5. Summary of the Muscles Involved in the Movements of the Wrist

Anatomic Movement	Prime Movers	Assistant Movers	Nerve Root Level	Normal Range of Motion
Flexion	Flexor carpi radialis Flexor carpi ulnaris	Palmaris longus Flexor digitorum profundus Flexor digitorum superficialis Extensor indices Extensor digiti minimi	C7 to T1	0°–80°
Extension	Extensor carpi longus Extensor carpi radialis brevis Extensor carpi ulnaris	Extensor digitorum	C6 to C7	0°–70°

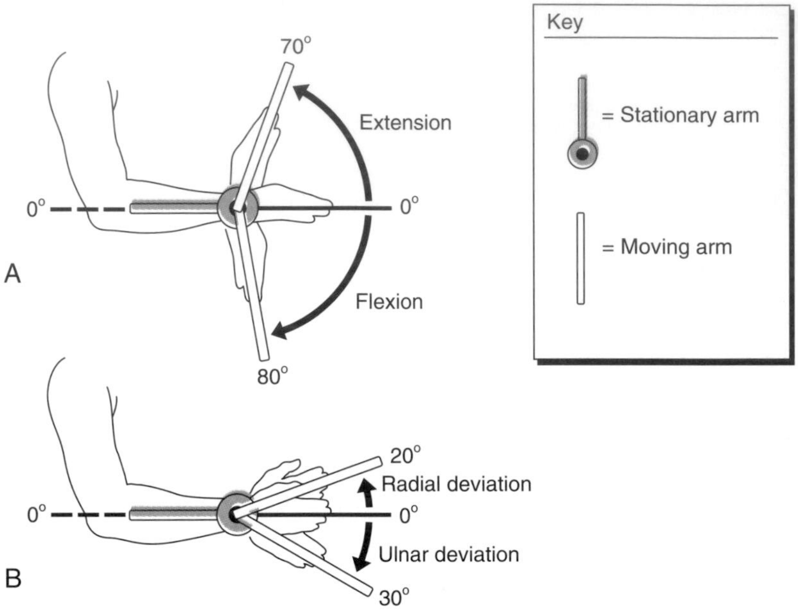

FIGURE 10–4. Measuring the range of motion of the wrist.

Measuring the Range of Motion of the Wrist

To measure wrist radial flexion[3] (Fig. 10–4), the examiner places the stationary arm of the goniometer along the midline of the back of the forearm between the ulna and the radius (pointing toward the lateral epicondyle of the humerus). The moving arm is placed along the metacarpophalangeal joint of the third digit. For wrist radial and ulnar deviation, the examiner places the stationary arm along the lateral midline of the ulna (pointing toward the medial epicondyle of the humerus). The moving arm is placed parallel to the fifth metacarpal bone.

WRIST AND HAND STRETCHES

Closed Wave (Fig. 10–5)

Prime movers: flexor carpi radialis, flexor carpi ulnaris, extensor carpi radialis longus, extensor carpi radialis brevis, and extensor carpi ulnaris.

- With the hand in a loose fist, slowly flex the wrist and hold
- Slowly extend the wrist and hold

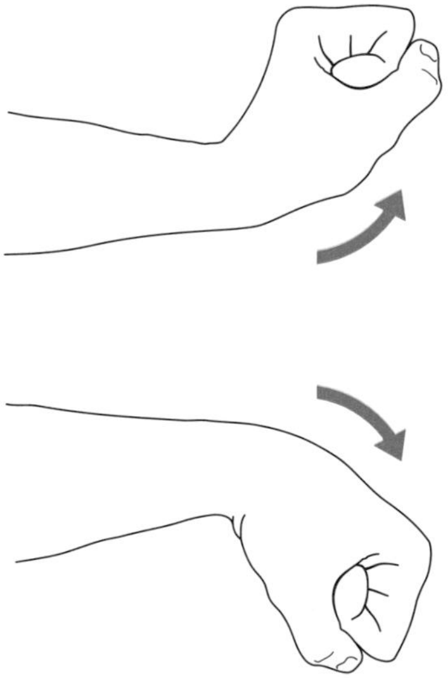

FIGURE 10–5. Closed wave.

Hand Spread (Fig. 10–6)

Prime movers: interossei dorsales, abductor digiti minimi, interossei palmaris, abductor pollicis longus, abductor pollicis brevis, and adductor pollicis.

- Spread the fingers apart (finger abduction); hold
- Slowly bring the fingers together

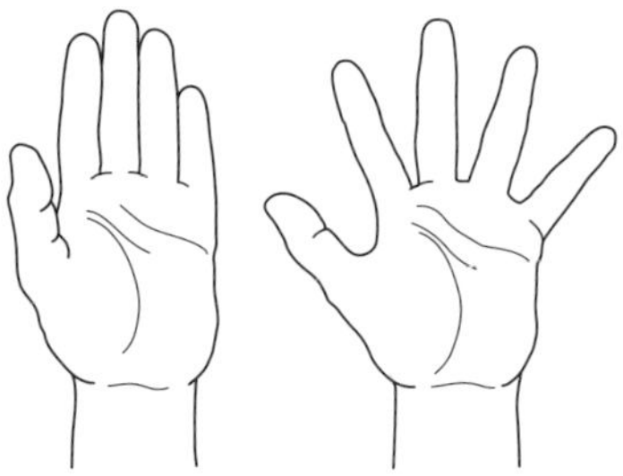

FIGURE 10–6. Hand spread.

Closed and Open Hands (Fig. 10–7)

Prime movers: same muscles as in Hand Spread, plus flexor digitorum superficialis, flexor digitorum, profundus, extensor digitorum, extensor indices, extensor digiti minimi, opponens pollicis, and opponens digiti minimi.

- Spread the fingers apart as far as possible; hold
- Slowly bring the fingers together and make a tight fist

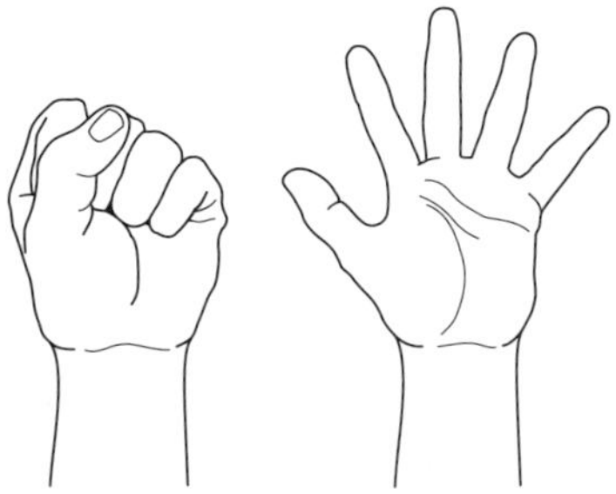

FIGURE 10–7. Closed and open hands.

Palm Stretch (Fig. 10–8)

Prime movers: flexor carpi radialis, flexor carpi ulnaris, flexor digitorum superficialis, and flexor digitorum profundus.

- Hold the involved hand in front of the body with the palm up
- Flex the elbow and rest it against the side of the body
- Use the opposite hand to stretch the wrist and fingers into extension; hold
- Gradually deepen the stretch; hold, then relax

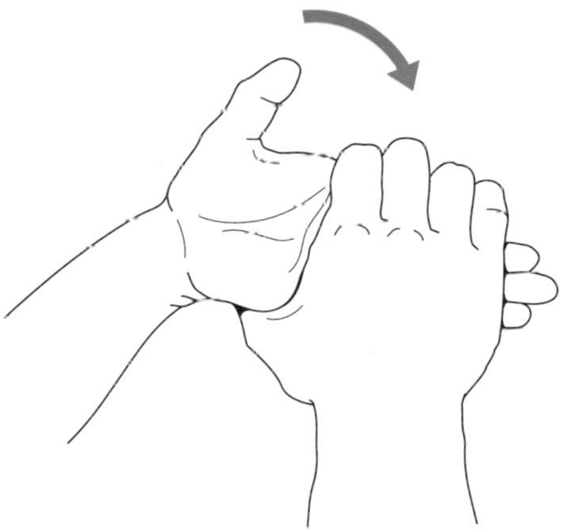

FIGURE 10–8. Palm stretch.

Praying Hands (Fig. 10–9)

Prime movers: flexor carpi radialis, flexor carpi ulnaris, flexor digitorum superficialis, flexor digitorum profundus, biceps, and deltoids.

- Place the palms of the hands together close to the body, with the fingers up
- Lift the elbows upward while lowering the hands
- Hold, then relax

Reverse Praying Hands (Fig. 10–10)

Prime movers: extensor carpi radialis longus, extensor carpi radialis brevis, and extensor carpi ulnaris.

- Place the dorsal surfaces (backs) of the hands together close to the body, with the fingers down
- Pull the elbows downward while raising the hands to chest level
- Hold, then relax

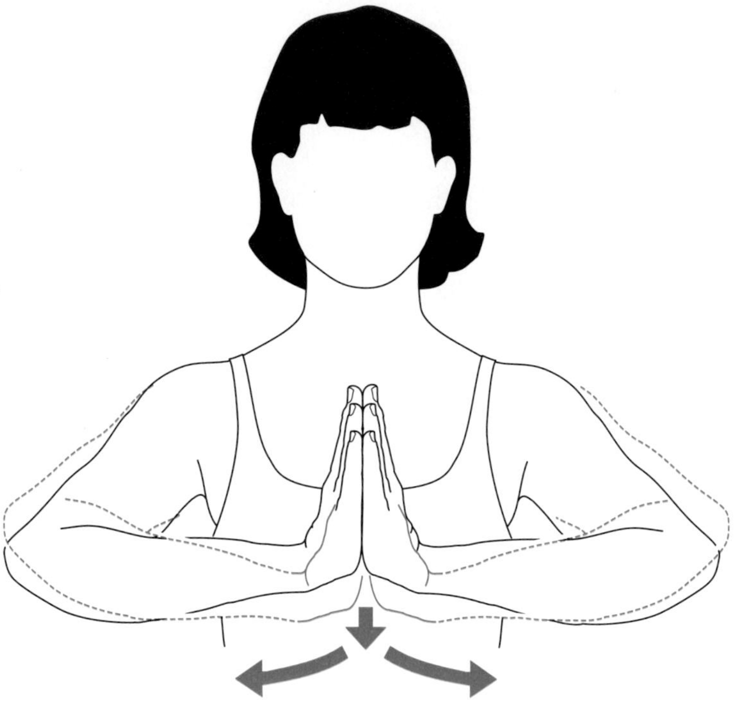

FIGURE 10–9. Praying hands.

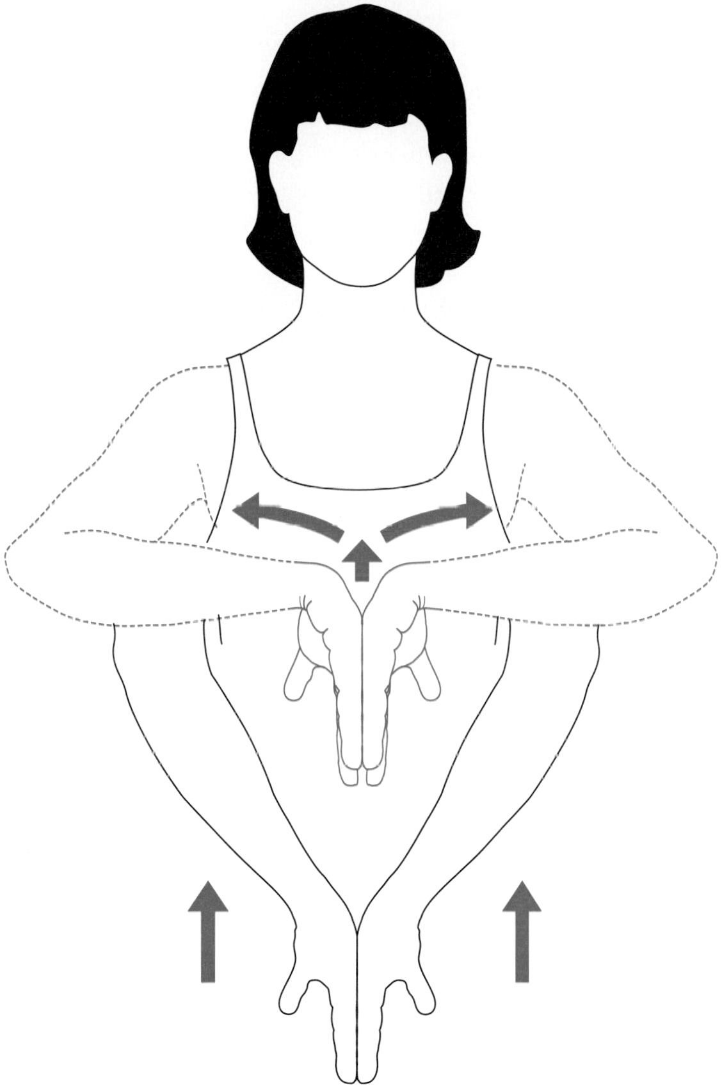

FIGURE 10–10. Reverse praying hands.

Supinator Stretch (Fig. 10–11)

Prime movers: supinator and biceps brachii.

- Flex the elbow of the involved hand to 90°
- Hold the elbow against the side with the palm down
- Place the uninvolved hand with the palm down on the dorsal surface of the (pronated) involved hand
- Use the uninvolved hand to gently turn the palm of the involved hand up and over (into more pronation)

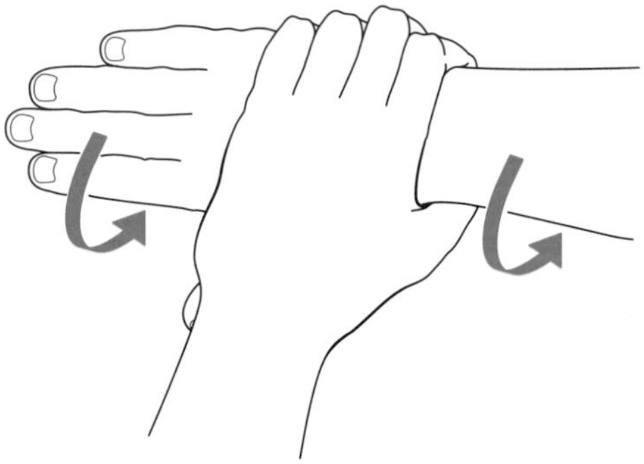

FIGURE 10–11. Supinator stretch.

Pronator Stretch (Fig. 10–12)

Prime movers: pronator quadratus and pronator teres.

- Flex the elbow of the involved hand to 90°
- Hold the elbow against the side with the palm up
- Place the uninvolved hand with the palm up on the dorsal surface of the (supinated) involved hand and grasp with the fingers on the medial border of the index finger
- Use the uninvolved hand to gently turn the palm of the involved hand up and over (into more supination)

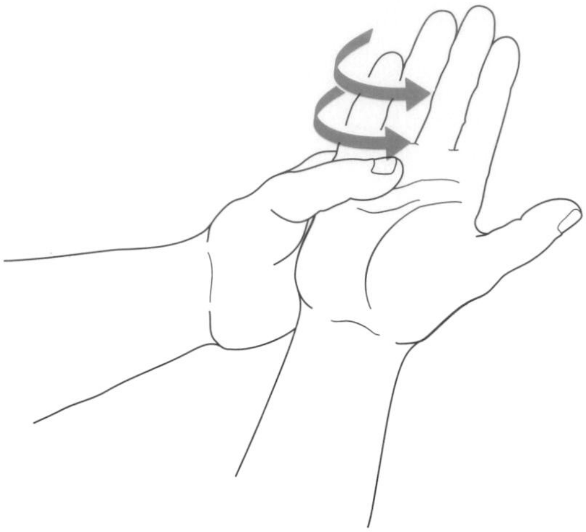

FIGURE 10–12. Pronator stretch.

Finger Tuck (Fig. 10–13)

Prime movers: lumbricals, flexor digitorum superficialis, and flexor digitorum profundus.

- Raise the hands
- Keeping the large knuckles straight, curl the small joints (middle and distal phalanges) downward
- Hold, then relax

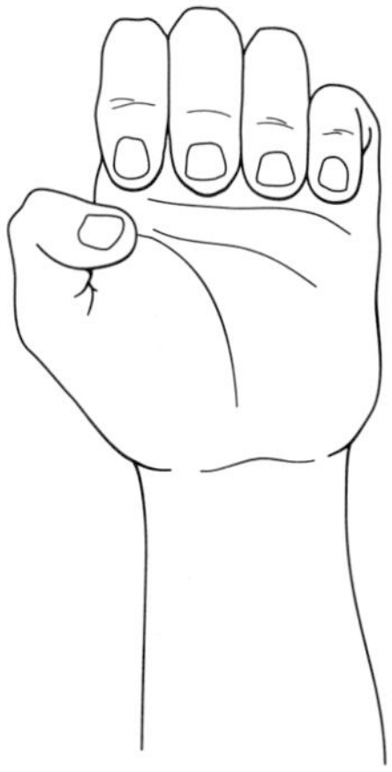

FIGURE 10–13. Finger tuck.

WRIST AND HAND EXERCISES

Wrist Circles (Fig. 10–14)

Prime movers: wrist flexors, wrist extensors, flexor digitorum superficialis, flexor digitorum profundus, biceps, triceps, and deltoids.

- Hold the arms out at the sides
- Keeping the forearms still, slowly make clockwise circles with the wrists
- Repeat in the counterclockwise direction

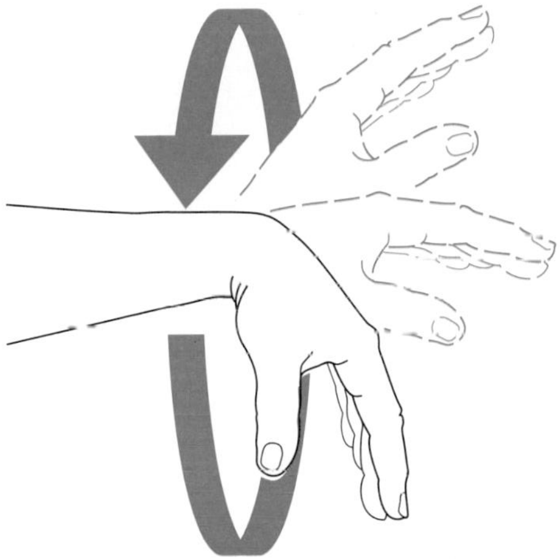

FIGURE 10–14. Wrist circles.

Thumb Movements (Fig. 10–15)

Prime movers: flexor pollicis brevis, flexor pollicis longus, extensor pollicis brevis, extensor pollicis longus, abductor pollicis longus, abductor pollicis brevis, adductor pollicis, opponens pollicis, and opponens digiti minimi. The exercise is performed in three parts:

Part A

Touch the thumb to the tip of each finger, forming the letter "o" each time (thumb opposition).

Part B

Make a large clockwise circle with the thumb; repeat in the counterclockwise direction (thumb circumduction).

Part C

Use the thumb to touch the base of each metacarpal (thumb opposition).

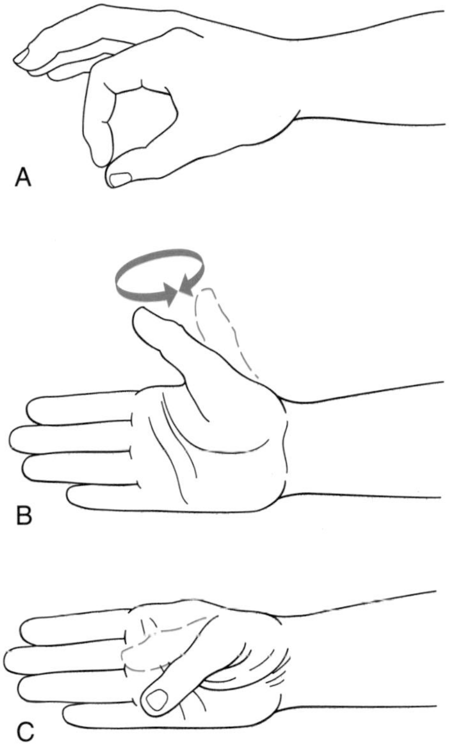

FIGURE 10–15. Thumb movements. *A* and *C*, Thumb opposition. *B*, Thumb circumduction.

Wrist Extension (Fig. 10–16)

Prime movers: extensor carpi radialis longus, extensor carpi radialis brevis, and extensor carpi ulnaris.

- Hold on to a flotation bell with the involved hand, the palm facing up toward the surface of the water and the elbow flexed to 90°
- Use the uninvolved hand to hold on to the forearm
- Slowly extend the wrist as far as possible toward the bottom of the pool
- Return to the original position
- Repeat

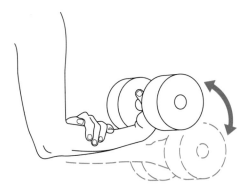

FIGURE 10–16. Wrist extension.

Wrist Flexion (Fig. 10–17)

Prime movers: flexor carpi radialis and flexor carpi ulnaris.

- Hold on to a flotation bell with the involved hand, the palm facing down toward the bottom of the pool and the elbow flexed to 90°
- Use the uninvolved hand to hold onto the forearm
- Slowly flex the wrist as far as possible toward the bottom of the pool
- Return to the original position

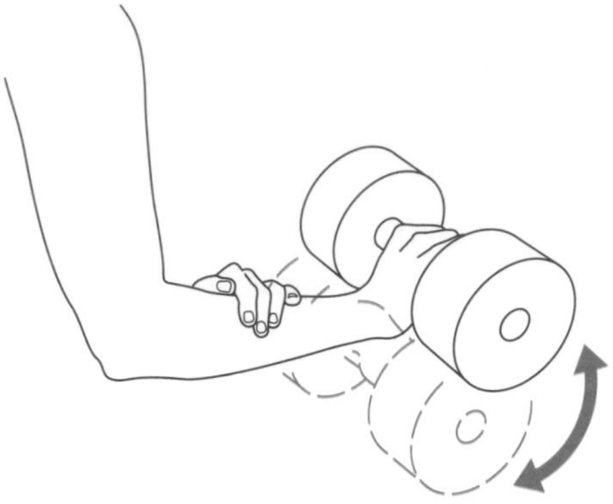

FIGURE 10–17. Wrist flexion.

Wrist Radial and Ulnar Deviation (Fig. 10–18)

Prime movers: flexor carpi radialis, extensor carpi radialis longus, extensor carpi radialis brevis, flexor carpi ulnaris, and extensor carpi ulnaris.

- Hold the elbow of the involved hand against the side, flexed to 90°
- Grasp a flotation bell with the thumb pointed up in a neutral position
- Move the hand upward as far as possible and then downward as far as possible without moving the forearm

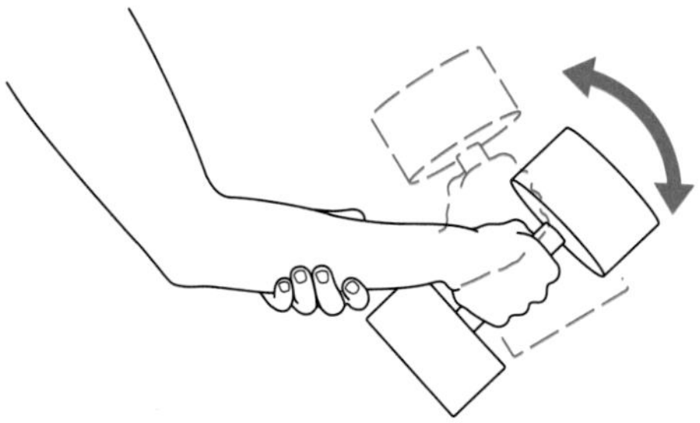

FIGURE 10–18. Wrist radial and ulnar deviation.

Wrist Rotation (Fig. 10–19)

Prime movers: supinator, pronator quadratus, and teres.

- Hold on to a flotation bell with the involved hand, the palm up and the elbow flexed
- Keeping the resistive device underwater, rotate the forearm until the palm of the hand is facing down
- Return to starting position

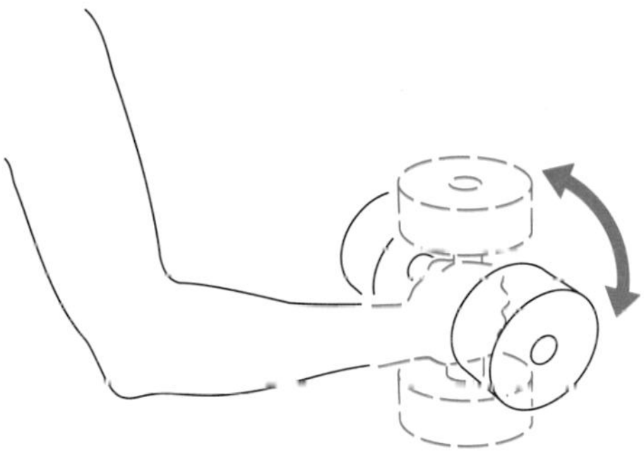

FIGURE 10–19. Wrist rotation.

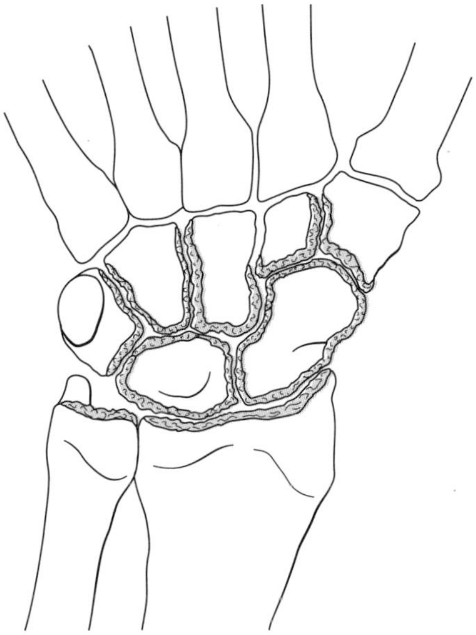

FIGURE 10–20. Wrist arthritis.

COMMON CONDITIONS OF THE WRIST AND HAND

Arthritis of the Wrist and Hand

The wrist and hand are common areas of the body in which arthritis occurs.

Origin

Rheumatoid arthritis is seen most often in the hands. Osteoarthritis in this area is usually the result of many years of heavy labor involving the hands.

Pathology

Any number of the joints involving the carpal bones, metacarpal bones, and phalanges may be affected (Fig. 10–20). Chapter 7 outlines the pathologic processes that may be responsible for this condition.

Signs and Symptoms

Pain, stiffness, and swelling are common symptoms. There may be periods of acute exacerbation as well as periods during which the symptoms subside.

Body Parts Affected

- Bones (carpals, metacarpals, phalanges)
- Joint surfaces (articular cartilage)
- Soft tissues (joint capsules, muscles, tendons, tendon sheaths, ligaments)

Exercise Priorities

- Controlled exercise program (be careful that the patient does not overdo it)
- Maximize range of motion
- Strengthen all wrist and hand muscles

Wrist Fracture

The two most common types of wrist fractures are the Colles fracture (involving the distal radius and ulna) and the scaphoid fracture (Fig. 10–21).

Origin

The typical mechanism of injury involves a fall on an outstretched hand.

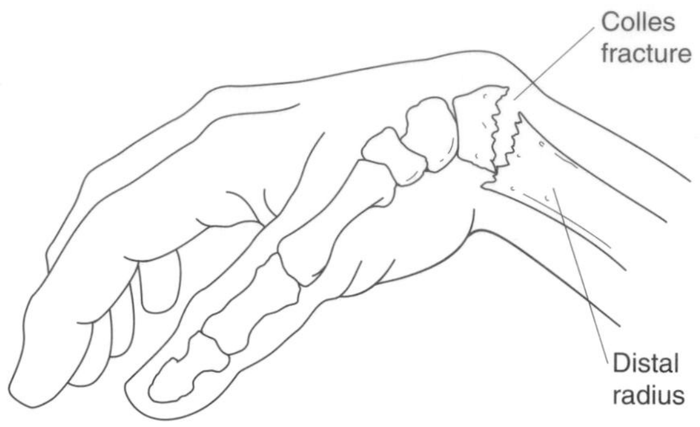

FIGURE 10–21. Wrist fracture. (Redrawn from Arnheim D. Modern Principles of Athletic Training, 8th ed. St. Louis: Times Mirror/Mosby College Publishing, 1993.)

Pathology

Although Colles fractures are often reduced surgically, the patient can be left with a swan-neck deformity of the wrist in which the distal radius and ulna are slightly curved. This is not usually a major problem, but the patient may not be able to achieve full range of motion because of the altered angle of the distal radius.

Scaphoid fractures may not be visible on X-ray until 2 to 3 weeks after injury. These fractures take longer to heal than the average fracture because of the poor blood supply to this small bone.

Signs and Symptoms

Wrist pain and stiffness are the dominant characteristics of these fractures. The fingers may also become stiff from being in a cast. This type of injury is one of the most common incidents precipitating the development of reflex sympathetic dystrophy.

Body Parts Affected

- Bones (radius, ulna, carpals, metacarpals)
- Articular cartilage
- Soft tissues (joint capsule, tendons, ligaments)
- Nerves (damage may have occurred during the injury)

Exercise Priorities

- Maximize range of motion (including pronation and supination)
- Strengthen all wrist muscles
- Practice functional hand movements

Wrist Tendonitis

Like elbow tendonitis, wrist tendonitis involves the muscles that flex and extend the wrist. The difference is that wrist tendonitis involves the long sections of tendons that attach at the wrist, whereas elbow tendonitis involves the attachments of the muscles at the elbow.

Origin

Tendonitis in this area of the body is most often the result of overuse. It is a common work-related injury.

Pathology

The pathology of this condition is described in Chapter 7. The tendons of the wrist flexors or extensors may be involved. It is also common for a tenosynovitis (inflammation of the tendon sheath) to develop (Fig. 10–22).

Signs and Symptoms

Although range of motion may be full, stretching of the affected tendon causes pain. Pain also in-

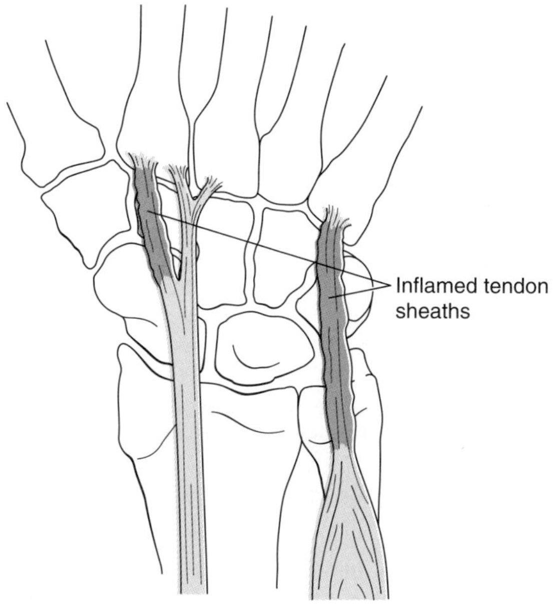

FIGURE 10–22. Wrist tendonitis.

creases with increased activity. If a tenosynovitis is present, there is often crepitus as the tendon tries to slide within its sheath.

Body Parts Affected

- Flexor and extensor tendons of the wrist
- Muscles (wrist flexors and extensors, muscles of the fingers and thumb)

Exercise Priorities

- Stretch injured tendons
- Establish a controlled strengthening program

Wrist Sprain

A wrist sprain involves an injury to one or more ligaments of the wrist joint.

Origin

The most common mechanism of injury is a fall onto an outstretched hand. A wrist sprain may also occur as the result of a sports injury or an automobile accident. If the wrist is forced into hyperflexion, the ligaments on the dorsal side of the wrist are injured. Conversely, hyperextension injures the ligaments on the volar side of the wrist.

Pathology

The pathology of this injury is outlined in Chapter 7. There are numerous ligaments in the wrist that may be involved (Fig. 10–23).

Signs and Symptoms

This is a very painful injury. Range of motion is very limited, especially in the direction that stretches the injured ligament. Swelling in the area may cause the symptoms of carpal tunnel syndrome as the nerves and vessels passing through the tunnel are compressed.

Body Parts Affected

- Ligaments of the wrist
- Joint capsule
- Wrist and finger muscles
- Nerves and vessels passing through the carpal tunnel

Exercise Priorities

- Restore range of motion
- Establish a program of controlled strengthening of wrist and finger muscles

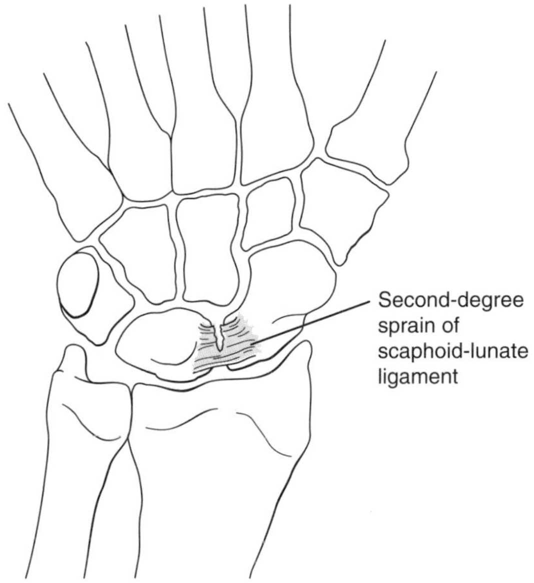

FIGURE 10–23. Wrist sprain.

- Restore functional activities involving the wrist and fingers

Wrist Dislocation

The term "wrist dislocation" can refer to the dislocation of the entire proximal row of carpal bones with respect to the distal end of the radius, or it can be applied if the lunate alone is subluxed.

Origin

As with many other wrist injuries, a fall onto an outstretched hand is the most common mechanism of injury.[4]

Pathology

A wrist dislocation is essentially the result of a third-degree sprain. A hyperflexion or hyperextension incident stretches ligaments beyond their normal limits, usually tearing those ligaments. A fracture of the radius may occur at the same time (Fig. 10–24).

Signs and Symptoms

The bony defect at the time of injury is visually obvious. After the dislocation has been reduced,

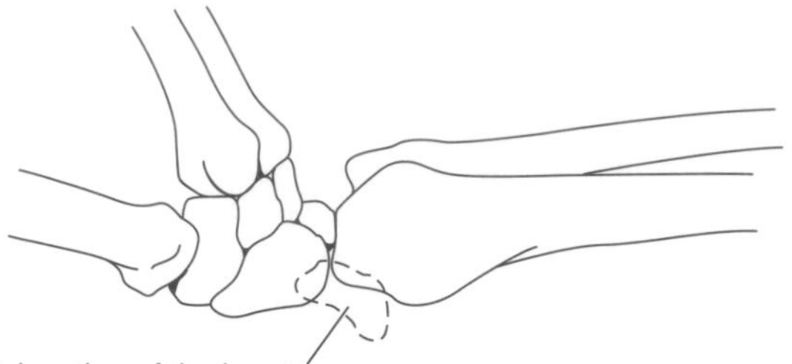

FIGURE 10–24. Wrist dislocation.

pain and apprehension on moving the wrist into the position in which the subluxation took place are the predominant symptoms.

Body Parts Affected

- Wrist ligaments
- Joint capsule
- Nerves and vessels of the area (may be damaged)
- Muscles and tendons of the wrist and fingers

Exercise Priorities

- Restore range of motion
- Establish a controlled strengthening routine

THE AQUATIC EXERCISE THERAPY PROTOCOL FOR CONDITIONS OF THE WRIST AND HAND

Phase One

Warm-up

Perform each exercise for 2 minutes.

- Bent Arm Pull (see Fig. 5–2)
- Breast Stroke (see Fig. 5–14)
- Side Stepping (push water with arms) (see Fig. 5–23)

Stretch

Perform six repetitions each, holding 10 seconds.

- Closed Wave (see Fig. 10–5)
- Finger Tuck (see Fig. 10–13)
- Closed and Open Hands (see Fig. 10–7)
- Hand Spread (see Fig. 10–6)

Strengthen

Perform one set of 8 to 12 repetitions. Use resistance of the water only.

- Wrist Flexion (see Fig. 10–17)
- Wrist Extension (see Fig. 10–16)
- Wrist Radial and Ulnar Deviation (see Fig. 10–18)

Phase Two

Warm-up

Perform same exercises as in Phase One, emphasizing wrist movement (full range of motion).

Stretch

Perform five repetitions each, holding 20 seconds. Perform same exercises as in Phase One, and add the following:

- Palm Stretch (see Fig. 10–8)
- Supinator Stretch (see Fig. 10–11)
- Pronator Stretch (see Fig. 10–12)

Strengthen

Perform two sets of 8 to 12 repetitions. Perform the exercises of Phase One but with small resistive paddles. Then add the following:

- Wrist Circles (holding onto float under the water) (see Fig. 10–14)
- Wrist Rotation (see Fig. 10–19)
- Thumb Movements (see Fig. 10–15)

Phase Three

Warm-up

Same as in Phase Two.

Stretch

Perform five repetitions each, holding 20 seconds. Perform same exercises as in Phase Two, then add the following:

- Praying Hands (see Fig. 10–9)
- Reverse Praying Hands (see Fig. 10–10)

Strengthen

Perform three sets of 8 to 12 repetitions. Use small hand paddles or hand floats to increase the resistance.

- Wrist Flexion (see Fig. 10–17)
- Wrist Extension (see Fig. 10–16)

- Wrist Radial and Ulnar Deviation (see Fig. 10–18)
- Wrist Circles (see Fig. 10–14)
- Wrist Rotation (see Fig. 10–19)
- Thumb Movements (see Fig. 10–15)

Phase Four

Warm-up

Perform same exercises as in Phase Two, but use small hand paddles or webbed gloves to push and pull the water.

Stretch

Perform five repetitions each, holding 30 seconds. Perform same exercises as in Phase Three, then add the following:

- Forearm Stretch (see Fig. 9–9)

Strengthen

Perform four sets of 8 to 12 repetitions. Perform the same exercises as in Phase Three. Increase the resistance by increasing the speed and range of movement and also by using larger paddles, flotation bells, or stretch bands.

REFERENCES

1. Magee D. Orthopedic Physical Assessment. Philadelphia: W.B. Saunders, 1987.
2. Green W, Heckman J. Rosemont, IL: The Clinical Measurement of Joint Motion. American Academy of Orthopaedic Surgeons, 1994.
3. Arnheim D. Modern Principles of Athletic Training, 8th ed. St. Louis: Times Mirror/Mosby College Publishing, 1993.
4. Gould J, Davis G. Orthopaedic and Sports Physical Therapy. St. Louis: C.V. Mosby, 1985.

Aquatic Rehabilitation for Disorders of Gait and Balance

Chapter 11

GAIT

Walking Re-education

The human foot is designed to absorb shock for the entire body. One of the greatest benefits of exercising in the water is the ability to eliminate shock or impact forces. Walking in the water is also easier than walking on land because of buoyancy. Injured limbs are able to perform partial weight-bearing exercises sooner, with less pain, and with less risk of further damage to the healing structures.

Gait re-education is often necessary after disease or trauma of a lower extremity.[1, 2] Re-education is also very important to correct abnormal gait patterns that, if uncorrected, may develop into pathologic conditions over time. Walking is a complex movement pattern that must be corrected gradually. In the beginning, it is important to focus on one particular aspect of the gait cycle. After that has improved, the therapist can move to the next stage, until the walking pattern is acceptable.[1]

The Gait Cycle

The gait cycle is a sequence of movements that characterize an individual's walking pattern. There are three recognized phases in the gait cycle: the stance phase, the swing phase, and the double stance phase. Each of these phases can be broken down into subphases (Table 11–1).

The Swing Phase

The swing phase constitutes 40% of a normal gait cycle.[3] During this phase, the foot does not bear weight as it moves forward. The quadriceps are the prime muscles used for swinging the legs. This phase may be broken down into three subphases (see Table 11–1).

Initial Swing

During this subphase, the dorsiflexors lift the toes off the floor to prevent them from dragging. The

TABLE 11–1. The Gait Cycle and the Influence of the Water on the Lower Limbs

		Swing Phase (40%)			Stance Phase (60%)			
		Initial Swing	*Midswing*	*Terminal Swing*	*Heel Strike*	*Flat Foot*	*Midstance*	*Push-off*
		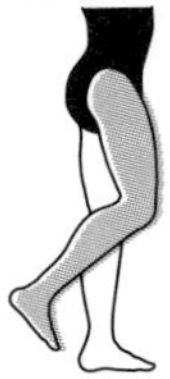	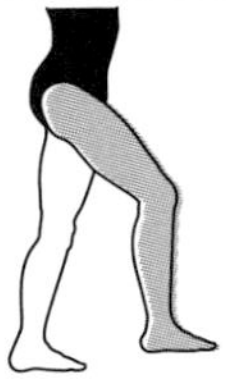	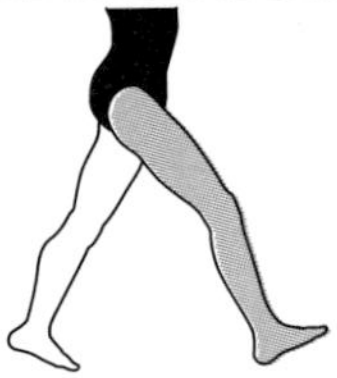	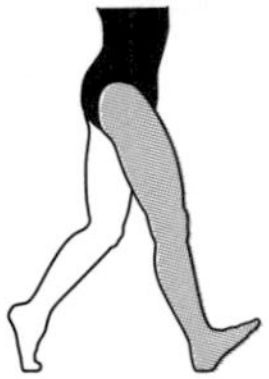	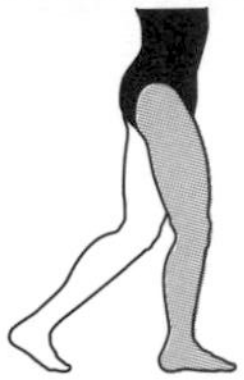	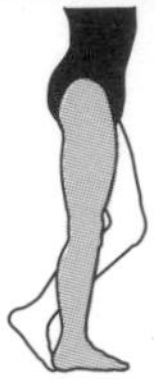	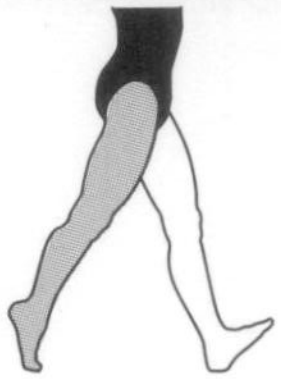
Influence of the Water	*Assisted*	• hip flexion • knee flexion 60°	• hip flexion	• hip flexion	• hip flexion* • ankle dorsiflexion	• hip flexion* • knee flexion 10°		• hip extension full
	Resisted	• ankle plantar flexion	• knee as it swings through and begins to extend	• knee extension to 0°	• knee extension full		• hip extension • ankle plantar flexion	• ankle plantar flexion† • metatarso-phalangeal extension†
	Suppported	• neutral foot	• neutral ankle and foot	• neutral ankle and foot	• neutral foot	• neutral ankle • neutral foot	• neutral knee, full extension • neutral foot	• neutral knee, full extension • neutral interphalangeals

*The trunk stays neutral throughout the cycle. As the hip begins to extend, buoyancy begins to offer some resistance to the movement.
†Buoyancy assists the upward thrust produced by ankle plantar flexion and metatarsophalangeal extension as the weight is shifted to the opposite leg.

knee flexes to about 60° in order to allow the leg to accelerate forward.

Midswing

During this subphase, the swing leg passes the weight-bearing leg. If the dorsiflexors are weak, the hip must flex more; this results in a high-stepping gait.[3]

Terminal Swing

During this subphase, the swing leg passes down before making contact with the floor. The quadriceps and hamstrings work together to control the speed of the swing.[3]

The Stance Phase

The stance phase constitutes 60% of a normal gait cycle.[3] During this phase, the foot is in contact with the floor and is bearing weight. The foot performs multiple functions during stance. Its most obvious roles are those of shock absorption and support.[4] The stance phase can be broken down into four subphases (see Table 11–1).

Heel Strike

The heel strike is characterized by the contraction of the dorsiflexors of the ankle, which keeps the toes up as the foot makes initial contact with the floor. The knee should be fully extended. Weak knee muscles cause the knee to buckle during weight acceptance.[4, 5]

Flat Foot

In this subphase, the contact foot is getting ready to absorb the weight of the body. If the ankle dorsiflexors are weak, the foot is allowed to "flop" down.

Midstance

This subphase is characterized by even weight distribution over the whole foot. One leg must balance the weight of the body during single-leg stance. Weak hip abductors allow the pelvis to tip down on the opposite side. Look for lack of hip extension here.

Push-off

During this subphase, the heel leaves the floor and the leg prepares for the swing phase. This requires adequate strength of the calf muscles.

The Double Stance Phase

The double stance phase is characterized by having both feet in contact with the floor. Double support occurs twice during a normal gait cycle as the body weight is shifted to the opposite leg. Normal gait parameters during this phase include the following:

1. The base width is 2 to 4 inches. A wider base of support indicates poor balance[3, 6] (Fig. 11–1).
2. The step length is 14 to 16 inches and should be equal bilaterally[3] (Fig. 11–2).
3. The lateral pelvic shift is 1 to 2 inches. This side-to-side movement centers the body's weight over the hips (Fig. 11–3).
4. The vertical pelvic shift is 2 inches. The high point occurs at midstance and the low point at heel strike (see Fig. 11–3).
5. The pelvic rotation is 4° forward on the swing leg and 4° backward on the stance leg.
6. The toes are angled outward 5° to 10°.

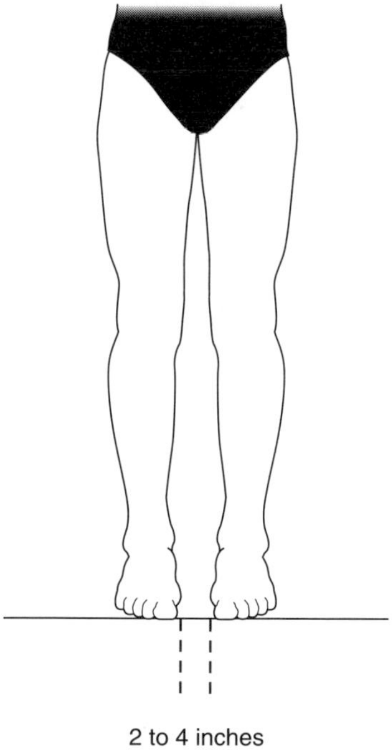

FIGURE 11–1. Double stance has a normal base width of 2 to 4 inches.

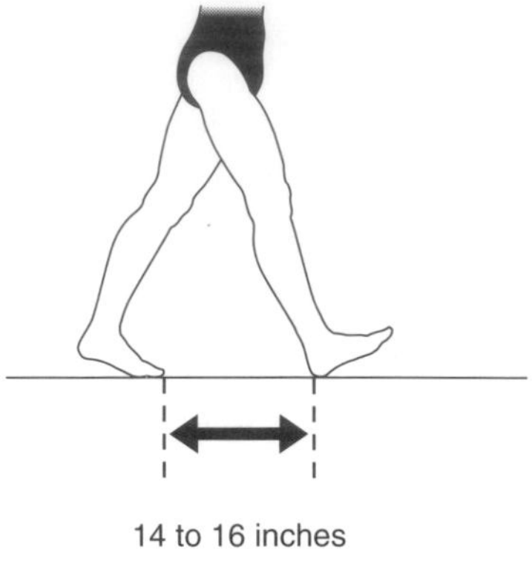

FIGURE 11–2. A normal step length is between 14 and 16 inches.

Gait Assessment

When walking forward in the water, the patient experiences weight transference from side to side and forward and backward. As the leg moves forward, buoyancy assists both the push-off by the calf muscles and flexion of the hip and knee. The hip extensors, on the other hand, have to work against buoyancy to lower the leg. This muscle work is different from that of walking on land, and it is therefore important to continue gait re-education on land.

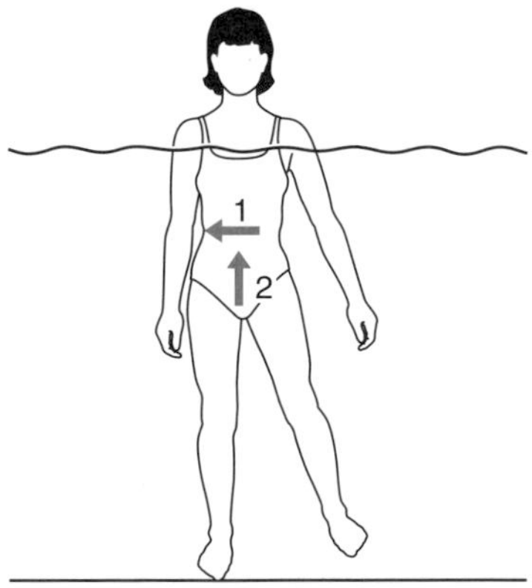

FIGURE 11–3. A normal gait pattern includes (1) a lateral and (2) a vertical pelvic shift.

On land, the therapist should observe the patient's gait pattern. It is important to check the following:

1. The trunk and joints of the lower limbs should be in proper position during each phase of the cycle.
2. The stride length should be even (it normally decreases with age[6]).
3. The weight transfer should be smooth and the position of the pelvis should be controlled.[1]
4. The muscles should be able to flex the hip and knee, extend the hip and knee, and dorsiflex and plantar flex the ankle.
5. The leg should undergo complete extension during push-off.
6. The base width during double stance should be normal.

Common Gait Abnormalities

Abnormal gait patterns can result from many kinds of injuries. It first must be decided whether the pattern is correctable. Problems that are not correctable include those caused by joint fusion, severe bony abnormality, or permanent nerve damage that has resulted in flaccidity or spasticity. Some of these problems may be correctable to a degree, but 100% normal gait may not be an attainable goal.

Gait abnormalities that result from many common orthopedic injuries may indicate specific problems to which rehabilitation exercises can be geared. The following is a list of several common problems and what they indicate. Although each person is different, analysis of gait often gives the therapist his or her first clues as to what the patient's primary problems may be.

WALKING WITH HIP OR KNEE STIFF. This may be a result of hip or knee pain. It may also indicate that the patient is afraid that pain or instability will occur. The original problem may have been corrected, but a habitual gait pattern may have developed. This gait may also indicate decreased range of motion in the hip or knee caused by swelling, muscle contractures, or a mechanical joint abnormality such as severe arthritis.

HYPEREXTENSION OF KNEE. It must first be determined whether hyperextension is abnormal for the patient (by observation of the movement of the *uninvolved* knee). Hyperextension may indicate joint instability. It may also occur if there is marked weakness of the quadriceps, whether from inactivity or from a neurologic problem (muscles not receiving the proper signals to control the knee joint).

CIRCUMDUCTION OF LEG DURING SWING PHASE. This may occur because there is an inability to flex the hip or knee due to stiffness, weakness, or pain. This compensatory pattern allows the patient to avoid catching the toes on the ground during swing phase. It may also be a habitual pattern that has never been pointed out to the patient before.

WALKING WITH LEG EXTERNALLY ROTATED. The most obvious reason for this gait is tightness in the hip external rotators. This gait may also stem from an inability to flex the hip because of stiffness, weakness, or pain. Patients who lack full dorsiflexion (eg, owing to a sprained ankle) also demonstrate this pattern.

TRENDELENBURG GAIT. This classic gait pattern is characterized by a dropping hip when the foot is lifted off the ground for the swing phase. It usually indicates weakness in the hip abductors of the opposite leg (from disuse or a neurologic problem). It may also be habitual; the patient may have grown accustomed to walking with a "waddling" gait.

FORWARD TILTING OF PELVIS ON INVOLVED SIDE WHEN TAKING A STEP. This is usually done to compensate for an inability to flex the hip (owing to stiffness or weakness). It is also commonly seen in people who have neurologic problems such as stroke. These patients may exhibit "patterned" or synergistic movements. Often, these patients cannot smoothly flex the hip and knee simultaneously.

ABNORMAL HEEL CONTACT. Normally, there is a distinct heel contact, followed by a smooth rocking forward onto the toes. Patients who lack normal dorsiflexion because of stiffness or weakness simply contact the floor with a flat foot. Weakness in the dorsiflexors may be caused by disuse or by a neurologic problem such as severe sciatica.

ABNORMAL PUSH-OFF. To have a normal push-off, the patient should be able to do Heel Raises (see Fig. 14–16). Factors that prevent this include disuse atrophy of the calf muscles, a strained or ruptured Achilles tendon, or an S1 disc bulge.

UNEQUAL STEP LENGTH. If the patient does not want to bear weight on the affected leg because of pain or fear of instability, the step length of the uninvolved leg will be shorter. Unequal step length may also be due to a lack of strength or flexibility in one leg. The normal gait pattern is disrupted because the involved leg cannot move as quickly or as smoothly as the uninvolved leg.

Gait Progressions

In many cases, patients can walk in the water before they are able to walk on land. Exercises to increase range of motion and strengthen weak muscles should be performed in addition to gait reeducation. The following exercises help to re-establish muscular strength and coordination before walking begins. The exercises that have not yet been described will be found in Chapters 12 through 14.

- Pelvic Movements (see Fig. 5–32)
- Hip Flexion (see Fig. 12–11)
- Hip Extension (see Fig. 12–12)
- Hip Abduction and Adduction (see Fig. 12–13)
- Resistive Knee Flexion and Extension (see Fig. 13–15)
- Squats (see Fig. 13–16)
- Heel Raises (see Fig. 14–16)
- Ankle Plantar Flexion (see Fig. 14–13)
- Ankle Dorsiflexion (see Fig. 14–12)
- Ankle Eversion and Inversion (see Fig. 14–14)
- Calf Stretch (see Fig. 14–7)
- Hamstring Stretch (see Fig. 13–10)
- Adductor Stretch (see Fig. 12–10)

Parallel bars are an important accessory in any therapy pool. The patient should begin with the feet 2 to 4 inches apart and the toes pointing forward. During the early stages of rehabilitation, the therapist should stand in front of the patient and offer support at the pelvis if necessary. This creates a wake that helps pull the patient forward toward the therapist. The patient should start with heel-to-toe walking. The involved leg should move forward in a straight line, and the heel should make contact with the floor. The patient should then roll onto the toe while lifting the heel of the uninvolved foot. The body's weight is then transferred onto the involved or injured foot.[6] The steps should be kept short so that the injured leg is bearing weight for only a short time. From this basic movement, the therapist can correct any gait abnormalities that may exist.

As the patient's condition improves, the therapist can begin to make gait training more difficult by

- supporting the patient from behind (ie, with no wake pulling the patient)
- having the patient walk without support of the therapist in the bars
- having the patient walk out of the parallel bars with the therapist supporting in front at the pelvis or shoulders
- having the patient walk out of the parallel bars holding onto a large float such as a flotation tube
- having the patient walk without a float
- having the patient walk with the use of a greater surface area of resistance, such as a tray

Gradually reducing the level of the water can be used to help the patient progress from partial weight bearing to full weight bearing at any time. However, it is important to continue gait training on land because the refraction of the water distorts the eye's perception of the lower limbs.

BALANCE

Balance allows the patient to maintain a position in space, to remain stable while moving, and to respond to external forces.[7] Injury or trauma to the lower extremities often results in some loss of proprioceptive feedback from the mechanoreceptors, especially in the ankle. Damage to the mechanoreceptors influences balance.[4]

Patients who have balance problems often have an extreme fear of falling. The water is an optimal medium in which to begin balance exercises because the water slows down movement. This, in turn, allows the patient time to respond to any unexpected movements.

Weight-bearing exercises help to rehabilitate muscle and joint function.[7, 8] The following exercises help restore proprioceptive function before the patient progresses to land. It is important to reinforce correct postural alignment throughout.

Straddle Standing (Fig. 11–4)

- Stand comfortably in a double stance position; hold
- Slowly progress to a normal base width

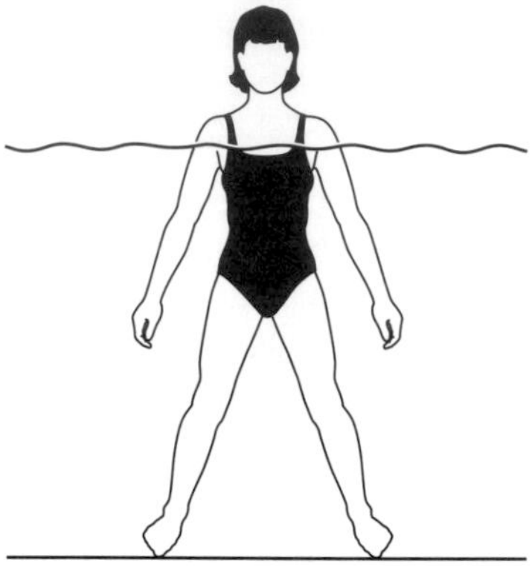

FIGURE 11–4. Straddle standing.

Side Stepping (Fig. 11–5)

- Stand upright with the legs straight
- Abduct one leg and contact the foot to the floor
- Adduct the opposite leg to the midline, returning to a standing position
- Repeat in the opposite direction

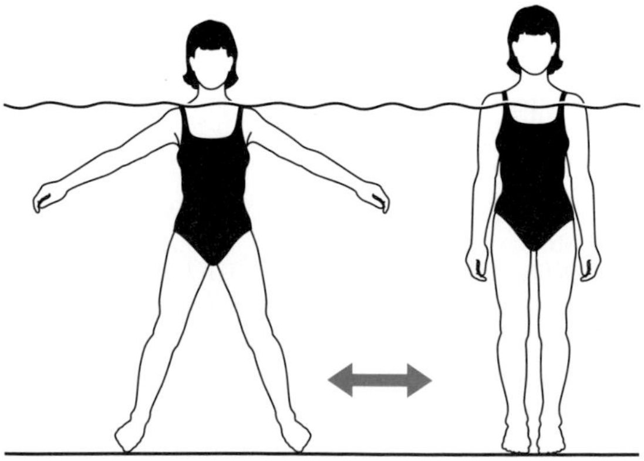

FIGURE 11–5. Side stepping.

Side-to-Side Weight Shifting (Fig. 11–6)

- Stand with the feet shoulder-width apart
- Shift the body weight from the left leg to the right leg
- Shift the body weight from the right leg to the left leg
- Slowly progress to a normal base width

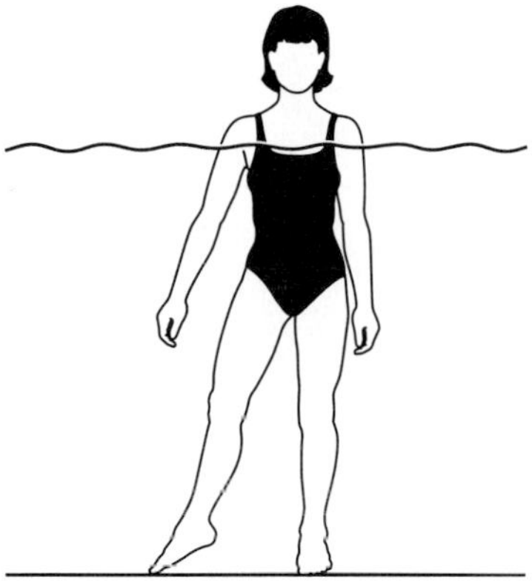

FIGURE 11–6. Side-to-side weight shifting.

Front-to-Back Weight Shifting (Fig. 11–7)

- Stand with one foot in front of the other
- Shift the body weight from the front leg to the back leg
- Shift the body weight from the back leg to the front leg
- Repeat with the other foot forward
- Gradually progress to a normal step length

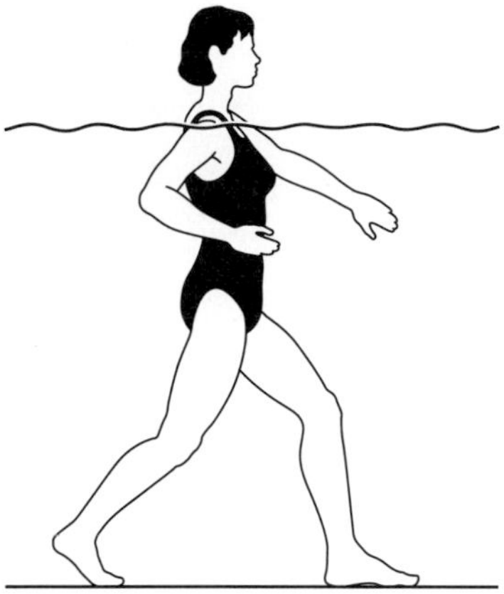

FIGURE 11–7. Front-to-back weight shifting.

Stork Stand (Fig. 11–8)

- Lift one leg by flexing the hip and knee
- Attempt to balance on the other leg, using the arms as necessary

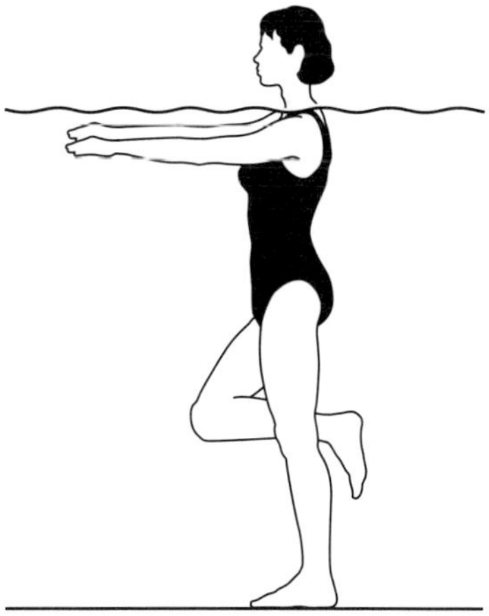

FIGURE 11–8. Stork stand.

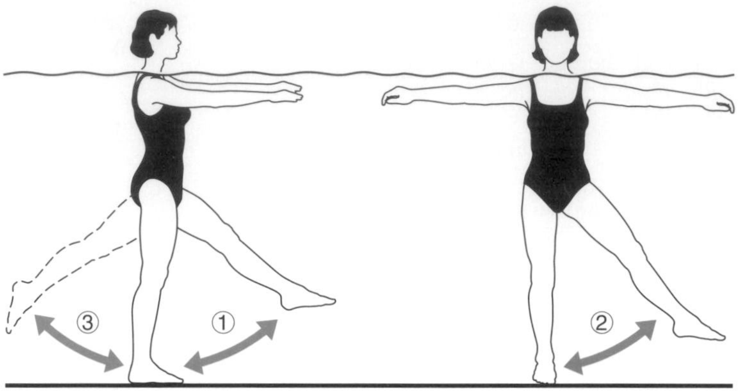

FIGURE 11–9. Leg balance exercises.

Leg Balance Exercises (Fig. 11–9)

- Stand on one leg with the arms underwater and gently move the other leg forward; hold 20 seconds
- Return to a neutral position (legs together)
- Move the non–weight-bearing leg to the side, hold, then return to a neutral position
- Move the non–weight-bearing leg backward, hold, then return to a neutral position
- Keep the trunk straight throughout; use the arms as necessary to assist balance
- Hold each position for 20 seconds before returning to neutral

Step-ups (Fig. 11–10)

- Stand in front of an aquatic step
- Flex the left hip and knee and place the left foot on the step
- Push off with the right foot and extend the left knee so that the body weight shifts onto the foot on top of the step
- Step down
- Repeat with other leg

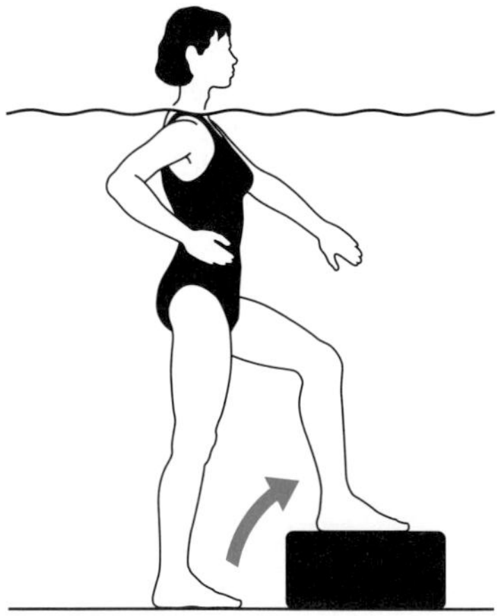

FIGURE 11–10. Step-ups.

Four-Corner Pivot (Fig. 11–11)

- From a double stance position, take one step forward with the left leg then one step with the right leg
- Pivot to the right on the right leg and take two more steps (with the left and then the right leg)
- Repeat the step-pivot pattern twice more, forming a square back to the original position
- Repeat the pattern, stepping off with right leg first

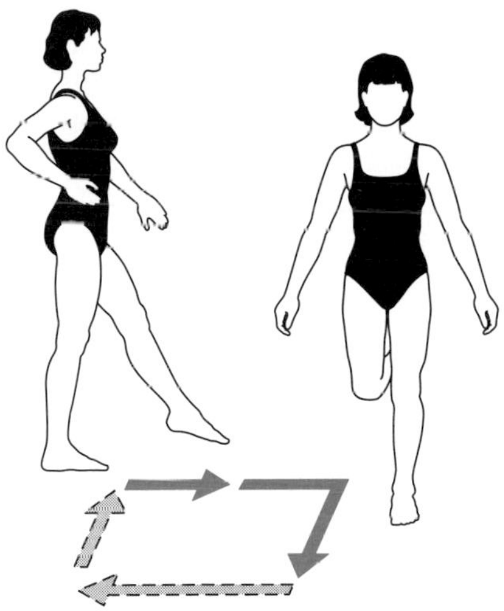

FIGURE 11–11. Four-corner pivot.

REFERENCES

1. Thomson A, Skinner A, Piercy J. Tidy's Physiotherapy. 12th ed. Toronto: Butterworth-Heinemann, 1991.
2. Messier SP, Loeser RF, Hoover JL, et al. Osteoarthritis of the knee: Effects on gait, strength, and flexibility. Arch Phys Med Rehabil 73:29–36, 1992.
3. Magee D. Orthopedic Physical Assessment. Philadelphia: W.B. Saunders, 1987.
4. Gould J, Davis G. Orthopedic and Sports Physical Therapy. St. Louis: C.V. Mosby, 1985.
5. Colborne GR, Olney SJ. Feedback of joint angle and EMG in gait of able-bodied subjects. Arch Phys Med Rehabil 71:478–483, 1990.
6. Wale J, ed. Tidy's Massage and Remedial Exercises. 11th ed. Bristol: John Wright & Sons, 1983.
7. Berg KO, Maki BE, Williams JI, et al. Clinical and laboratory measures of postural balance in an elderly population. Arch Phys Med Rehabil 73:1073–1080, 1992.
8. Perry J, Mulroy SJ, Renwick SE. The relationship of lower extremity strength and gait parameters in patients with post-polio syndrome. Arch Phys Med Rehabil 74:165–169, 1993.

CHAPTER 12

AQUATIC REHABILITATION OF THE HIP

THE STRUCTURE AND FUNCTION OF THE HIP

The Anatomic Parts

The hip joint is a multiaxial, ball-and-socket, synovial joint. The articulation is formed where the convex head of the femur inserts snugly into the concave acetabulum of the pelvic bone (Fig. 12–1).

The joint capsule is strong, and so are the muscles that control its movement. Although the hip joint is capable of movement similar to that of the shoulder, the range of mobility is sacrificed in the interest of stability.[1] The joint provides a reasonable range of movement and functions in both static and dynamic weight bearing. The ligaments that reinforce the joint capsule derive their names from the bony parts they connect. They are the iliofemoral, the pubofemoral, and the ischiofemoral ligaments (Fig. 12–2).

The acetabulum is made up of the fusion of the ilium, ischium, and pubic bones, and it is the legs' connection to the spine.

The Muscles and Their Actions

A muscle must cross a joint to act directly on that joint. The way in which a muscle crosses a joint affects the action. The muscles discussed in this section are primarily involved at the hip only or at the hip and knee. The hip joint permits the following movements (Fig. 12–3):

- flexion and extension (Tables 12–1 and 12–2)
- abduction and adduction (Table 12–3)
- internal (inward) and external (outward) rotation (Table 12–4)

Table 12–5 summarizes the muscles involved in the movements of the hip.

Measuring the Range of Motion of the Hip

To measure hip flexion and extension, the patient lies in a supine position[2] (Fig. 12–4), and the examiner places the stationary arm of the goniometer along a line through the crest of the ilium, femur, and greater trochanter. The moving arm is placed

Text continued on page 179

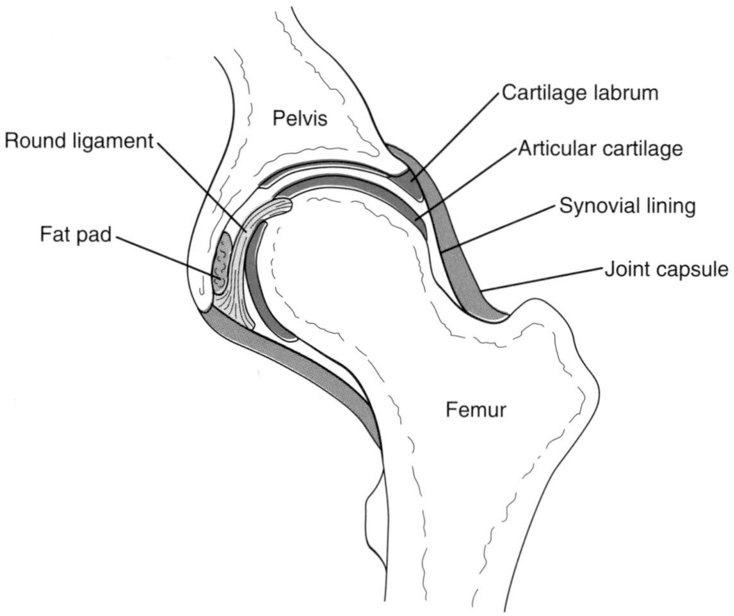

FIGURE 12–1. The bones of the hip joint.

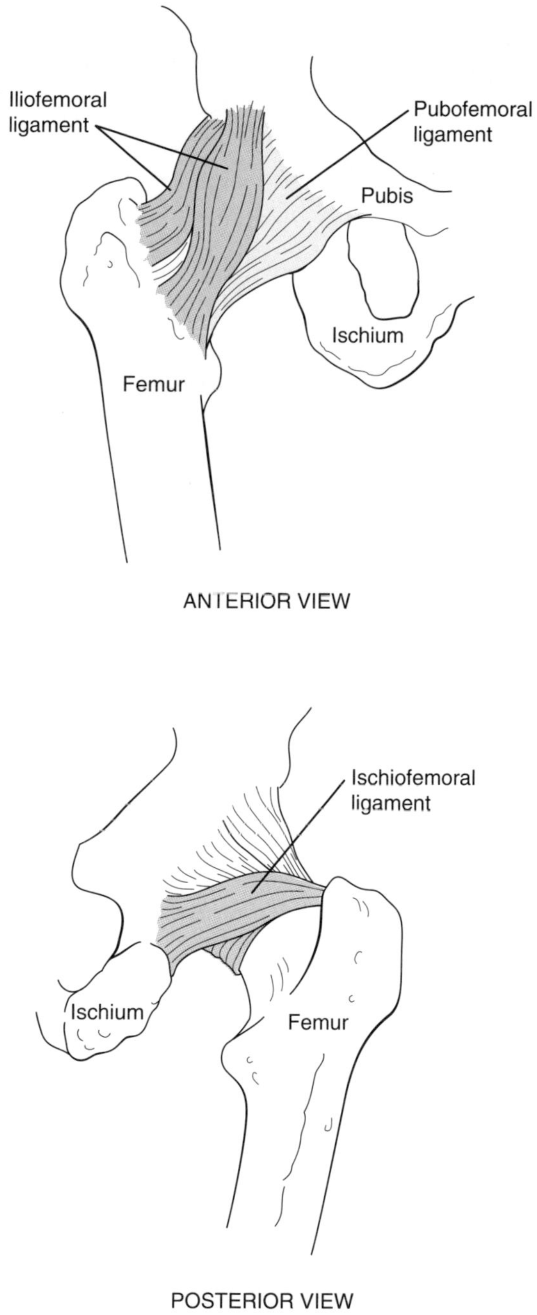

FIGURE 12–2. The ligaments of the hip joint.

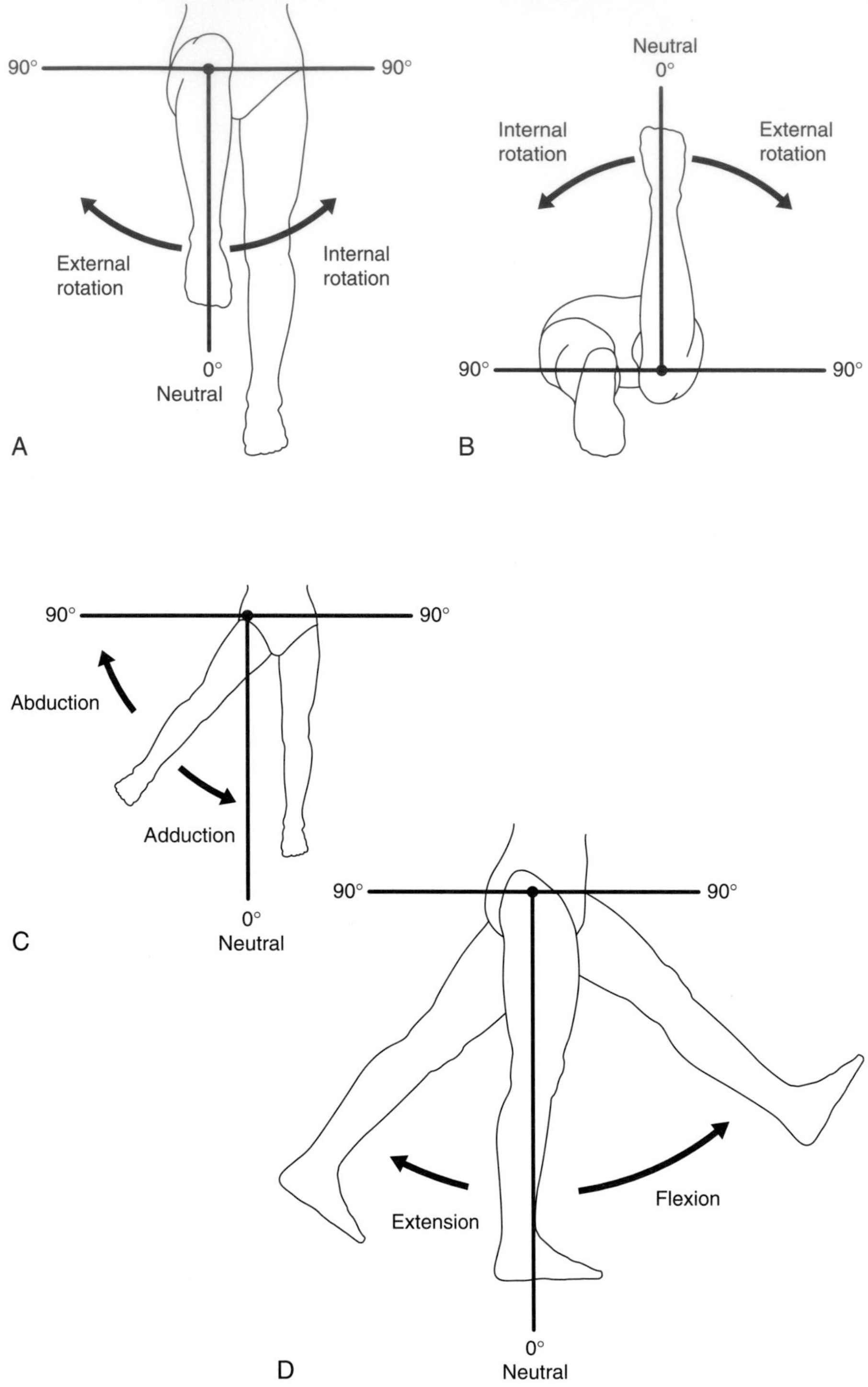

FIGURE 12–3. Movements of the hip joint showing normal range of motion. *A,* Hip rotation in flexion (standing). *B,* Hip rotation in extension (prone). *C,* Hip abduction and adduction (standing). *D,* Hip flexion and extension (standing). (Adapted from Green W, Heckman J. The Clinical Measurement of Joint Motion. Rosemont, IL: American Academy of Orthopaedic Surgeons, 1994.)

TABLE 12–1. The Muscles Involved in Hip Flexion

Muscle	Origin (O)	Insertion (I)	Action
Iliopsoas 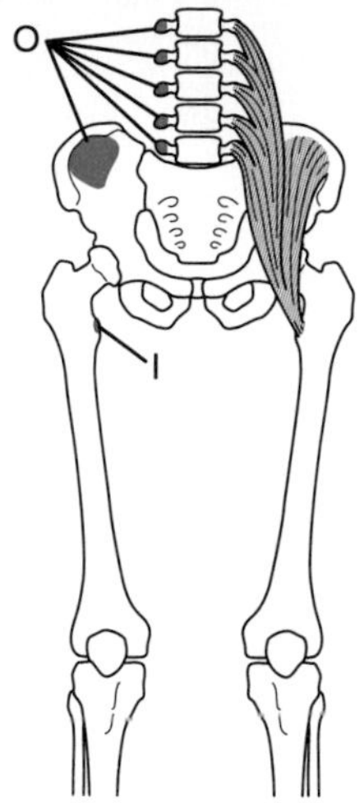	Psoas portion: Sides of the lumbar vertebrae Anterior sacrum Iliacus portion: Iliac fossa (inner)	Lesser trochanter of the femur	Flexes thigh at the hip Accessory movements: Rotates thigh outward Stabilizes hip
Sartorius 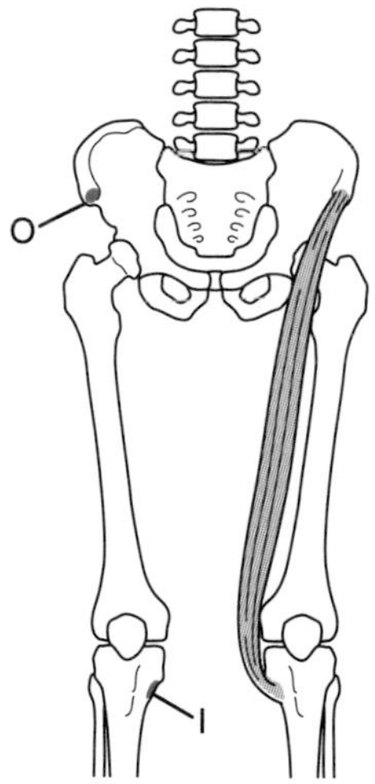	Anterior superior iliac spine	Front of the medial condyle of the tibia	Flexes the thigh at the hip Accessory movements: Flexes the leg at the knee Assists knee inward rotation Assists abduction Rotates the thigh outward

Table continued on following page

TABLE 12–1. The Muscles Involved in Hip Flexion *Continued*

Muscle	Origin (O)	Insertion (I)	Action
Pectineus 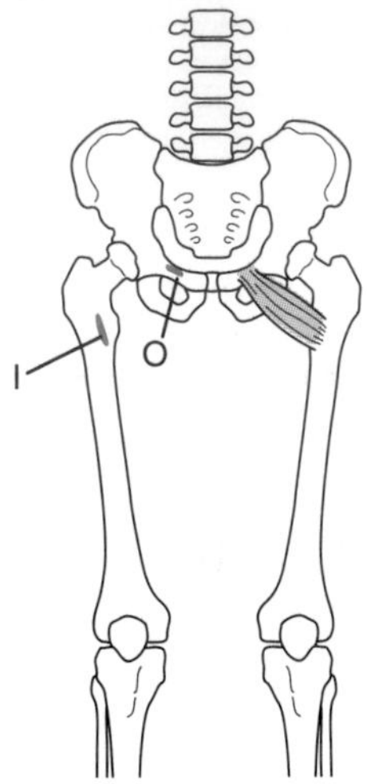	Pubic crest	Pectineal line of the femur	Flexes the thigh at the hip Accessory movements: Hip adduction Weak assistant for outward rotation
Rectus femoris 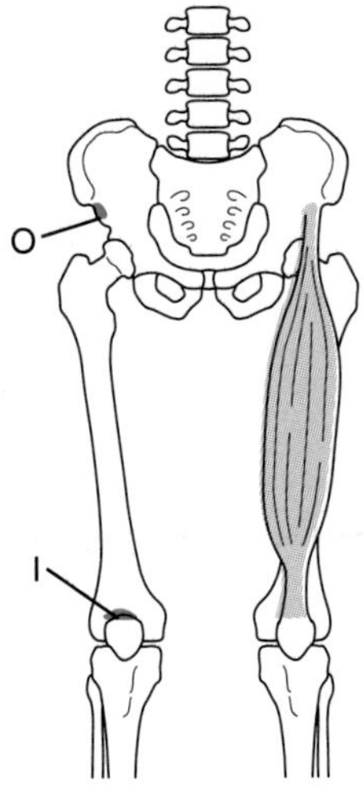	Anterior interior iliac spine	Top of the patella (via the patellar ligament to the tibial tuberosity)	Flexes the thigh at the hip Accessory movements: Assists hip abduction Extends the leg at the knee

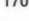

TABLE 12–2. The Muscles Involved in Hip Extension

Muscle	Origin (O)	Insertion (I)	Action
Gluteus maximus 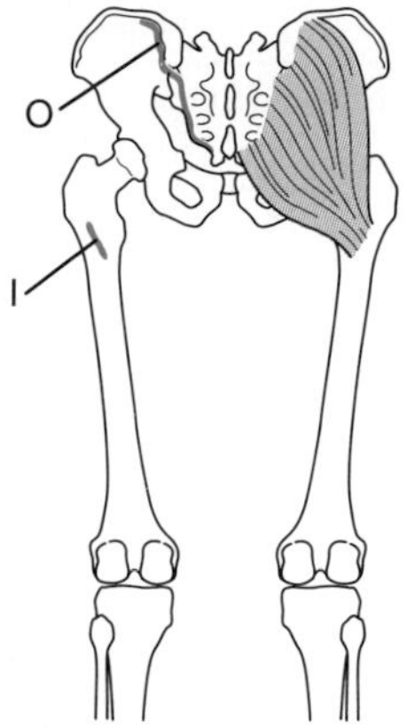	Posterior surface of the ilium, sacrum, and lumbar fascia	Gluteal line of the femur	Extends the thigh at the hip Accessory movements: Outward rotation Upper fibers assist abduction Lower fibers assist adduction
Semimembranosus 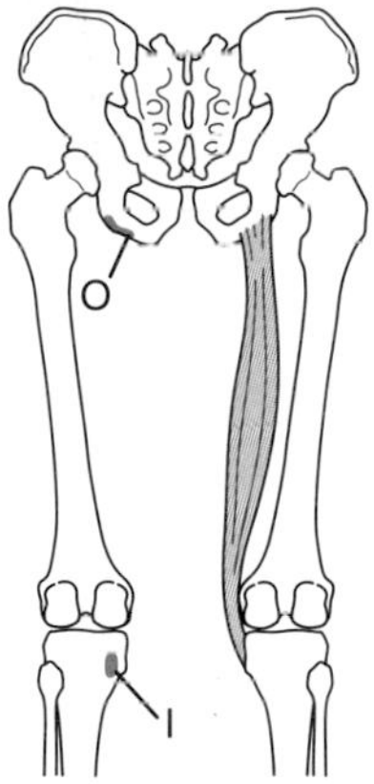	Tuberosity of the ischium	Front of the medial condyle of the tibia	Extends the thigh at the hip Accessory movements: Knee flexion Assists inward rotation
Semitendinosus 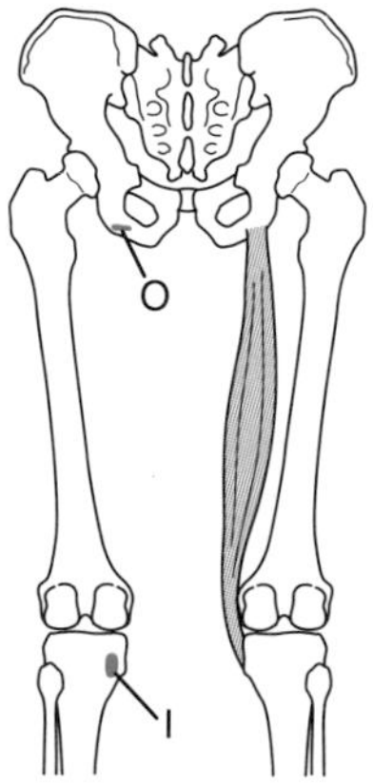	Tuberosity of the ischium	Front of the medial condyle of the tibia	Extends the thigh at the hip Accessory movements: Assists inward rotation Knee flexion Inward rotation of the knee

Table continued on following page

TABLE 12–2. The Muscles Involved in Hip Extension *Continued*

Muscle	Origin (O)	Insertion (I)	Action
Biceps femoris (long head) 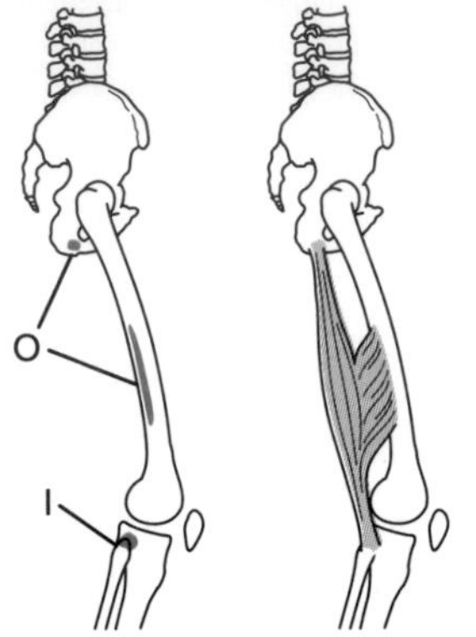	Tuberosity of the ischium Linea aspera (lateral lip)	Lateral condyle of the tibia and the head of the fibula	Extends the thigh at the hip Accessory movements: Assists outward rotation Knee flexion Knee outward rotation

TABLE 12–3. The Muscles Involved in Hip Abduction and Adduction

Muscle	Origin (O)	Insertion (I)	Action
Adductor magnus 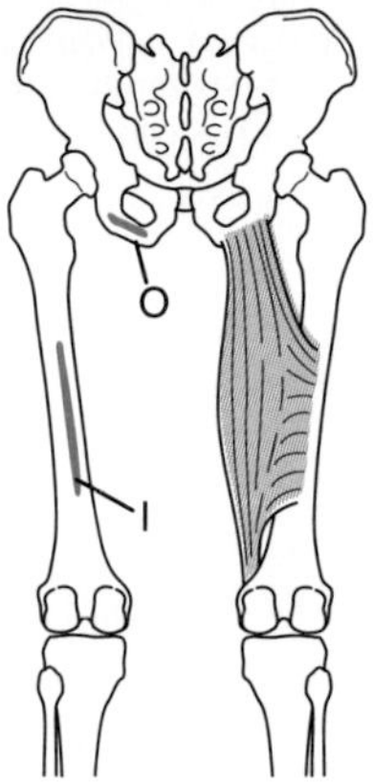	Ramus of pubis and ischium	Linea aspera Adductor tubercle	Adducts the thigh at the hip Accessory movements: Upper fibers assist outward rotation and hip flexion Lower fibers assist inward rotation and hip extension
Adductor longus 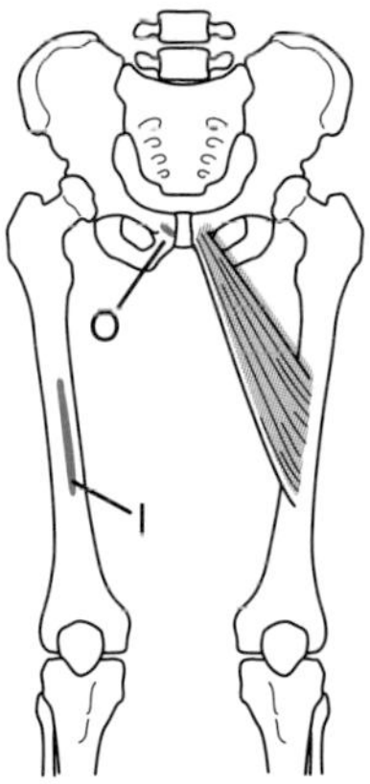	Crest of the pubis	Middle portion of the linea aspera	Adducts the thigh at the hip Accessory movements: Assists hip flexion Assists outward rotation

Table continued on following page

TABLE 12–3. The Muscles Involved in Hip Abduction and Adduction *Continued*

Muscle	Origin (O)	Insertion (I)	Action
Adductor brevis 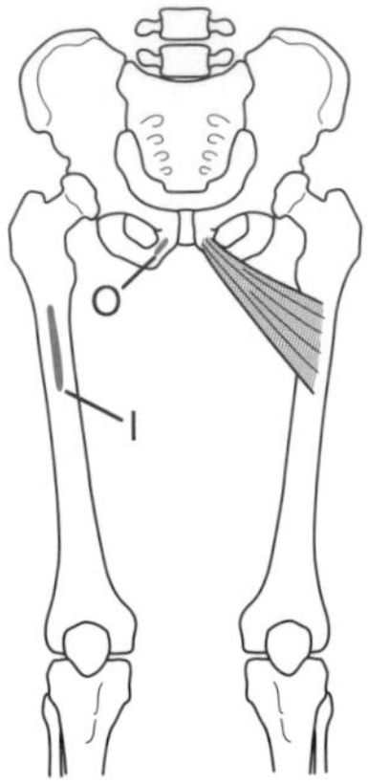	Inferior crest of the pubis (below longus)	Upper portion of the linea aspera	Adducts the thigh at the hip Accessory movements: Assists hip flexion Assists outward rotation
Gracilis 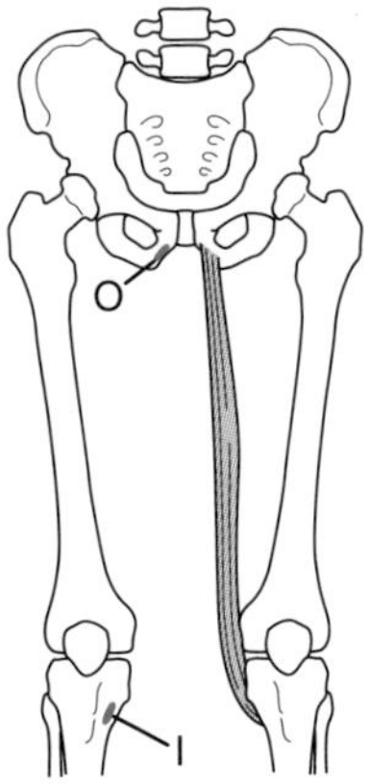	Descending pubic ramus	Front of medial condyle of the tibia	Adducts the thigh at the hip Accessory movements: Assists flexion and inward rotation of the hip Assists knee flexion and inward rotation

TABLE 12–4. The Muscles Involved in Hip Internal and External Rotation

Muscle	Origin (O)	Insertion (I)	Action
Gluteus minimus 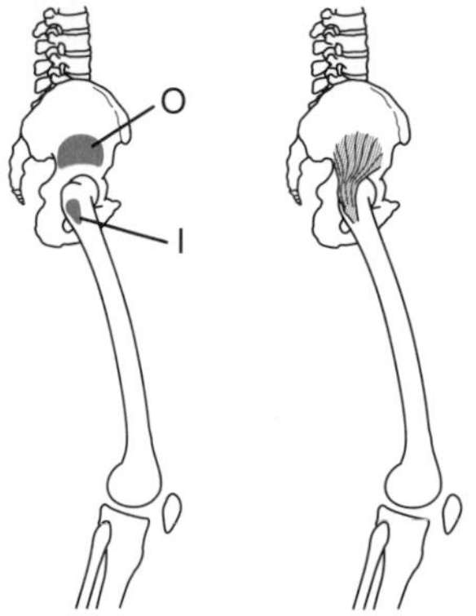	Outer surface of the ilium (under gluteus medius)	Greater trochanter of the femur	Rotates the thigh inward (anterior fibers) Accessory movements: Assists abduction Assists outward rotation (posterior fibers) Assists extension
Tensor fasciae latae 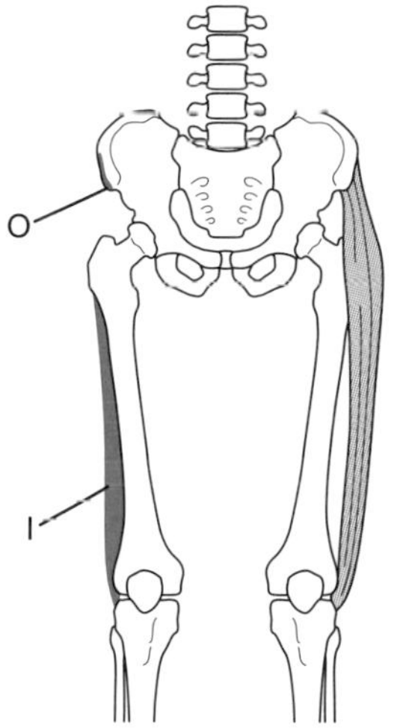	Anterior iliac fossa just below the crest	Fascia of the thigh (iliotibial tract)	Rotates the thigh inward Accessory movements: Flexes the thigh at the hip Hip abduction (from flexed position)

Table continued on following page

TABLE 12–4. The Muscles Involved in Hip Internal and External Rotation *Continued*

Muscle	Origin (O)	Insertion (I)	Action
Six Deep Lateral Rotators 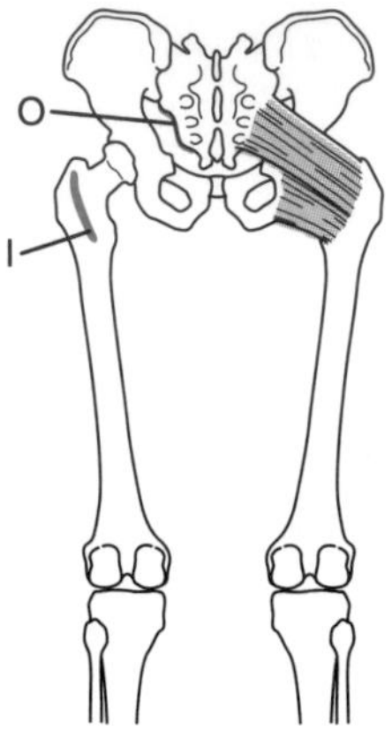 **1. Obturator externus** **2. Obturator internus** **3. Quadratus femoris** **4. Piriformis** **5. Gemellus superior** **6. Gemellus inferior**	Posterior pelvis on the sacrum, ischium, and obturator foramen	Greater trochanter of the femur	Outward rotation of the thigh

TABLE 12–5. Summary of the Muscles Involved in the Movements of the Hip

Action	Prime Movers	Assistant Movers	Nerve Root Level	Normal Range of Motion
Flexion	Iliopsoas Rectus femoris Pectineus	Tensor fascia latae Gracilis Adductor longus Adductor magnus	L1 to S3	110°–120°
Extension	Gluteus maximus Biceps femoris Semitendinosus Semimembranosus	Gluteus medius Gluteus minimus	L4 to S3	10°–15°
Abduction	Gluteus medius	Iliopsoas Sartorius Rectus femoris Tensor fasciae latae Gluteus	L4 to S1	30°–50°
Adduction	Pectineus Gracilis Adductor longus Adductor brevis Adductor magnus		L1 to S4	30°
Internal rotation	Gluteus minimus	Tensor fasciae latae Semitendinosus Semimembranosus Hip adductors	L4 to S2	30°–40°
External rotation	Gluteus maximus	Sartorius Iliopsoas Biceps femoris Six deep lateral rotators	L1 to S3	40°–60°

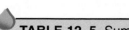

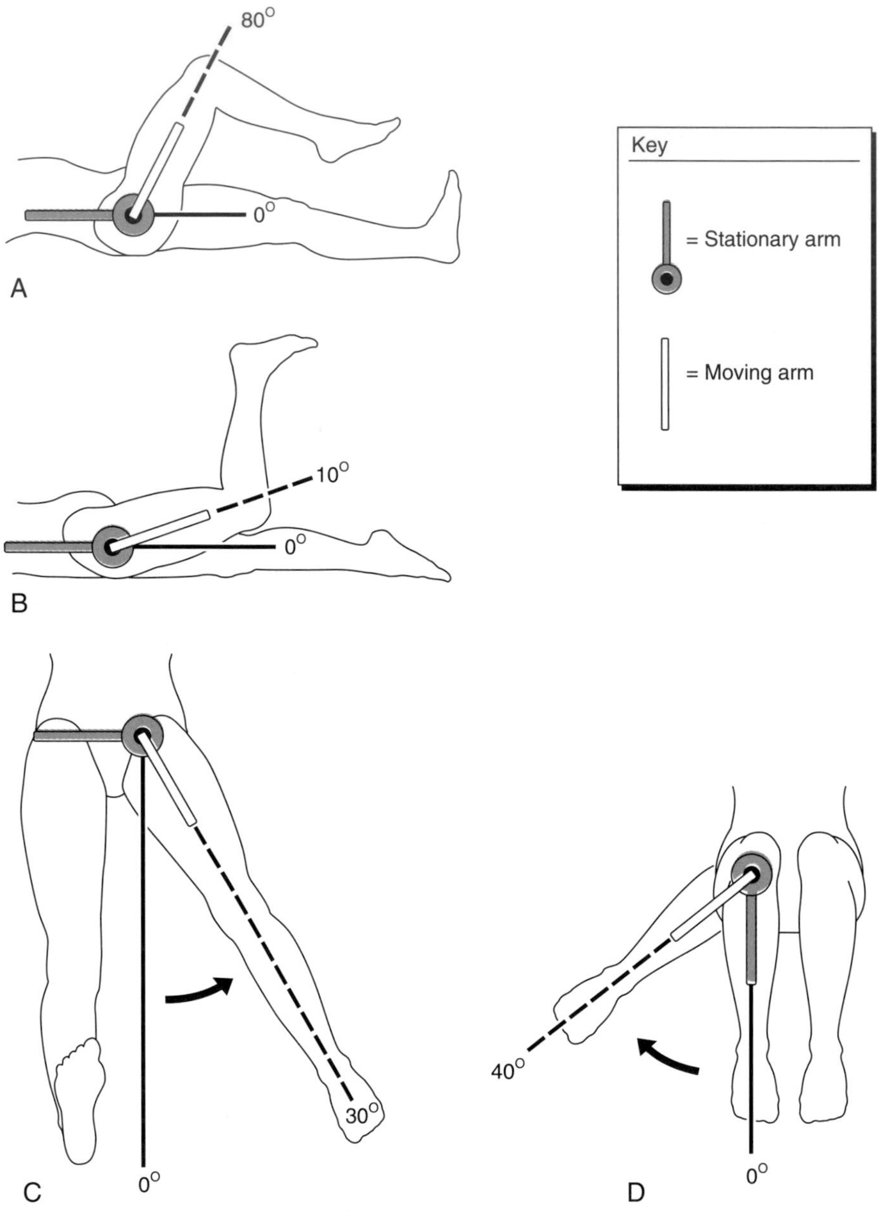

FIGURE 12–4. Measuring the range of motion of the hip joint. *A,* Hip flexion (supine). *B,* Hip extension (prone). *C,* Hip abduction (sitting). *D,* Hip external rotation (sitting). (Adapted from Green W, Heckman J. The Clinical Measurement of Joint Motion. Rosemont, IL: American Academy of Orthopaedic Surgeons, 1994.)

in line with the femur, pointing toward the lateral condyle of the femur. Hip extension is measured in the same way but with the patient in a prone position.[3]

To measure hip abduction and adduction, the patient lies in a supine position, and the examiner places the stationary arm of the goniometer at the anterior superior iliac spine. The moving arm is placed parallel to the anterior aspect of the femur, pointing toward the middle of the patella.[3]

To measure hip internal and external rotation, the patient sits, and the examiner places the center of the goniometer in the midpatellar region, with the stationary arm along the middle of the tibia. The moving arm is placed along the middle of the tibia.

HIP STRETCHES

Hip Flexor Stretch (Fig. 12–5)

Prime movers: iliopsoas, rectus femoris, pectineus, tensor fascia latae, and Achilles tendons.

- Step forward with the uninvolved leg and flex the knee, keeping the knee of the involved leg straight
- Press the hip of the involved leg forward while keeping the trunk upright; feel the stretch in the front of the hip
- Hold, then relax

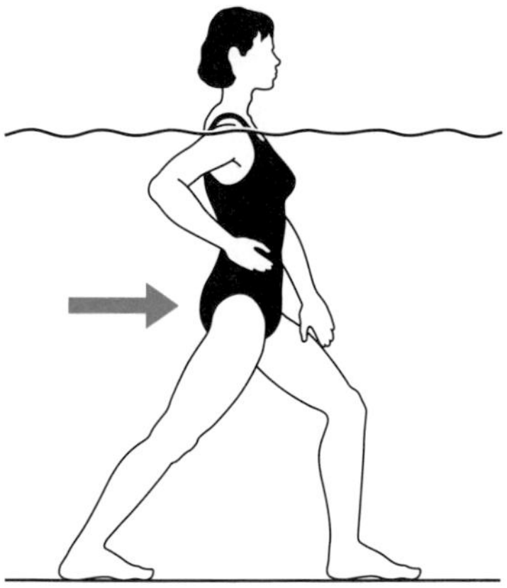

FIGURE 12–5. Hip flexor stretch.

Hip Tensor Stretch (Fig. 12–6)

Prime movers: tensor fasciae latae and gluteus medius.

- Stand sideways at arm's length away from the edge of the pool, with one hand on the pool edge and the other hand on the hip.
- Cross the leg that is closest to the side of the pool behind the other leg
- Press the hip toward the pool wall, keeping the arm straight
- Do not bend forward at the waist
- Feel the stretch over the outside of the hip
- Hold, then relax

CAUTION: This exercise is contraindicated for patients with total hip replacement

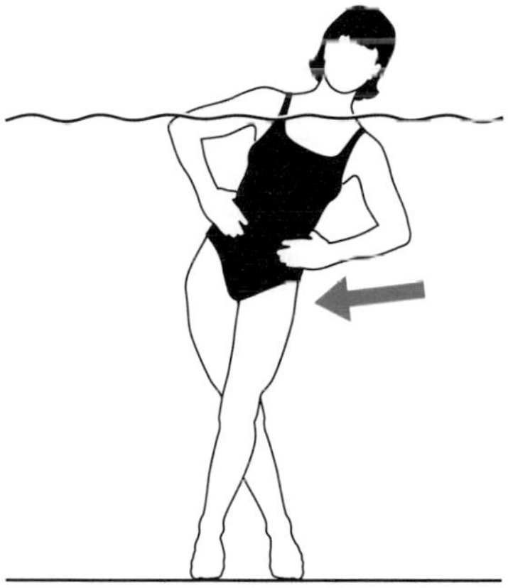

FIGURE 12–6. Hip tensor stretch.

Hip External Rotation Stretch
(Fig. 12–7)

Prime movers: hip flexors, gluteus medius, gluteus minimus, adductors, and tensor fascia latae.

- Stand with the back against the pool wall (or hold on to parallel bar with one hand)
- Flex the knee and hip of the involved leg, then place the sole of the foot on the shin of the support leg (or on the pool wall)
- Gently press the knee of the involved leg laterally (outward)
- Feel the stretch on the inside of the hip
- Hold, then relax

CAUTION: This exercise is contraindicated for patients with total hip replacement

Hip Internal Rotation Stretch
(Fig. 12–8)

Prime movers: gluteus medius, obturator internus, obturator externus, quadratus femoris, piriformis, and sartorius.

- Stand with the back against the pool wall (or hold on to a parallel bar with one hand)
- Flex the knee and hip of the involved leg, then place the sole of foot on the shin of the support leg (or on the pool wall)
- Gently press the knee of the involved leg medially (inward) toward the opposite knee; do not cross the midline
- Hold, then relax

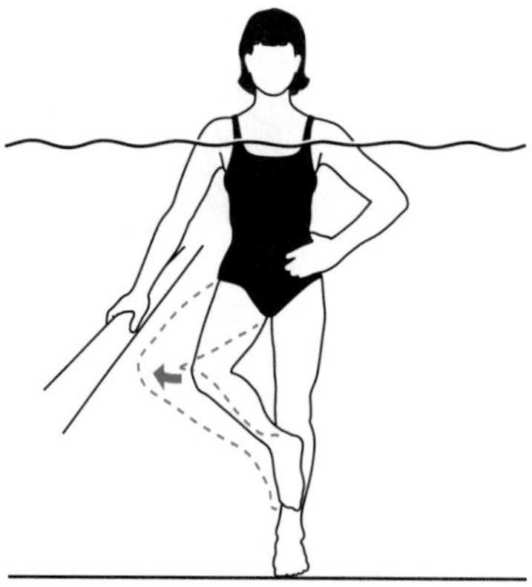

FIGURE 12–7. Hip external rotation stretch.

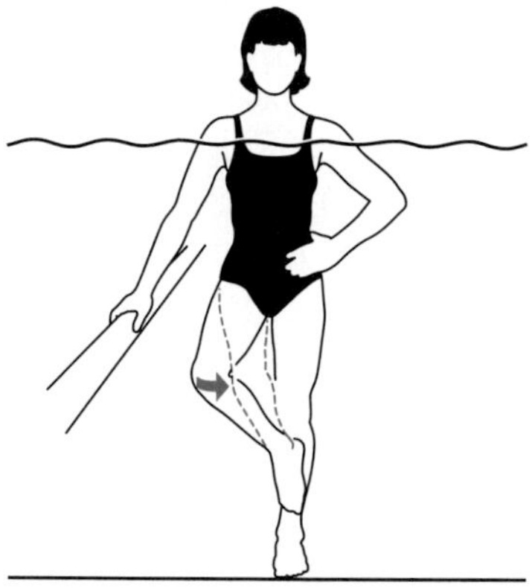

FIGURE 12–8. Hip internal rotation stretch.

Groin Stretch (Fig. 12–9)

Prime movers: hip adductors, hip abductors, hip flexors, gluteus maximus, hip rotators, quadriceps, and hamstrings.

- Hang vertically in an inner tube
- Place the soles of the feet together, externally rotating the hips
- Gently pull the heels upward until a stretch is felt in the groin and inner thigh
- Hold, then relax

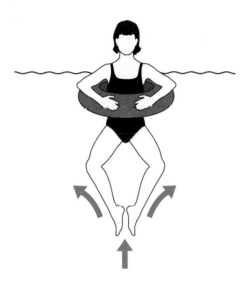

FIGURE 12–9. Groin stretch.

Adductor Stretch (Fig. 12–10)

Prime movers: adductor longus, adductor brevis, adductor magnus, gracilis, and pectineus.

- Stand with the feet more than shoulder-width apart
- Bend the left knee while shifting the weight to the left leg
- Keep the right leg straight and the trunk facing forward; feel the stretch in the right groin area
- Do not let the knee bend past the toes
- Hold, then return to the original position

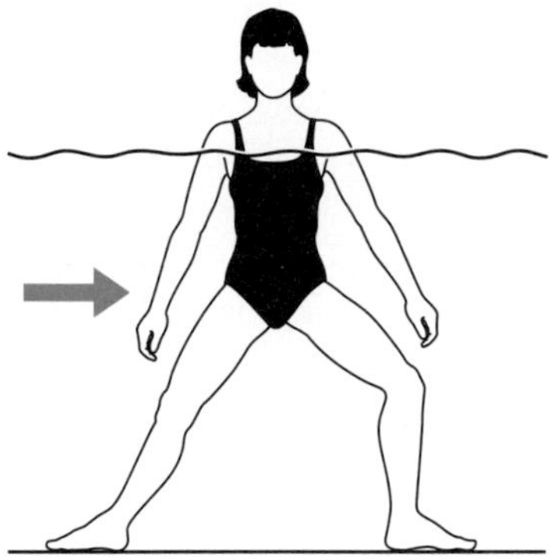

FIGURE 12–10. Adductor stretch.

HIP EXERCISES

Hip Flexion (Fig. 12–11)

Prime movers: quadriceps, hip flexors, gluteus maximus, hamstrings, and hip adductors.

- Stand with the feet together and with one side toward the pool wall, holding on with the near arm
- Gently raise the opposite leg straight out in front of the body, flexing only from the hip
- Keep the trunk upright and the head forward; the knee of the support leg should be slightly bent
- Return to the starting position

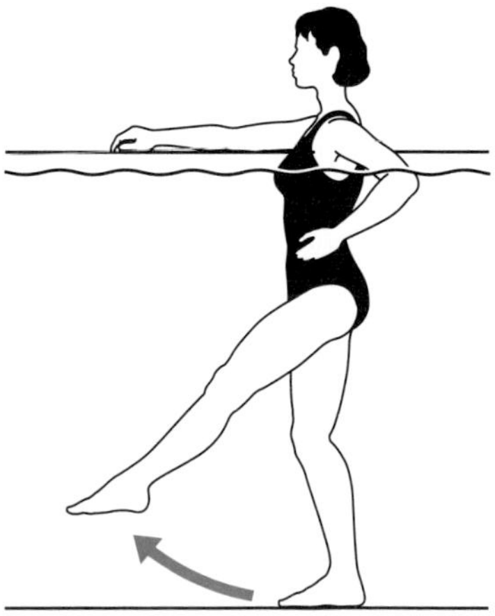

FIGURE 12–11. Hip flexion.

Hip Extension (Fig. 12–12)

Prime movers: gluteus maximus, hamstrings, quadriceps, hip flexors, erector spinae, and hip adductors.

- Stand with the feet together and with one side toward the pool wall, holding on with the near arm
- Gently press the opposite leg straight backward, extending only from the hip, tightening the buttock
- Keep the trunk upright and the head forward; the knee of the support leg should be slightly bent
- Return to the starting position

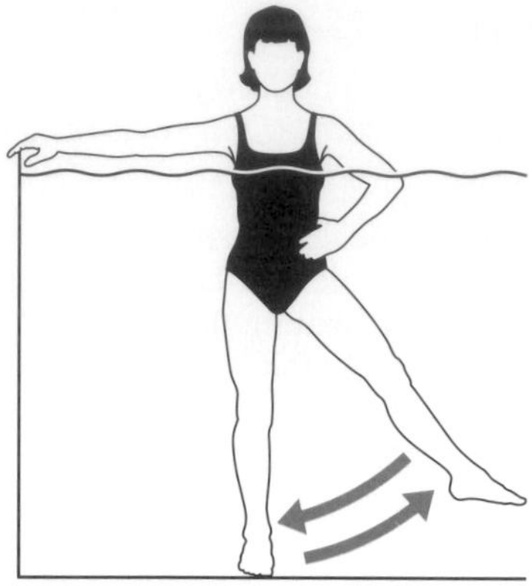

FIGURE 12–13. Hip abduction and adduction.

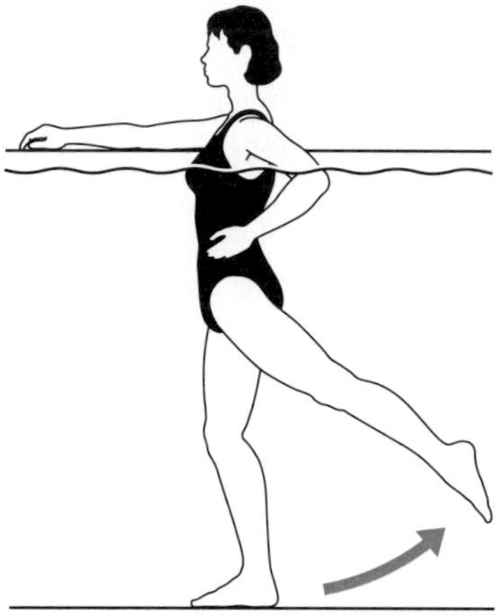

FIGURE 12–12. Hip extension.

Hip Abduction and Adduction (Fig. 12–13)

Prime movers: gluteus medius, pectineus, gracilis, adductor longus, adductor brevis, and adductor magnus.

- Stand holding on to the pool wall, an arm's length away
- Gently raise (abduct) the right leg straight out to the side
- Return (adduct) to the starting position (midline)

Hip Circumduction (Fig. 12–14)

Prime movers: hip abductors, hip adductors, gluteus maximus, hip flexors, and abdominals.

- Stand holding on to the pool wall, an arm's length away
- Gently raise one leg to the side
- Move the leg in a clockwise circular pattern from the hip, keeping the leg straight
- Keep the trunk upright and the head forward
- Repeat in a counterclockwise direction

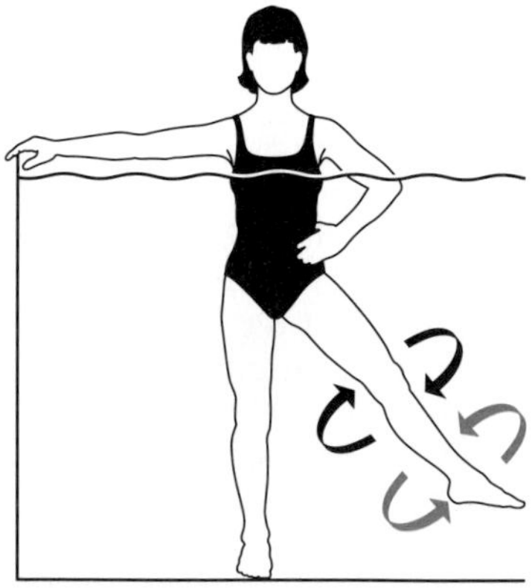

FIGURE 12–14. Hip circumduction.

Hip Rotation (Fig. 12–15)

Prime movers: gluteus maximus and gluteus minimus.

- Stand with the back against the pool wall or parallel bar
- Flex one hip and knee to 90°
- Gently rotate the hip by moving the ankle laterally (internal rotation) and then medially (external rotation)
- Keep the knee and hip in a horizontal line

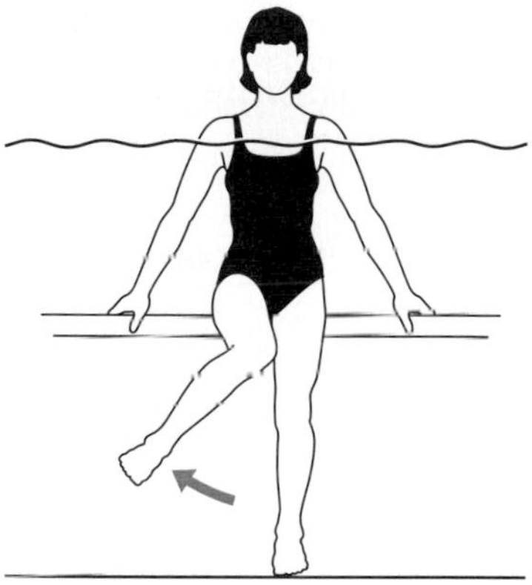

FIGURE 12–15. Hip rotation.

Straight Leg Kick (Fig. 12–16)

Prime movers: hip flexors, gluteus maximus, hamstrings and quadriceps

- Lie prone on the water and use a kickboard for support (or lie supine, holding on to an inner tube for support)
- Keeping the legs straight, alternately flex and extend the hips, producing a gentle fluttering motion

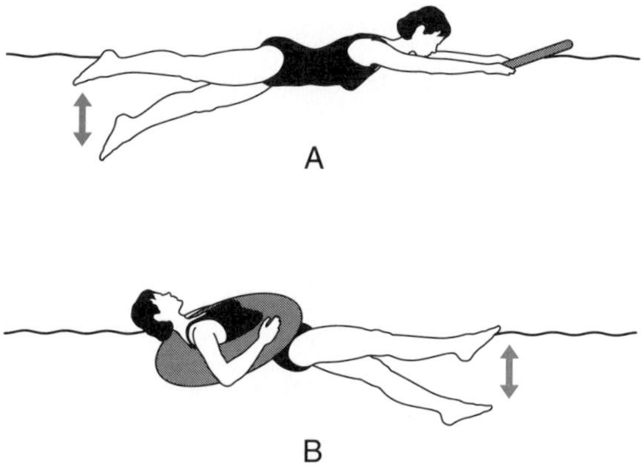

FIGURE 12–16. Straight leg kick. *A,* Prone. *B,* Supine.

Stride Jump (Fig. 12–17)

Prime movers: hip abductors, hip adductors, gluteus maximus, quadriceps, hamstrings, pectoralis, deltoid, rhomboids, trapezius, and triceps.

- Stand with the feet together and the arms at the sides
- Hop upward and simultaneously abduct hips and arms, landing in a stride position with the arms out to the sides
- Hop upward and adduct the hips and arms, returning to the starting position

VARIATION: Cross-Stride Jump is performed like Stride Jump, except that the hips adduct past the midline (legs cross)

CAUTION: This exercise is contraindicated for patients with total hip replacement

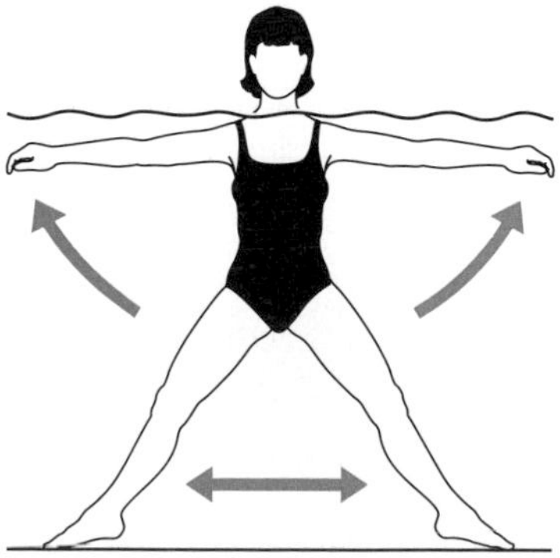

FIGURE 12–17. Stride jump.

Standing Bum Squeeze (Fig. 12–18)

Prime mover: gluteus maximus.

- Isometrically contract the buttocks, squeezing them tightly together
- Hold, then relax

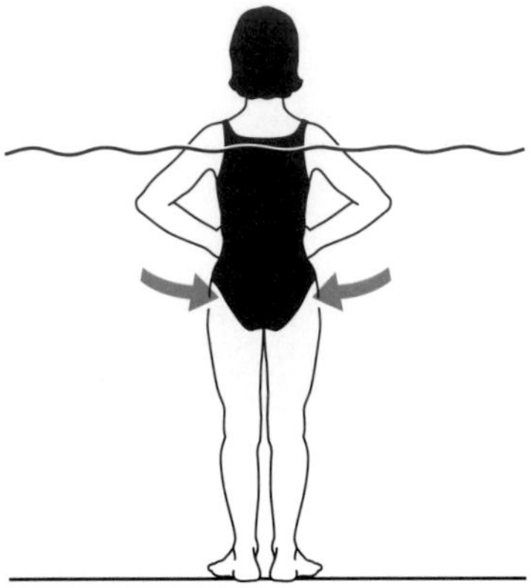

FIGURE 12–18. Standing bum squeeze.

Bent Knee Hip Rotation (Fig. 12–19)

Prime movers: adductor longus, adductor brevis, gluteus medius, gluteus maximus, gluteus minimus, tensor fascia latae, obturator internus, obturator externus, piriformis, and sartorius.

- Stand with one side toward the pool wall; flex the opposite hip and knee to 90°
- Move the leg outward horizontally, maintaining flexion
- Return to the starting position and lower the leg
- Flex the hip and knee again and move the leg inward (toward the opposite knee)
- Return to the starting position and lower the leg

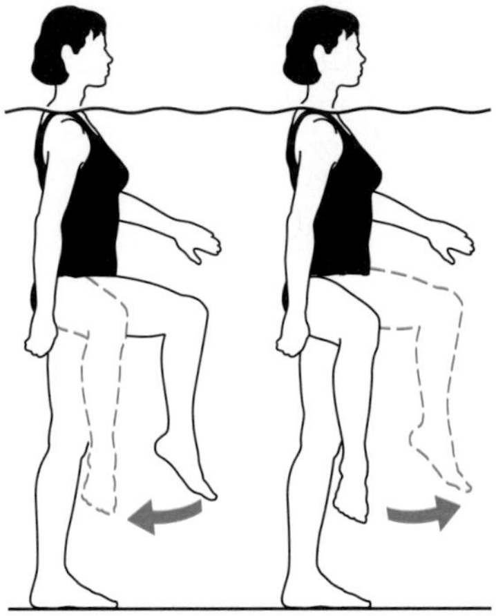

FIGURE 12–19. Bent knee hip rotation.

COMMON CONDITIONS OF THE HIP

Hip Arthritis

The hip joint is often affected by arthritis because it is a weight-bearing joint (Fig. 12–20).

Origin

The most common cause of hip arthritis is simply wear and tear. Consequently, this condition usually affects people older than 50 years of age. If it presents in a younger patient, there is usually a predisposing factor, such as a fracture that has damaged a joint surface.

Pathology

Osteoarthritis is the most common form of arthritis affecting the hip joint. As depicted in Figure 12–20, the joint surfaces of both the femur and the acetabulum are affected. Exercise cannot reverse this degeneration, but it can help to improve function.

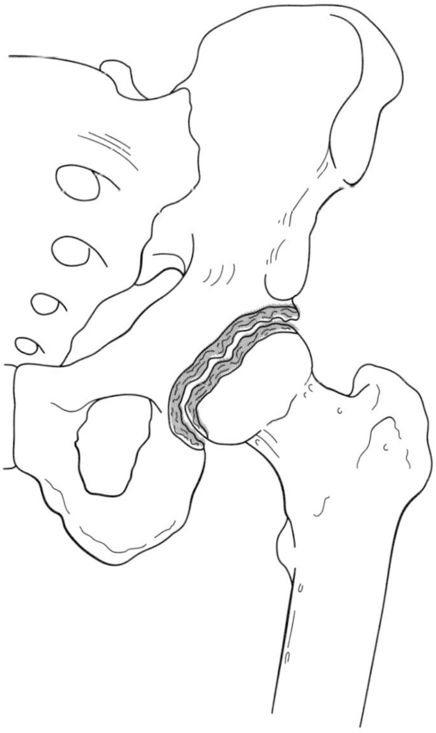

FIGURE 12–20. Hip arthritis.

Signs and Symptoms

Pain from the hip is often referred into the groin area or into the knee. Pain becomes worse during weight-bearing activities. Crepitus may also be present as the hip moves through its range of motion.

Body Parts Affected

- Bones (femur, pelvis)
- Joint surfaces (articular cartilage)
- Soft tissues (joint capsule, muscles, tendons, ligaments)

Exercise Priorities

- Establish a controlled exercise program (be careful that the patient does not overdo it)
- Maximize range of motion
- Strengthen all hip muscles

Groin Strain

The term "groin strain" refers to an injury of the hip flexors in the groin or upper thigh region (Fig. 12–21).

Origin

These muscles can be injured if a sudden burst of activity is required (eg, during a sporting event) and either the muscles are not warmed up or they are fatigued.

Pathology

The pathology of this condition is described in Chapter 7. The injury may occur because the muscle is overstretched during the activity. It may also be the result of the muscle's own forceful contraction. The iliopsoas is the most commonly involved muscle.

Signs and Symptoms

Pain increases when the involved muscles are stretched or when the patient tries to run. If the injury is chronic, the pain may be intermittent; the patient may be free of pain for weeks before pain recurs. It is therefore important to continue with rehabilitation exercises even after the pain has subsided.

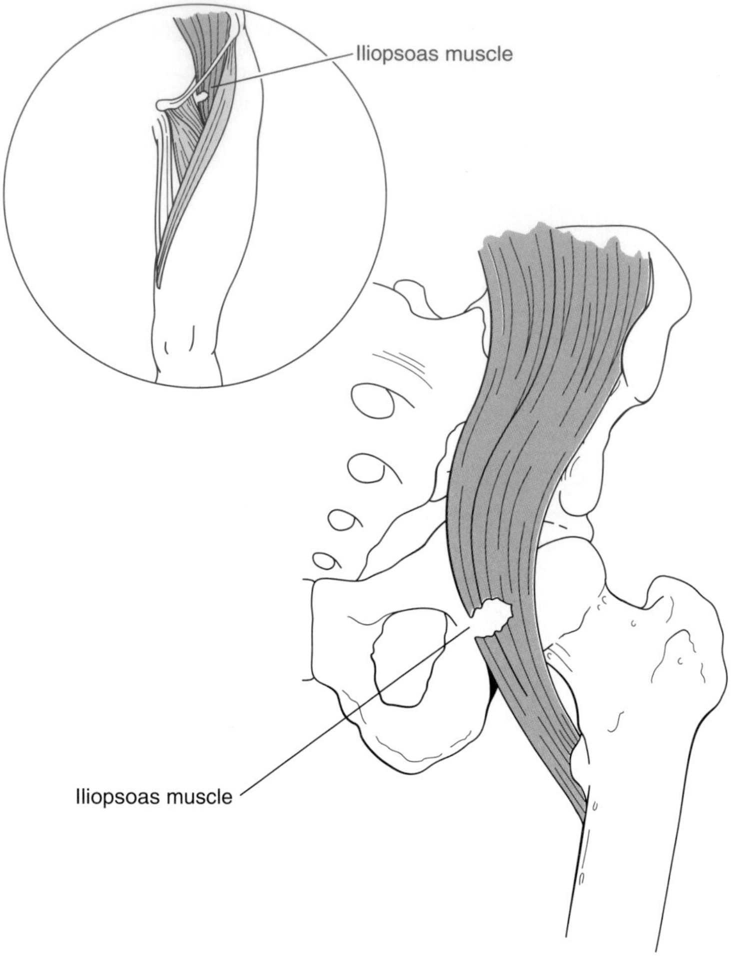

FIGURE 12–21. Groin strain (partial muscle tear).

Body Parts Affected

- Muscles of the groin (iliopsoas, rectus femoris, adductor longus, adductor magnus)
- Adjacent muscles (quadriceps, hamstrings, gluteals)

Exercise Priorities

- Stretch the involved muscles
- Increase the strength and endurance of all hip muscles
- Gradual return to normal activities

Hip Bursitis

This condition involves the inflammation of one of the bursae of the hip joint (Fig. 12–22).

Origin

Bursitis in the hip area is caused by friction between the femur and the overlying muscles and tendons.

Pathology

The psoas bursa, trochanteric bursa, or ischial bursa may be involved. The pathology of bursitis is outlined in Chapter 7.

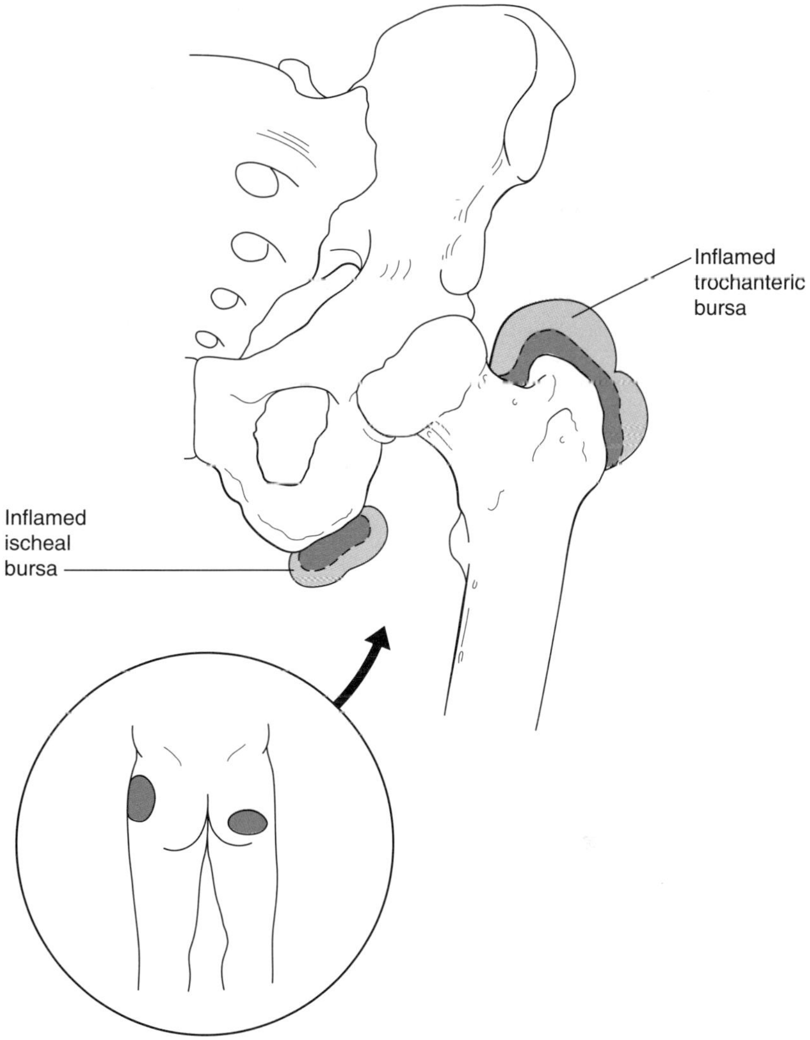

FIGURE 12–22. Hip bursitis.

Signs and Symptoms

The pain that occurs with this condition often varies without any apparent cause. It is common for the hip's range of motion to be full.

Body Parts Affected

- Hip bursae (psoas, trochanteric, and ischial bursae)
- Muscles (gluteus minimus, medius, and maximus; tensor fascia latae; hamstrings; quadriceps)

Exercise Priorities

- Stretch tight muscles
- Strengthen all hip muscles
- Correct gait abnormalities

Hip Fracture

A fractured neck of the femur is a common injury among elderly people (Fig. 12–23).

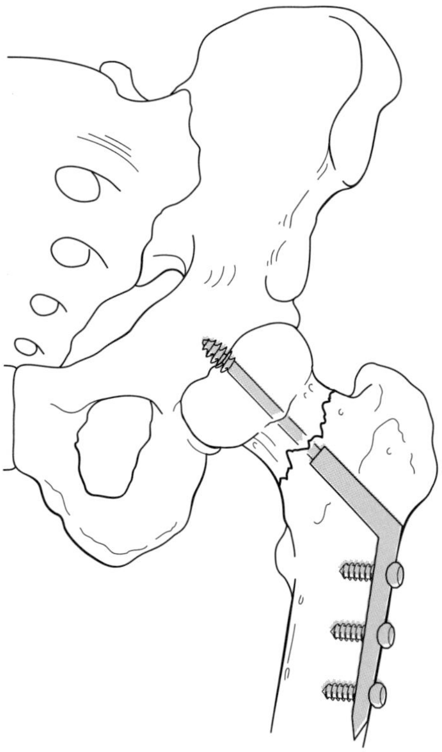

FIGURE 12–23. Hip fracture repaired by internal fixation.

Origin

This injury is almost always caused by a fall onto the hip.

Pathology

Elderly patients with osteoporosis are at high risk to sustain this type of fracture. As shown in Figure 12–23, internal fixation is often used so that early mobilization is possible. This is especially important in the elderly population, because elderly patients are also susceptible to postoperative complications such as pneumonia.

Signs and Symptoms

At the time of injury, the patient is unable to bear weight because of pain. Within a few days of surgery, weight bearing is possible with some form of walking aid. If the pain persists several months after the original injury, X-rays should be taken to rule out avascular necrosis of the femoral head.

Body Parts Affected

- Bones (femur, pelvis)
- Joint surfaces (articular cartilage)
- Soft tissues (joint capsule, muscles, tendons, ligaments)

Exercise Priorities

- Restore full range of motion
- Strengthen all hip muscles
- Correct gait abnormalities

Fractured Pelvis

A fractured pelvis involves at least one break in the pelvic ring (Fig. 12–24).

Origin

A substantial force is necessary to fracture the pelvis. Fracture usually occurs as a result of an automobile accident or a fall from a significant height.

Pathology

Pelvic fractures occur in varying degrees. The simplest type is a single bone fracture, such as a chip off the iliac crest. If the femur is driven through the acetabulum, the hip joint eventually develops arthritis to some extent. Fractures that disrupt the integrity of the pelvic ring may be severe

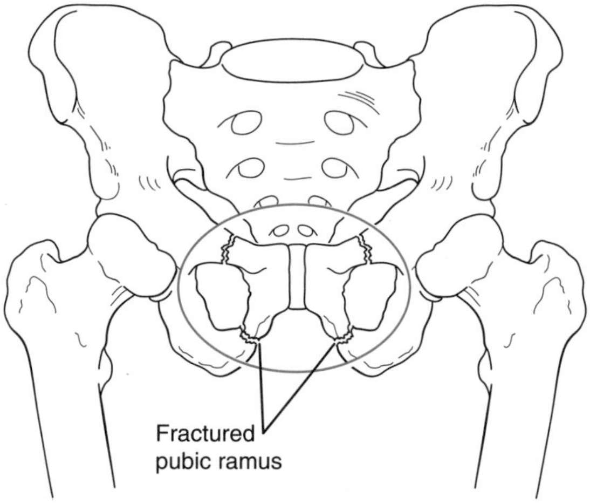

FIGURE 12–24. Fractured pelvis.

enough to necessitate external fixation to assist the healing process.

Signs and Symptoms

The amount of pain and disability varies with the severity of the injury. Because patients with this injury are often restricted in weight bearing for several months, aquatic exercise therapy can play a major role in rehabilitation of these patients.

Body Parts Affected

- Bones (pelvis, femur)
- Soft tissues (hip joint capsule, leg muscles, low back muscles)
- Nerves, vessels, and internal organs (may have been injured at the time of the accident)

Exercise Priorities

- Restore range of motion for hip and knee (within restrictions set by doctor)
- Strengthen lower extremity
- Correct gait abnormalities

Hip Dislocation

In this serious injury, the femoral head pops out of its socket (the acetabulum) (Fig. 12–25).

Origin

The hip joint is so strong that a major traumatic incident, such as an automobile accident, is required to dislocate a hip. Posterior dislocation occurs if the leg is internally rotated and adducted at the time of the accident, and internal rotation should be avoided during rehabilitation of such an injury. Anterior dislocation occurs if the leg is externally rotated and abducted; therefore, external rotation after such an injury should be avoided.

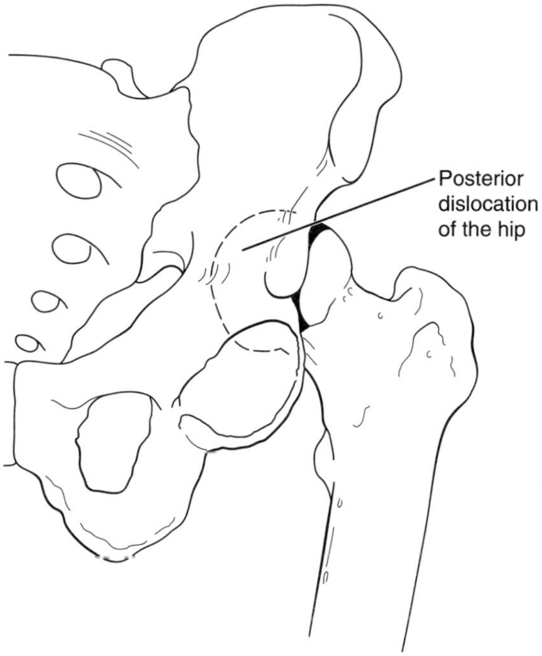

FIGURE 12–25. Hip dislocation.

Pathology

This injury is often accompanied by a fracture of the acetabulum. The joint capsule and the ligaments of the hip are always torn to some extent. In addition, several nerves and arteries may be affected. The sciatic nerve may be damaged, or the femoral artery may be severed. Avascular necrosis of the femoral head may develop.

Signs and Symptoms

At the time of injury, the patient is in severe pain. There is also a visible defect in the hip joint. No therapy should begin until the patient has been seen by an orthopedic surgeon. Even after reduction, pain and muscle spasm combine to limit range of motion for several months.

Body Parts Affected

- Bones (pelvis, femur)
- Soft tissues (joint capsule, ligaments, muscles)
- Nerves and vessels

Exercise Priorities

- Restore range of motion (stay within the limits prescribed by the doctor, and attempt no internal rotation with posterior dislocations and no external rotation with anterior dislocations)
- Strengthen all hip muscles

Total Hip Replacement

In this surgery, the hip joint is replaced with an artificial joint (Fig. 12–26).

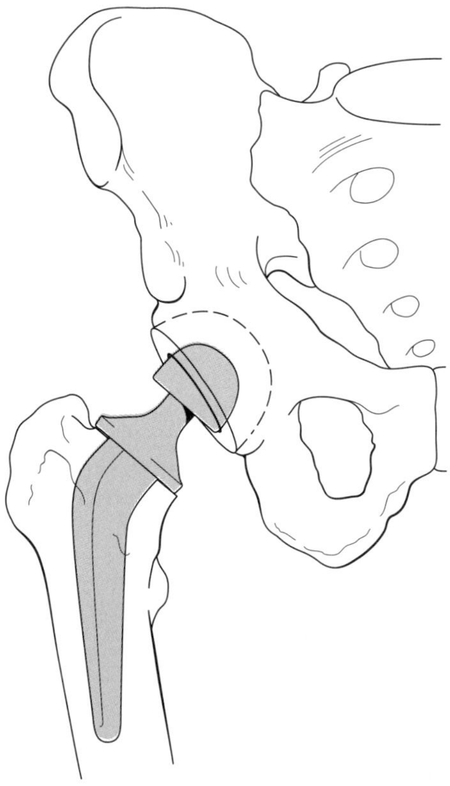

FIGURE 12–26. Total hip replacement.

Origin

Total hip replacement is necessary if the hip joint has degenerated to the point that activities of daily living (especially walking) have become painful. This degeneration may be caused by natural wear and tear or by a previous injury.

Mechanics

The femoral component consists of a metal ball connected to a stem that fits into the femoral shaft. The pelvic component consists of a high-density plastic cup. These components may be cemented into place, or they may be designed to have the bone grow around them. Weight bearing can begin earlier if cement is used, but it is debatable which type of junction lasts longer. It must be stressed to the patient that the replacement is performed so that activities of daily living will be less painful, not so that the patient can return to high-level sports. Some common restrictions placed on the patient by the surgeon include no adduction past neutral, no hip flexion past 90°, no external rotation, and no crossing of the legs.

Body Parts Affected

- Bones (femur, pelvis)
- Hip and knee muscles (gluteal muscles, hamstrings, tensor fascia latae, quadriceps, groin muscles)

Exercise Priorities

- Increase range of motion (stay within prescribed limits)
- Increase strength of hip and leg muscles (especially hip extensors and abductors, which are important for walking)
- Correct gait abnormalities

THE AQUATIC EXERCISE THERAPY PROTOCOL FOR CONDITIONS OF THE HIP

Phase One

Warm-up

Perform each exercise for 2 minutes.

- Forward Walking (see Fig. 5–21)
- Backward Walking (see Fig. 5–22)
- Side Stepping (do not cross legs) (see Fig. 5–23)

Stretch

Perform five repetitions of each exercise, holding for 10 seconds. These exercises are described in Chapter 13.

- Passive Quadriceps Stretch (see Fig. 13–6)
- Hamstring Stretch (do not exceed 90° of hip flexion for patients with total hip replacement) (see Fig. 13–10)

Strengthen

Perform one set of 8 to 12 repetitions.

- Hip Flexion (do not exceed 90° for patients with total hip replacement or hip dislocation) (see Fig. 12–11)
- Hip Extension (see Fig. 12–12)
- Hip Abduction and Adduction (do not cross midline for patients with total hip replacement) (see Fig. 12–13)
- Standing Bum Squeeze (see Fig. 12–48)

Phase Two

Warm-up

Perform each exercise for 2 minutes.

- Forward Walking (see Fig. 5–21)
- Backward Walking (see Fig. 5–22)
- Stiff Leg Walking (see Fig. 5–25)
- Crossover Stepping (omit for patients with total hip replacement or hip dislocation) (see Fig. 5–24)
- Bicycle (see Fig. 5–31)

Stretch

Perform five repetitions of each exercise, holding for 20 seconds.

- Quadriceps Stretch (see Fig. 13–5)
- Active Hamstring Stretch (see Fig. 13–11)
- Hip Flexor Stretch (see Fig. 12–5)
- Hip Internal Rotation Stretch (see Fig. 12–8)
- Hip External Rotation Stretch (omit for patients with total hip replacement or hip dislocation) (see Fig. 12–7)
- Adductor Stretch (see Fig. 12–10)

Strengthen

Perform two sets of 8 to 12 repetitions.

- Hip Flexion (see Fig. 12–11)
- Hip Extension (see Fig. 12–12)
- Hip Abduction and Adduction (see Fig. 12–13)
- Hip Rotation (internal rotation only for patients with total hip replacement) (see Fig. 12–15)
- Hip Circumduction (do not cross midline for patients with total hip replacement) (see Fig. 12–14)

Phase Three

Warm-up

Perform each exercise for 2 minutes. Ankle cuffs may be used to increase resistance.

- Marching (see Fig. 5–28)
- Backward Walking (see Fig. 5–22)
- Crossover Stepping (omit for patients with total hip replacement or hip dislocation) (see Fig. 5–24)
- Bicycle (see Fig. 5–31)
- Pelvic Movements (for patients with total hip replacement or hip dislocation, use forward and backward movements only) (see Fig. 5–32)

Stretch

Perform five repetitions of each exercise, holding for 30 seconds.

- Hip Tensor Stretch (omit for patients with total hip replacement or hip dislocation) (see Fig. 12–6)
- Groin Stretch (see Fig. 12–9
- Quadriceps Stretch (see Fig. 13–5)
- Hip Flexor Stretch (see Fig. 12–5)
- Hip Internal Rotation Stretch (see Fig. 12–8)
- Hip External Rotation Stretch (see Fig. 12–7)

Strengthen

Perform three sets of 8 to 12 repetitions.

- Straight Leg Kick (see Fig. 12–16)
- Lunges (see Fig. 13–17)
- Squats (see Fig. 13–16)
- Hip Rotation (internal rotation only for patients with total hip replacement) (see Fig. 12–15)
- Hip Circumduction (do not cross midline for patients with total hip replacement) (see Fig. 12–14)

Phase Four

Warm-up

Perform each exercise for 2 minutes.

- Marching (see Fig. 5–28)
- Backward Walking (see Fig. 5–22)

- Bicycle (see Fig. 5–31)
- Leg Exchange (see Fig. 5–29)
- Jogging (see Fig. 5–30)

Stretch

Perform five repetitions of each exercise, holding for 30 seconds. Perform the exercises from Phase Three, concentrating on movements that help achieve full range of motion.

Strengthen

Perform four sets of 8 to 12 repetitions. Perform the exercises from Phase Three, using ankle cuffs or resistance boots to increase resistance as appropriate. Then add the following:

- Lunges (see Fig. 13–17)
- Squats (see Fig. 13–16)
- Straight Leg Kick (see Fig. 12–16)
- Stride Jump (see Fig. 12–17)
- Bent Knee Hip Rotation (patients with total hip replacement or hip dislocation should avoid hip flexion greater than 90° and avoid external rotation) (see Fig. 12–19)
- Deep water lower extremity exercises (see Chapter 6) (see Figs. 6–12 through 6–16, 6–18 through 6–23, 6–25, and 6–29)

REFERENCES

1. Magee D. Orthopedic Physical Assessment. Philadelphia: W.B. Saunders, 1987.
2. Green W, Heckman J. The Clinical Measurement of Joint Motion. Rosemont, IL: American Academy of Orthopaedic Surgeons, 1994.
3. Arnheim, D. Modern Principles of Athletic Training. Toronto, Times Mirror/Mosby College Publishing, 1985.

Aquatic Rehabilitation of the Knee

Chapter 13

THE STRUCTURE AND FUNCTION OF THE KNEE

The Anatomic Parts

The knee is an atypical hinge joint with two bony articulations. The tibiofemoral joint is formed where the femoral condyles join the tibial condyles. Because the rounded condyles of the femur do not fit well on the tibial condyles, two semilunar cartilages or menisci are present to improve the fit medially and laterally[1, 2] (Fig. 13–1). The medial meniscus is fixed, but the lateral meniscus is able to slide. This freedom allows lateral rotation of the tibia during the final degrees of extension of the knee.[1, 2]

The joint relies on the surrounding ligaments and muscles for its strength and stability. Anterior and posterior stability is provided by two strong ligaments inside the knee, the anterior and posterior cruciate ligaments. Medial and lateral stability is provided by the collateral ligaments (Fig. 13–2).

The patellofemoral joint is the articulation between the patella and the intercondylar (trochlear) groove on the anterior aspect of the distal portion of the femur. The patella is in the quadriceps tendon, which protects the joint capsule anteriorly and helps improve the mechanics of the knee.

The Muscles and Their Actions

A muscle must cross a joint to act directly on that joint. The way in which a muscle crosses a joint affects the action. The muscles discussed in this section are responsible for movement of the knee. The knee joint permits the following movements:[3]

- flexion and extension (Fig. 13–3 and Tables 13–1 and 13–2)
- internal (medial) rotation of the tibia on the femur

Table 13–3 summarizes the muscles involved in the movements of the knee.

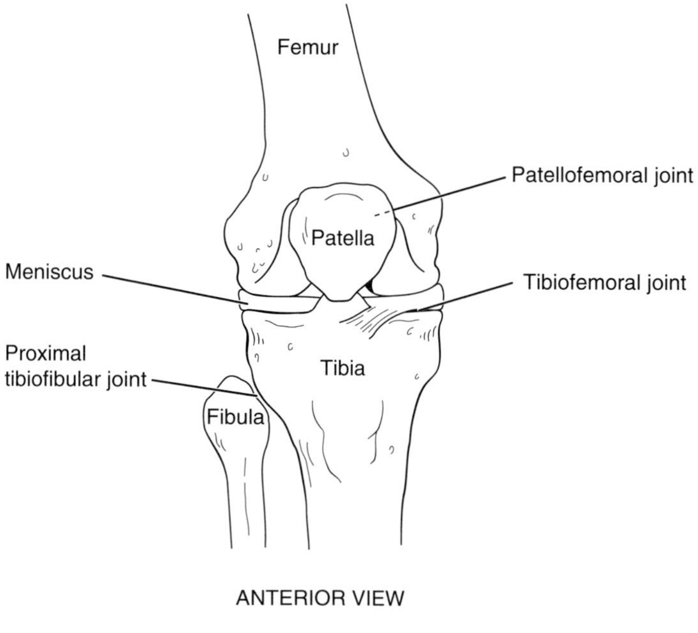

FIGURE 13–1. The bones and joints of the knee (anterior view).

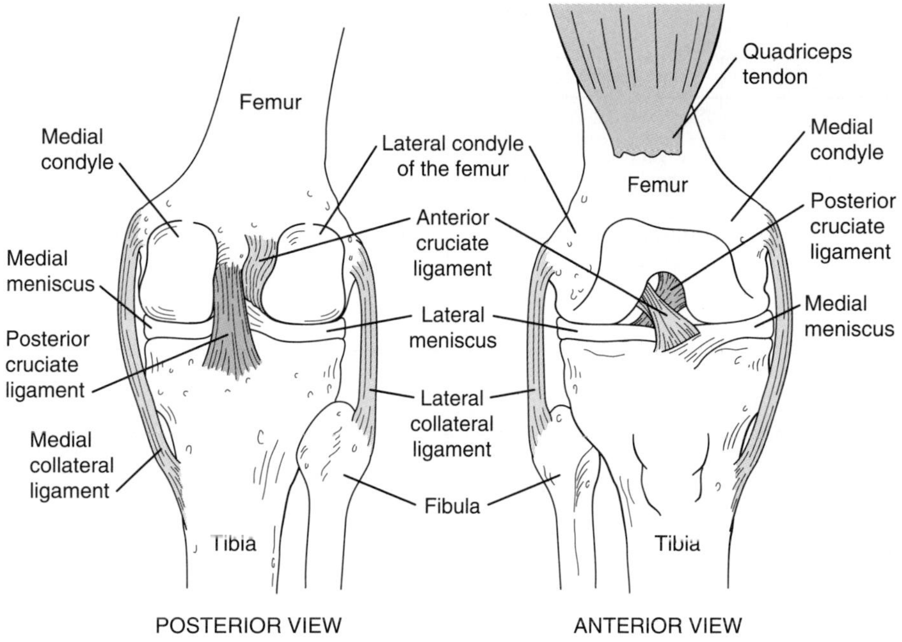

FIGURE 13–2. The ligaments supporting the knee joint.

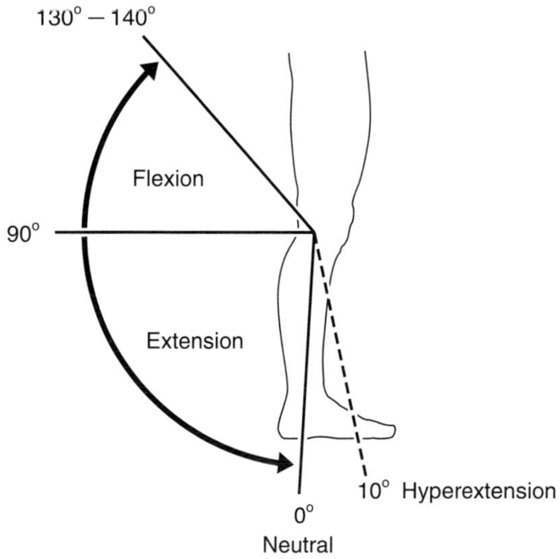

FIGURE 13–3. Movements of the knee joint showing normal range of motion.

TABLE 13–1. The Muscles Involved in Knee Flexion

Muscle	Origin (O)	Insertion (I)	Action
Semitendinosus	See Table 12–2	See Table 12–2	Knee flexion
Semimembranosus	See Table 12–2	See Table 12–2	Knee flexion
Biceps femoris	See Table 12–2	See Table 12–2	Knee flexion
Popliteus 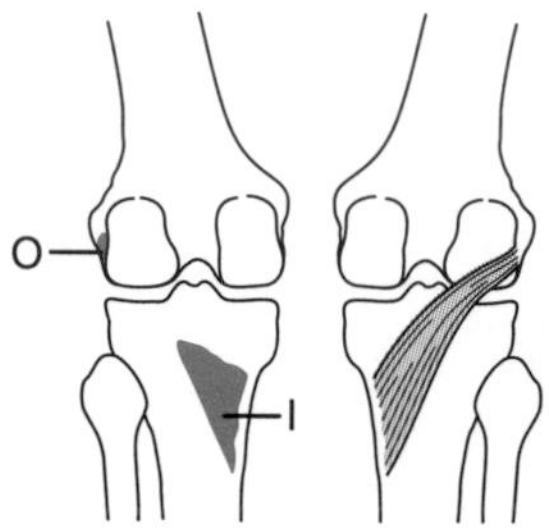	Posterior lateral condyle of the femur	Posterior tibia below the medial condyle of the femur	Knee flexion

TABLE 13–2. The Muscles Involved in Knee Extension

Muscle	Origin (O)	Insertion (I)	Action
Quadriceps: **1. Rectus femoris**	See Table 12–1	All four muscles of the quadriceps insert in the top of the patella via the patella ligament to the tibial tuberosity	Knee extension
2. Vastus lateralis 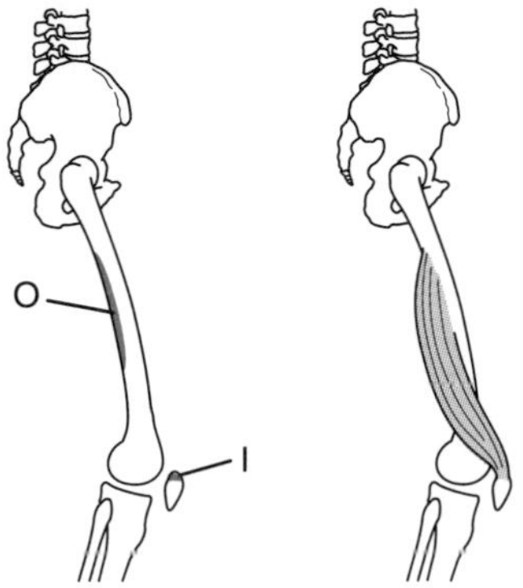	2. Lateral lip of the linea aspera		Knee extension
3. Vastus intermedius **4. Vastus medialis** 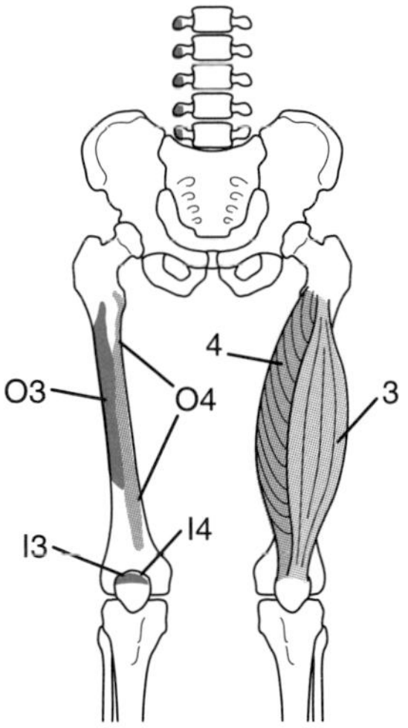	3. Anterior surface shaft of the femur 4. Medial lip of the linea aspera		Knee extension

TABLE 13–3. Summary of the Muscles Involved in the Movements of the Knee

Anatomic Movement	Prime Movers	Assistant Movers	Nerve Root Level	Normal Range of Motion
Flexion	Semitendinosus Semimembranosus Biceps femoris	Sartorius Gracilis Gastrocnemius Plantaris	L2 to S3	0°–140°
Extension	Rectus femoris Vastus lateralis Vastus intermedius Vastus medialis		L2 to L4	0°–10°
Internal rotation	Semitendinosus Semimembranosus	Sartorius Gracilis Popliteus	L2 to S5	20°–30°
External rotation	Biceps femoris		L5 to S3	30°–40°

Measuring the Range of Motion of the Knee

To measure knee flexion and extension, the examiner places the stationary arm of the goniometer along the lateral side of the femur, pointing toward the lateral condyle of the greater trochanter[4] (Fig. 13–4). The moving arm is placed parallel to the lateral midline of the fibula, pointing toward the lateral malleolus.[4]

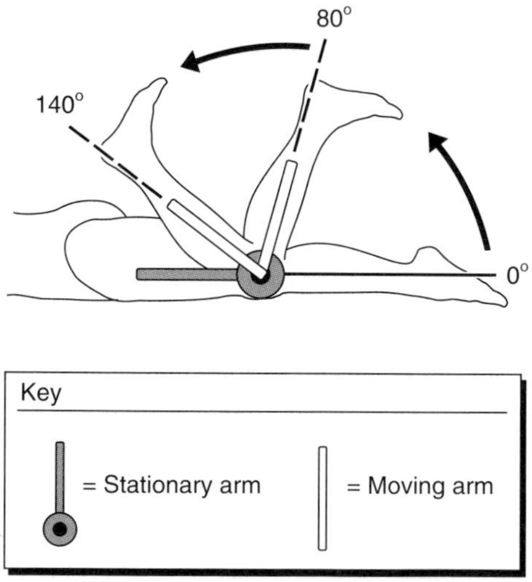

FIGURE 13–4. Measuring the range of motion of the knee.

KNEE STRETCHES

Quadriceps Stretch (Fig. 13–5)

Prime movers: quadriceps muscles and hip flexor muscles.

- Stand holding on to the pool wall
- Flex the involved knee and grasp the ankle with the hand of the same side
- Pull the heel out and toward the buttock until a stretch is felt in front of involved thigh
- Maintain hip extension
- Hold, then relax and lower the foot

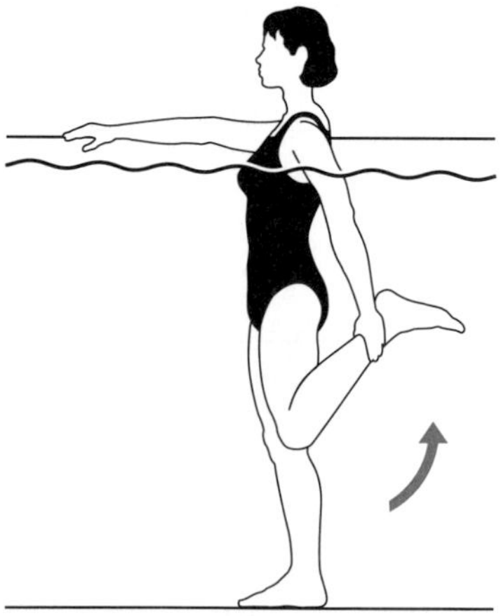

FIGURE 13–5. Quadriceps stretch.

Passive Quadriceps Stretch (Fig. 13–6)

Prime movers: quadriceps muscles and hip flexor muscles. This exercise is for restricted knee flexion muscles.

- Place a flotation device around the ankle of the involved leg
- Stand facing the pool wall with the fronts of the thighs and hips touching the wall
- Keep the trunk upright with the knees and hips in vertical alignment
- Gently flex the knee as far as possible, pressing the heel toward the buttock
- Hold, then relax and lower the leg

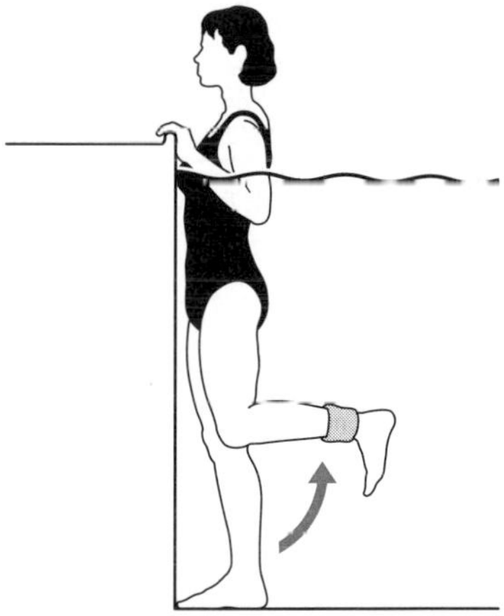

FIGURE 13–6. Passive quadriceps stretch.

Seated Knee Flexion Stretch (Fig. 13–7)

Prime mover: quadriceps.

- Sit with the knees over one parallel bar, holding on to the bar behind
- Cross the uninvolved calf over the shin of the involved leg and press the involved leg back until a stretch is felt
- Hold, then relax

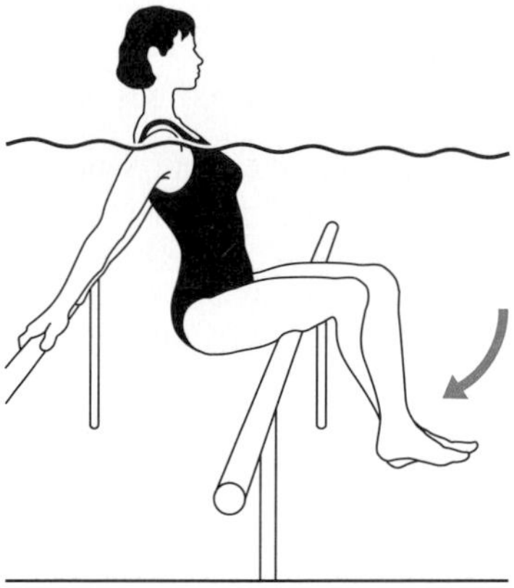

FIGURE 13–7. Seated knee flexion stretch.

Seated Knee Extension Stretch (Fig. 13–8)

Prime movers: hamstrings.

- Sit with knees over one parallel bar, holding on to the bar behind
- Place the uninvolved foot under the ankle of the opposite leg
- Straighten the uninvolved leg to assist knee extension of the involved leg
- Hold, then relax

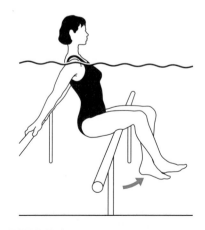

FIGURE 13–8. Seated knee extension stretch.

Lunge Stretch (Fig. 13–9)

Prime movers: gluteus maximus and hamstrings.

- Stand facing the pool ladder; grasp the ladder with both hands and place the foot of the involved leg on a rung of the ladder at a comfortable level
- Press the hips forward, lunging the knee into flexion
- Keep the heel of the support leg on the ground and supporting the hip in extension
- Hold, then relax

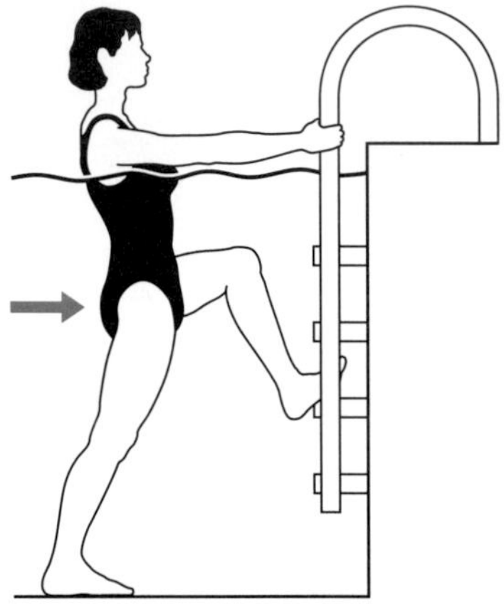

FIGURE 13–9. Lunge stretch.

Hamstring Stretch (Fig. 13–10)

Prime movers: hamstrings and gluteus maximus.

- Place the heel of the involved foot on the floor (or face the ladder, hold on with both hands, and place the involved foot on the ladder at a comfortable height) with the involved ankle in dorsiflexion
- Bend forward at the hips, keeping the head and trunk positioned forward over the legs and stretching the hamstring muscles of the involved leg
- Hold, then relax

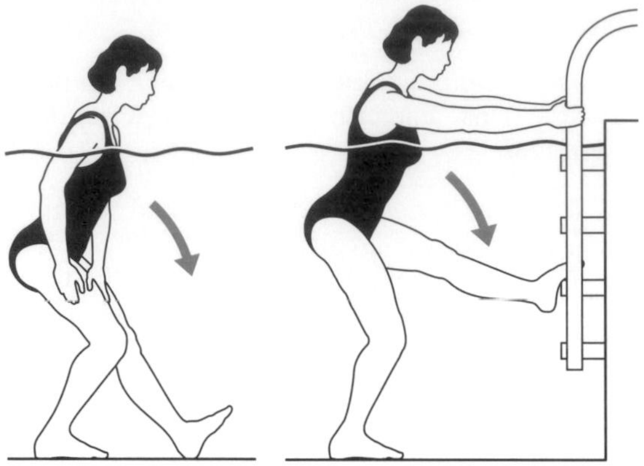

FIGURE 13–10. Hamstring stretch.

Active Hamstring Stretch (Fig. 13–11)

Prime movers: hamstrings, gluteus maximus, gastrocnemius, and soleus.

- Stand facing the pool wall and place the involved foot on the wall at a comfortable height with the forefoot on the wall and the knee slightly bent
- Slowly straighten the involved leg without locking the knee
- Maintain proper spinal alignment by lifting the chest
- Hold, then flex the knee and relax

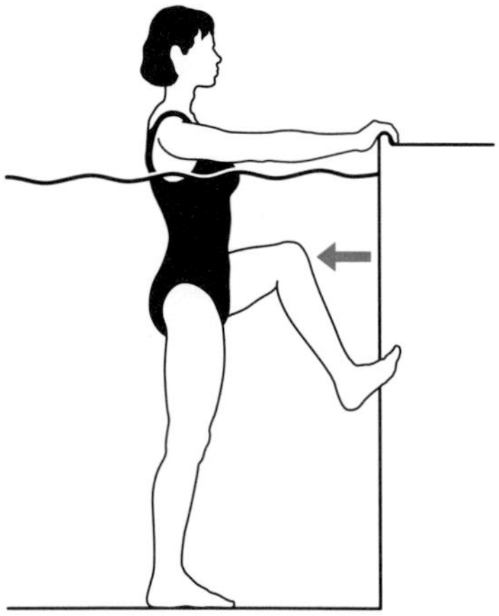

FIGURE 13–11. Active hamstring stretch.

KNEE EXERCISES

Single-Leg Bicycle (Fig. 13–12)

Prime movers: hamstrings, quadriceps, gluteus maximus, hip flexors, and hip adductors.

- Holding on to the pool wall, stand on the uninvolved leg
- Flex and extend the involved leg, performing a cycling action
- Reverse the direction and repeat

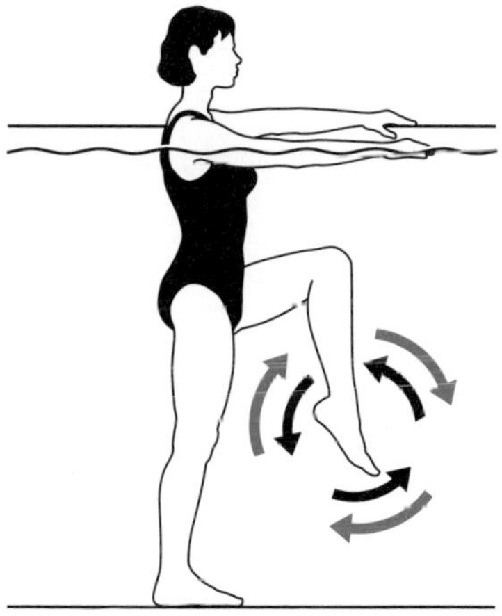

FIGURE 13–12. Single-leg bicycle.

Thigh Extension (Fig. 13–13)

Prime movers: quadriceps, hamstrings, and gastrocnemius.

- Place a flotation device around the ankle of involved leg
- Stand with the stomach against the pool wall, holding on to the edge
- Slowly flex and extend the involved knee backward, maintaining neutral hip alignment

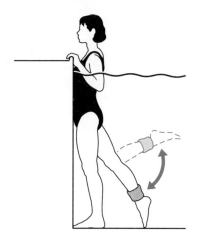

FIGURE 13–13. Thigh extension.

Hamstring Pull-back (Fig. 13–14)

Prime movers: hip flexors, quadriceps, hamstrings, and gastrocnemius.

- Stand with the back against the pool wall, hold on to the wall, and flex the hip of the involved leg to 90°
- Flex and extend the knee while maintaining hip flexion

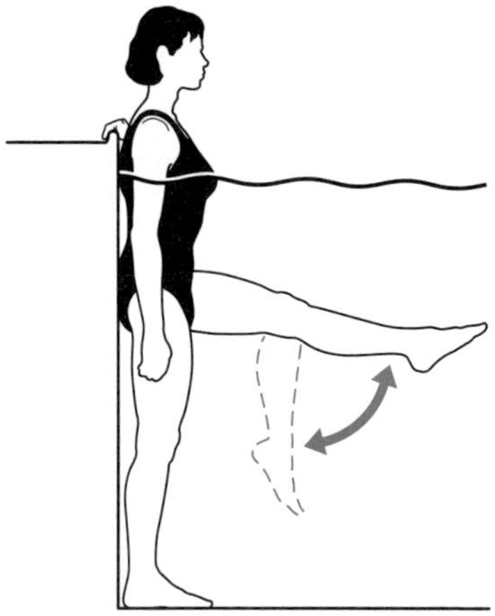

FIGURE 13–14. Hamstring pull-back.

Resistive Knee Flexion and Extension
(Fig. 13–15)

Prime movers: quadriceps and hamstrings.

- Place a resistive device on the ankle of the involved leg
- Stand with the involved knee over one of the parallel bars so that the lower end of the thigh is resting on the bar
- Holding on to the bar behind, flex and extend the involved knee

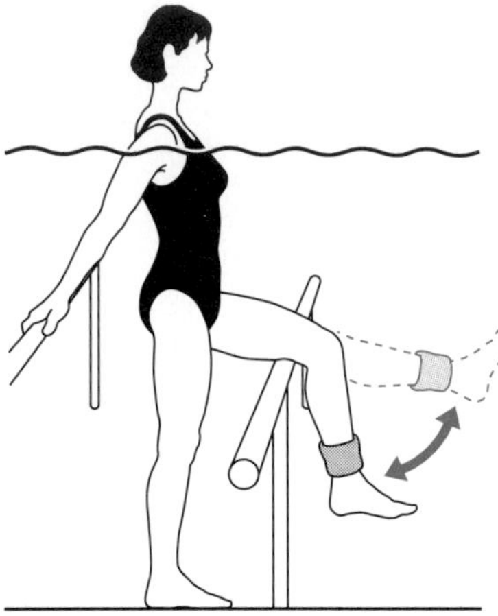

FIGURE 13–15. Resistive knee flexion and extension.

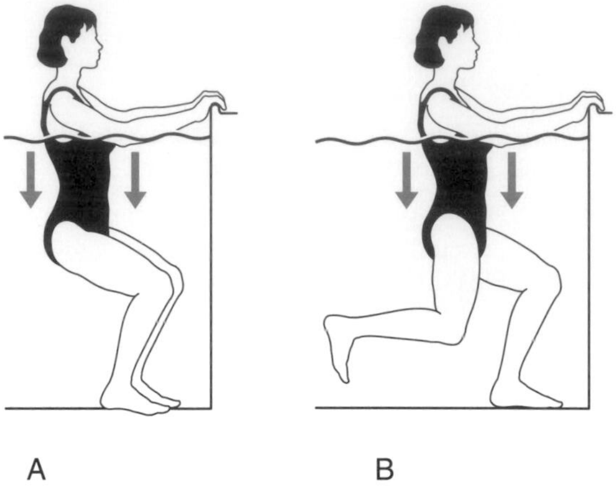

FIGURE 13–16. Squats. *A,* Double-leg. *B,* Single-leg.

Squats (Fig. 13–16)

Prime movers: quadriceps, hip adductors, gluteus maximus, hamstrings, and hip abductors.

- Stand facing pool wall with the feet shoulder-width apart
- Slowly bend the knees and lower the torso until the thighs are almost parallel to pool floor; the hips should be no lower than knee level
- Extend the legs without arching the back, and return to the starting position

VARIATION: Single-Leg Squat (same as squat but use one leg only)

VARIATION: Jump Squat (same as squat but extend the legs forcefully enough to hop off the pool floor)

Lunges (Fig. 13–17)

Prime movers: quadriceps, hip flexors, gluteus maximus, hamstrings, and hip adductors.

- Stand with the feet together and the pelvis tilted back
- Take a step forward with the involved leg, bending the front knee and landing on the foot with the toes pointing forward; the back should remain straight
- Straighten the forward leg with a backward pushing motion originating from the heel, and return to the starting position

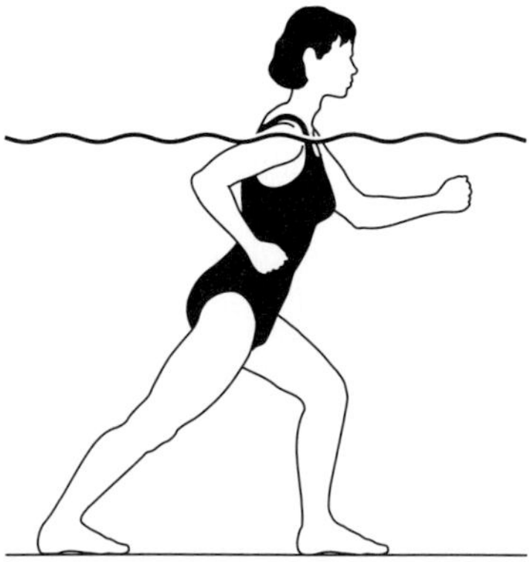

FIGURE 13–17. Lunges.

Fin Kicks (Fig. 13–18)

Prime movers: quadriceps, hamstrings, hip flexors, gluteus maximus, and hip adductors.

- Lie prone, holding on to the side of the pool or a flotation device, with swim fins on both feet
- Alternately flex and extend at the knees, performing a kicking action

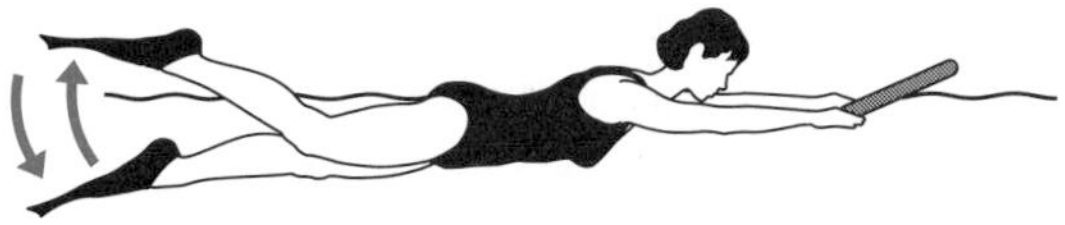

FIGURE 13–18. Fin kicks.

Pliés (Fig. 13–19)

Prime movers: hip rotators, quadriceps, hamstrings, and hip abductors.

- Stand with the feet wider than shoulder-width apart, toes turned outward, and arms out at the sides
- Keeping the back straight and the head upright, bend the knees to a half-squat position; keep the heels on the floor
- Return to a standing position by pushing with the thigh muscles; maintain the pelvic tilt throughout
- Rise up on the toes and hold momentarily, then relax

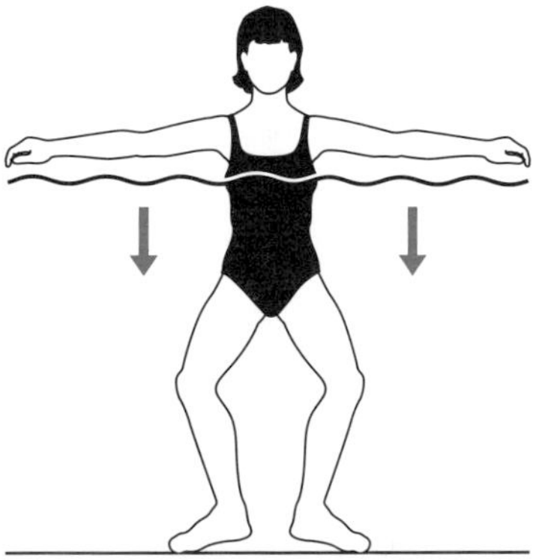

FIGURE 13–19. Pliés.

Step-ups (Fig. 13–20)

Prime movers: gluteus maximus, quadriceps, and gastrocnemius.

- Stand in front of an aquatic step
- Flex the hip and knee of the involved leg and place the foot on the step
- Step up onto the platform with the involved leg (buoyancy will assist) and then bring up the uninvolved leg
- Step down to the pool floor with the involved leg, then the uninvolved leg

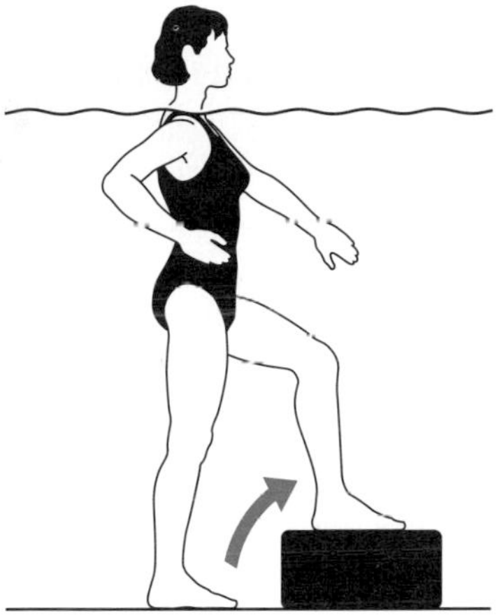

FIGURE 13–20. Step-ups.

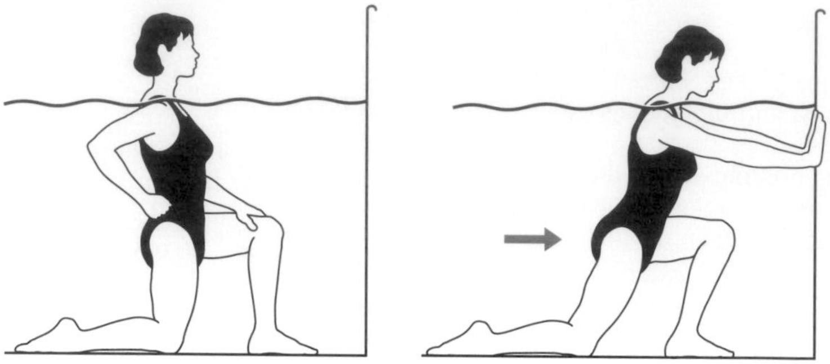

FIGURE 13–21. Kneeling forward flexion.

Kneeling Forward Flexion (Fig. 13–21)

Prime movers: gluteus maximus, quadriceps, hamstrings, gastrocnemius, and soleus.

- In shallow water near the pool wall, kneel on uninvolved leg and place the other foot on the floor; flex the hip and knee of the involved leg to 90° (if possible)
- Placing the hands on the pool wall, move the trunk as far forward as possible over the involved leg, forcing the forward knee into greater flexion
- Perform small rocking movements forward and backward within a pain-free range of motion

COMMON CONDITIONS OF THE KNEE

Knee Arthritis

The knee is commonly afflicted by many of the types of arthritis described in Chapter 7.

Origin

Osteoarthritis of the knee is often caused simply by wear and tear (Fig. 13–22). There also may be some predisposing factor, such as a previous injury.

Pathology

The various pathologic processes are described in Chapter 7.

Signs and Symptoms

Pain, swelling, and decreased range of motion occur in varying degrees. As the arthritis advances, walking becomes difficult.

Body Parts Affected

- Bones (femur, tibia, fibula)
- Joint surfaces (articular cartilage)
- Soft tissues (joint capsule, muscles, tendons, ligaments)

Exercise Priorities

- Establish a controlled exercise program (be careful that the patient does not overdo it)
- Maximize range of motion
- Strengthen all knee muscles

Damaged articular cartilage

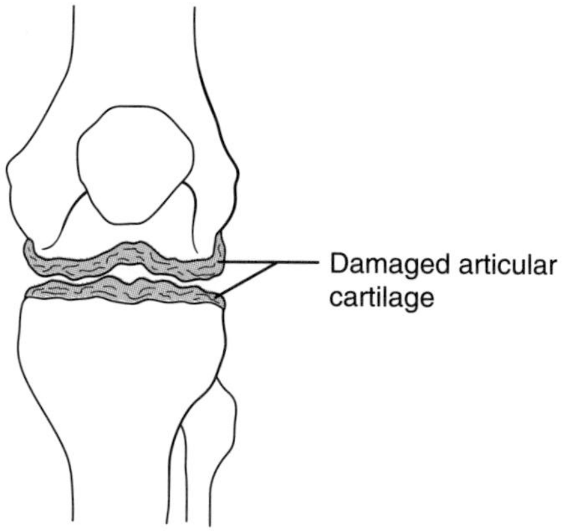

FIGURE 13–22. Knee arthritis.

Knee Fracture

Fracture of any bone of the lower extremity close to the knee joint may be called a knee fracture. This may include fractures of the femur, tibia, fibula, or patella (Fig. 13–23).

Origin

Fractures near the knee occur as the result of many different kinds of accidents.

Pathology

The various types of fractures are described in Chapter 7. Because many fractures near the knee are repaired with internal fixation, aquatic exercise therapy can begin as soon as the incisions have healed. It is still important, however, to check for the doctor's restrictions on weight bearing.

Signs and Symptoms

The amount of pain, stiffness, and weakness varies from person to person. Often, it is the swelling of the knee joint that limits movement.

Body Parts Affected

- Bones (femur, tibial, patella, fibula)
- Knee joint (capsule, ligaments, menisci)
- Muscles (quadriceps, hamstrings, gastrocnemius)

Exercise Priorities

- Restore full range of motion
- Strengthen knee, hip, and ankle muscles
- Correct gait abnormalities

Knee Meniscus Injuries

The meniscus (also known as cartilage) between the tibia and the femur is a commonly injured tissue.

Origin

The medial meniscus is usually damaged because of a blow to the lateral aspect of the knee. Such an injury usually tears the medial collateral ligament first. Because the medial meniscus is attached to

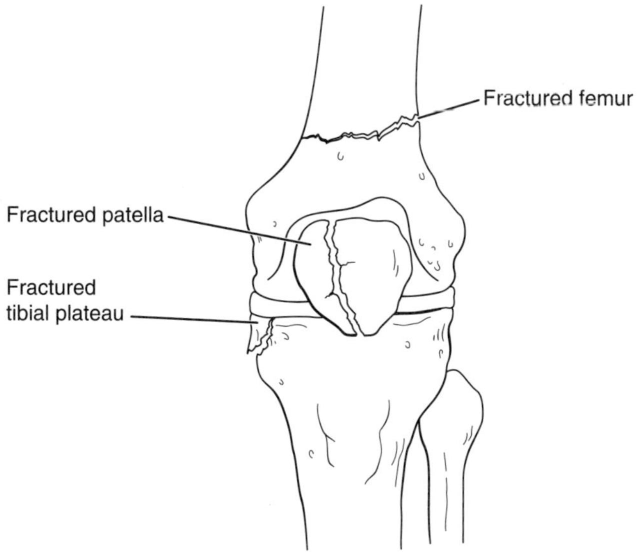

FIGURE 13–23. Fractures of the knee.

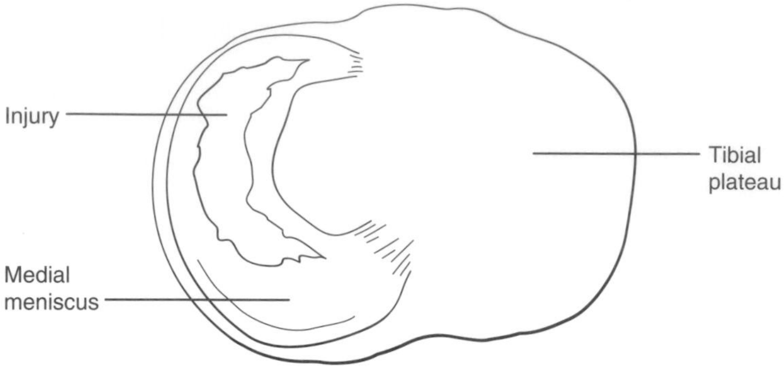

FIGURE 13–24. Bucket handle tear of the meniscus.

this ligament, it also is torn. A compression and rotation force can also injure the medial meniscus.

The lateral meniscus is usually injured by a hyperflexion force. This causes the meniscus to be pinched between the femur and the tibia.

Pathology

There are two common types of meniscal tears. The first, shown in Figure 13–24, is known as a bucket handle tear. It often occurs with medial collateral ligament sprains. The posterior horn tear, shown in Figure 13–25, is the second common type of tear. These injuries are often a constant source of inflammation until they are surgically repaired.

Signs and Symptoms

This injury causes pain along the joint line. Tears of the medial meniscus often prevent full extension, and lateral meniscal tears limit flexion. The patient may also experience a giving way of the knee or a catching or locking sensation.

Body Parts Affected

- Menisci (medial and lateral)
- Joint capsule (and knee ligaments)
- Muscles (quadriceps, hamstrings, gastrocnemius)

Exercise Priorities

- Restore range of motion
- Strengthen quadriceps, hamstrings, hip muscles, and gastrocnemius

Knee Strain

This term applies to an injury to any of the muscles or tendons that surround the knee.

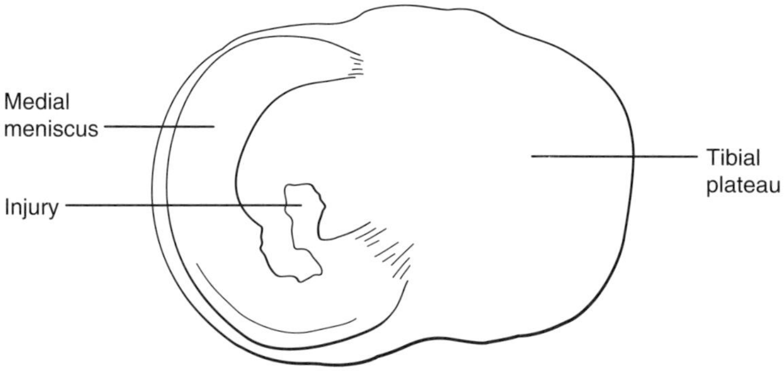

FIGURE 13–25. Posterior horn tear of the meniscus.

Origin

Tears of a muscle or tendon near the knee usually occur during some strenuous form of physical activity. Tendonitis in the knee region is brought on by a repetitive activity such as jumping, running, or climbing.

Pathology

The pathology of strains is outlined in Chapter 7. In the area of the knee, the quadriceps (Fig. 13–26), hamstrings, and gastrocnemius are the muscles usually involved.

Signs and Symptoms

Pain and swelling are the characteristics of strains. Pain is usually increased by stretching the involved muscle but actually decreases after the muscle is warmed up.

Body Parts Affected

- Muscles and tendons of the knee (quadriceps, hamstrings, gastrocnemius)
- Knee joint (capsule, meniscus, ligament, and articular cartilage involvement must be ruled out)

Exercise Priorities

- During the acute phase, stretch the involved muscles to restore range of motion
- Establish a controlled exercise program
- Advance strengthening exercises to return the patient to normal activity level

Knee Sprain

A knee sprain involves an injury to one or more ligaments of the knee.

Origin

This injury commonly occurs during contact sports, but it can occur any time an external force is applied to the knee. A blow to the lateral aspect of the knee damages the medial collateral ligament and may also injure the anterior cruciate ligament. A blow to the medial aspect of the knee damages the lateral collateral ligament and the anterior cruciate ligament. A blow to the front of the knee damages the posterior cruciate ligament, and a blow to the back of the knee injures the anterior cruciate ligament (Fig. 13–27). A twisting force, such as

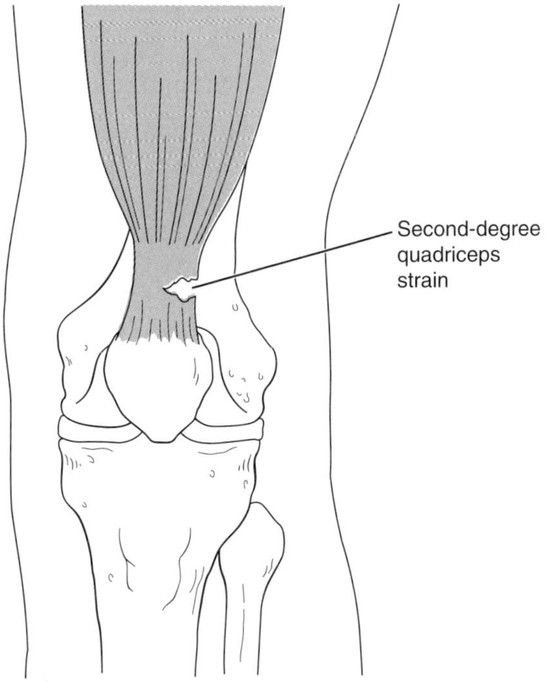

FIGURE 13–26. Quadriceps muscle strain.

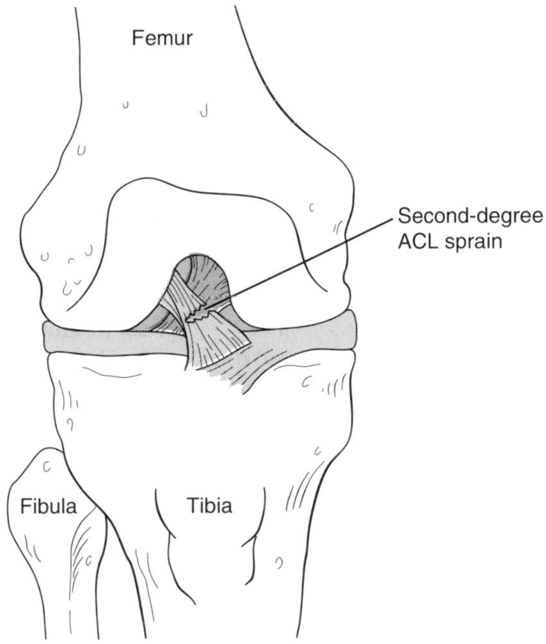

FIGURE 13–27. Anterior cruciate ligament sprain.

may occur while skiing, usually injures the medial collateral and anterior cruciate ligaments.

Pathology

The pathology of a sprain is outlined in Chapter 7. Knee sprains are often combined with a meniscal tear or an injury to the joint capsule. This is true of medial collateral ligament sprains in particular, because the ligament is attached to the medial meniscus. The joint capsule is involved because it is blended with the medial collateral ligament.

As described in Chapter 7, ligaments are slow-healing structures. Consequently, it is important that the healing ligament not be stressed during the long rehabilitation process. For this reason, resistive hip exercises should be performed with the resistive device attached above the knee. Attaching the device to the lower leg could put unwanted stress on an injured ligament.

Signs and Symptoms

A sprain of any of the knee ligaments may result in enough swelling to severely restrict range of motion. This swelling also contributes to the feeling of weakness and instability that many patients report. True instability, however, is present only with severe second- and third-degree sprains.

Body Parts Affected

- Knee ligaments (anterior cruciate, posterior cruciate, medial collateral, lateral collateral)
- Joint capsule
- Menisci
- Muscles of the knee (quadriceps, hamstrings, gastrocnemius)
- Adjacent muscles (gluteus muscles, tensor fascia latae, hip abductors, hip adductors)

Exercise Priorities

- Always check for doctor's orders for specific restrictions
- Treat a sprain of the anterior cruciate ligament with the same exercise routine as for an anterior cruciate repair (no isolated quadriceps exercises until the ligament is well healed)
- Strengthen all knee, hip, and ankle muscles
- Correct balance and gait abnormalities
- Return the patient to a functional level (for work or sport)

Anterior Cruciate Ligament Repair

This term refers to the surgical repair of a ruptured anterior cruciate ligament.

Origin

Third-degree sprains of the anterior cruciate ligament are most often caused by a blow to the side or back of the knee. They may also occur with a twisting injury, such as may occur while skiing.

Pathology

The pathology of a third-degree sprain is described in Chapter 7. Two of the most common surgical procedures to repair the torn ligament are the quadriceps tendon graft (Fig. 13–28) and the semitendinosus transfer. Both procedures can be done partly through an arthroscope to minimizing scarring, and they have similar courses of rehabilitation.

Signs and Symptoms

Postoperative stiffness and swelling are the norm. As the swelling subsides, range of motion increases. Many surgeons, however, do not want full extension to be achieved too soon. They feel that if the knee is slightly stiff going into extension, the repair may be stronger. Also, full extension stresses the ligament repair.

Body Parts Affected

- Knee joint structures (repaired ligament, other ligaments, joint capsule, menisci)
- Knee muscles (quadriceps, hamstrings, gastrocnemius)
- Adjacent muscles (gluteus muscles, tensor fascia latae, hip abductors, hip adductors)

Exercise Priorities

- Check with the surgeon for a specific protocol
- Increase knee flexion, but do not push for full extension until it is called for by the surgeon's protocol
- Initially strengthen the hip, hamstring, and calf muscles (attach resistive devices above the knee to avoid stress on the repaired ligament)
- Add quadriceps strengthening when ordered
- Work toward normal strength, endurance, balance, and coordination

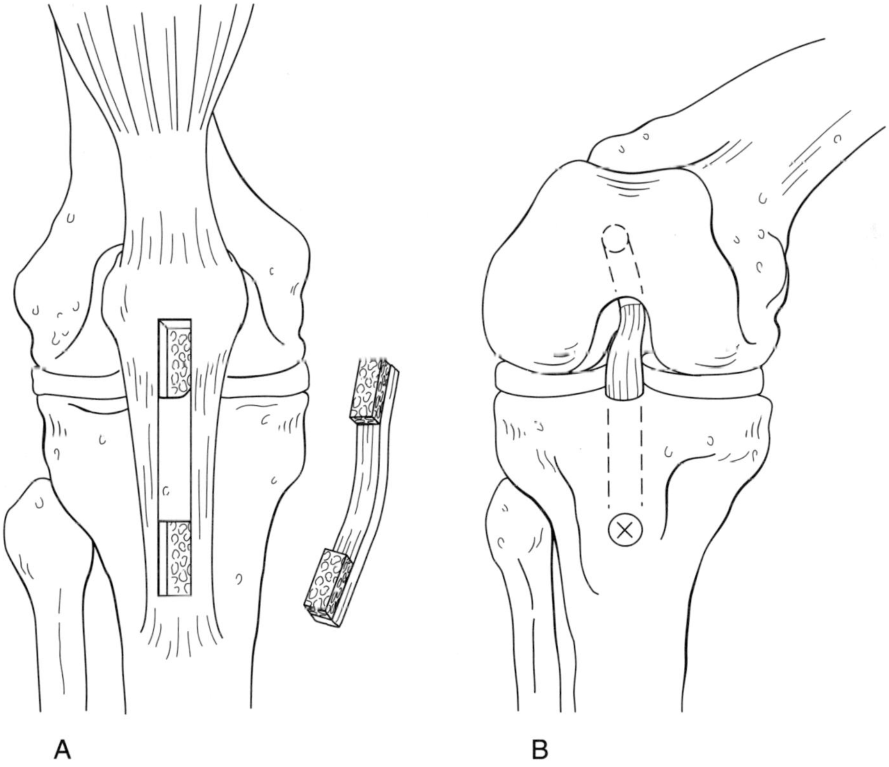

FIGURE 13–28. Anterior cruciate repair with quadriceps tendon graft. *A,* Donor site. *B,* Position of graft repair.

Total Knee Replacement

This surgical procedure involves the replacement of a painful, damaged knee joint with an artificial joint.

Origin

This operation is most often performed on knees that are severely affected by osteoarthritis or rheumatoid arthritis. It is done to alleviate pain, not to return the patient to high-level sports or other demanding activities.

Mechanics

The femoral component of the prosthesis is metal, and the tibial component is plastic (Fig. 13–29). As with hip replacements, these components may or may not be cemented into place. Cementing allows for earlier full weight bearing, but it is debatable which technique has better long-term results. Patients often experience a "clicking" sensation, which usually resolves spontaneously within a few months. During this rehabilitation period, patients are expected to attain between 90° and 110° of flexion. Because there are no knee ligaments remaining, attaining full flexion would result in an unstable joint.

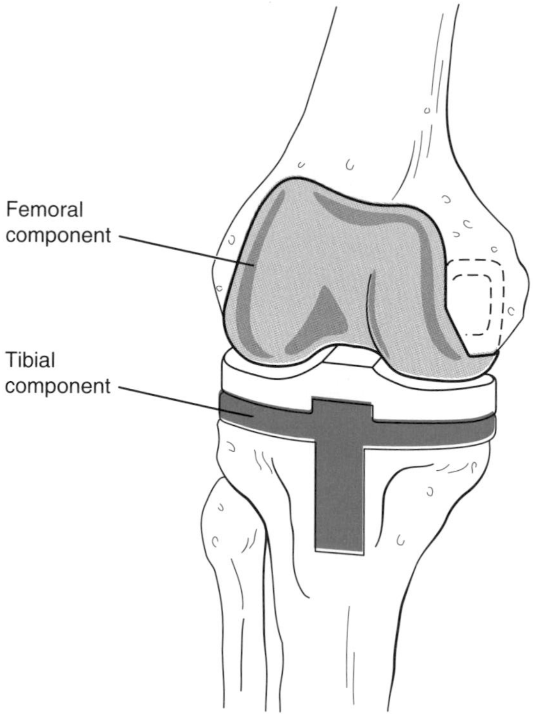

FIGURE 13–29. Total knee replacement.

Signs and Symptoms

After the postoperative pain and swelling have subsided, the patient must contend with stiffness and weakness. One of the most common problems encountered after this surgery is the formation of adhesions along the incision. This condition contributes to the stiffness and slows recovery. The scar tissue is best dealt with by massaging the area and continuing to stretch the knee into flexion.

Body Parts Affected

- Bones (femur, tibia, patella)
- Muscles (quadriceps, hamstrings, gastrocnemius)

Exercise Priorities

- Increase range of motion (the goal is full extension and 90° of flexion)
- Strengthen the knee and hip muscles
- Correct gait abnormalities (check with the surgeon for restrictions on weight bearing)

THE AQUATIC EXERCISE THERAPY PROTOCOL FOR CONDITIONS OF THE KNEE

Phase One

Warm-up

Perform each exercise for 2 minutes.

- Forward Walking (see Fig. 5–21)
- Backward Walking (see Fig. 5–22)
- Side Stepping (do not cross legs) (see Fig. 5–23)

Stretch

Perform five repetitions of each exercise, holding for 10 seconds.

- Passive Quadriceps Stretch (see Fig. 13–6)
- Hamstring Stretch (do not push for full extension after repair of the anterior cruciate ligament) (see Fig. 13–10)
- Calf Stretch (see Fig. 14–7)

- Seated Knee Flexion Stretch (see Fig. 13–7)
- Seated Knee Extension Stretch (see Fig. 13–8)

Strengthen

Perform one set of 8 to 12 repetitions.

- Single-Leg Bicycle (see Fig. 13–12)
- Squats (see Fig. 13–14)
- Hip Abduction and Adduction (see Fig. 12–13)
- Hip Flexion (see Fig. 12–11)
- Hip Extension (see Fig. 12–12)
- Resistive Knee Flexion and Extension (omit extension for patients with anterior cruciate ligament repair at this phase) (see Fig. 13–15)
- Hamstring Pull-back (see Fig. 13–14)

Phase Two

Warm-up

Perform each exercise for 2 minutes.

- Forward Walking (see Fig. 5–21)
- Backward Walking (see Fig. 5–22)
- Stiff Leg Walking (see Fig. 5–25)
- Bicycle (see Fig. 5–31)

Stretch

Perform five repetitions of each exercise, holding 20 seconds.

- Calf Stretch (see Fig. 14–7)
- Quadriceps Stretch (see Fig. 13–5)
- Active Hamstring Stretch (see Fig. 13–11)
- Lunge Stretch (see Fig. 13–9)

Strengthen

Perform two sets of 8 to 12 repetitions

- Thigh Extension (see Fig. 13–13)
- Hamstring Pull-back (see Fig. 13–14)
- Resistive Knee Flexion and Extension (use small resistance paddles) (see Fig. 13–15)
- Hip Flexion (use small resistance paddles) (see Fig. 12–11)
- Hip Extension (use small resistance paddles) (see Fig. 12–12)
- Hip Abduction and Adduction (use small resistance paddles) (see Fig. 12–13)
- Heel Raises (see Fig. 14–16)
- Side-to-Side Weight Shifting (see Fig. 11–6)
- Front-to-Back Weight Shifting (see Fig. 11–7)

Phase Three

Warm-up

Perform each exercise for 2 minutes. Ankle cuffs may be used to increase resistance.

- Marching (see Fig. 5–28)
- Backward Walking (see Fig. 5–22)
- Bicycle (see Fig. 5–31)

Stretch

Perform five repetitions of each exercise, holding for 30 seconds.

- Quadriceps Stretch (see Fig. 13–5)
- Active Hamstring Stretch (see Fig. 13–11)
- Calf Stretch (see Fig. 14–7)
- Lunge Stretch (see Fig. 13–9)

Strengthen

Perform three sets of 8 to 12 repetitions.

- Heel Raises (see Fig. 14–16)
- Resistive Knee Flexion and Extension (use larger paddles) (see Fig. 13–15)
- Lunges (see Fig. 13–17)
- Fin Kicks (see Fig. 13–18)
- Step-ups (see Fig. 13–20)
- Stork Stand (see Fig. 11–8)

Phase Four

Warm-up

Perform each exercise for 2 minutes. Ankle cuffs may be used to increase resistance.

- Marching (see Fig. 5–28)
- Backward Walking (see Fig. 5–22)
- Bicycle (see Fig. 5–31)
- Leg Exchange (see Fig. 5–29)
- Jogging (see Fig. 5–30)

Stretch

Perform five repetitions of each exercise, holding 30 seconds.

- Quadriceps Stretch (see Fig. 13–5)
- Active Hamstring Stretch (see Fig. 13–11)

- Calf Stretch (see Fig. 14–7)
- Lunge Stretch (see Fig. 13–9)

Strengthen

Perform four sets of 8 to 12 repetitions.

- Heel Raises (see Fig. 14–16)
- Resistive Knee Flexion and Extension (use resistance boots) (see Fig. 13–15)
- Lunges (see Fig. 13–17)
- Pliés (see Fig. 13–19)
- Kneeling Forward Flexion (see Fig. 13–21)
- Step-ups (see Fig. 13–20)
- Leg Balance Exercises (see Fig. 11–9)
- Deep water exercises for lower extremities (see Figs. 6–12 through 6–29)

REFERENCES

1. Magee D. Orthopedic Physical Assessment. Philadelphia: W.B. Saunders, 1987.
2. Gould J, Davis G. Orthopedic and Sports Physical Therapy. St. Louis: C.V. Mosby, 1985.
3. Green W, Heckman J. The Clinical Measurement of Joint Motion. Rosemont, IL: American Academy of Orthopaedic Surgeons, 1994.
4. Arnheim D. Modern Principles of Athletic Training. St. Louis: Times Mirror/Mosby College Publishing, 1985.

Aquatic Rehabilitation of the Ankle and Foot

CHAPTER 14

THE STRUCTURE AND FUNCTION OF THE ANKLE AND FOOT

The Anatomic Parts

THE LOWER LEG. The distal tibiofibular joint is the articulation between the lower ends of the tibia and fibula (Fig. 14–1). It is a fibrous joint joined by an interosseous membrane, with anterior and posterior tibiofibular ligaments binding the bones firmly together.

THE ANKLE. The talocrural joint (ankle) is a synovial hinge joint formed by the articulation of the convex superior surface of the talus, the concave distal end of the tibia (medial malleolus), and the lateral malleolus of the fibula[1, 2] (see Fig. 14–1). These surfaces fit well and allow dorsiflexion and plantar flexion of the ankle. The medial and lateral malleolus and the strong collateral ligaments supporting the joint permit little or no sideways movement. The ligament supporting the capsule medially is the fan-shaped deltoid or medial ligament. The lateral side of the capsule is supported by three ligaments: the anterior and posterior talofibular ligaments and the calcaneofibular ligament (Fig. 14–2). The ligamentous support of the ankle is so strong that the fibula and even the tibia may fracture before the ligaments tear.

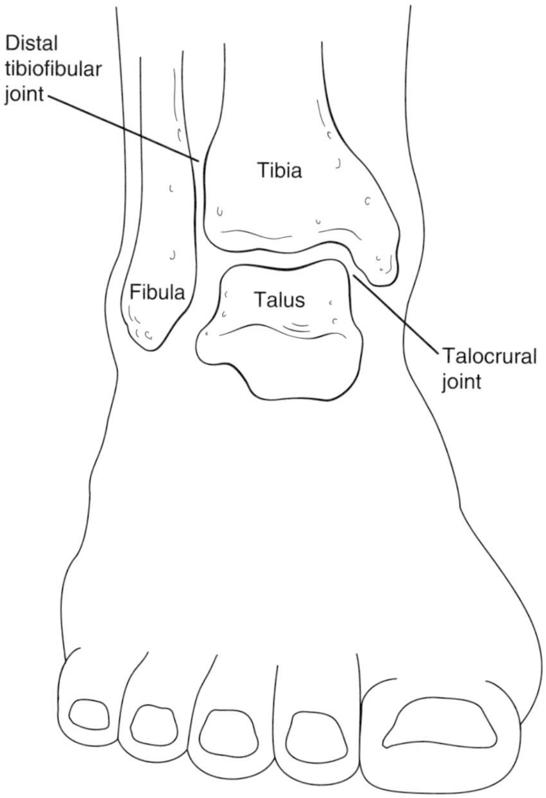

FIGURE 14–1. The bones and joints of the lower leg and ankle.

The subtalar joint is a uniaxial synovial joint with the articulation occurring between the talus and the calcaneus (Fig. 14–3). This joint is supported by the medial and lateral collateral ligaments, the interosseous ligament, and the talocalcaneal ligaments. The subtalar joint permits supination and pronation of the ankle.

THE MIDFOOT. The midfoot comprises seven bones. The midtarsal joints include the following:

- the talocalcaneonavicular joint, which is the articulation between the talus and the navicular
- the cuneonavicular joint, which are the articulations between the medial, intermediate, and lateral cuneiform and the navicular
- the cubiodeonavicular joint, which is the articulation between the cuboid and the navicular
- the intercuneiform joints, which are the articulations between the medial, the intermediate, and lateral cuneiform bones
- the cuneocuboid joint, which is the articulation between the cuneiform and the cuboid
- the calcaneocuboid joint, which is the articulation between the calcaneus and the cuboid (Fig. 14–4).

THE FOREFOOT. The metatarsophalangeal joints (see Fig. 14–4) are condyloid synovial joints similar to the metacarpophalangeal joints of the hand. They permit flexion, extension, abduction, and adduction.

The interphalangeal joints of the toes are hinged synovial joints that are supported by the collateral and plantar ligaments. The movements permitted at this joint are flexion and extension.

The Muscles and Their Actions

A muscle must cross a joint to act directly on that joint. The way in which a muscle crosses a joint affects the action. The muscles discussed in this section are involved at the ankle and foot. The

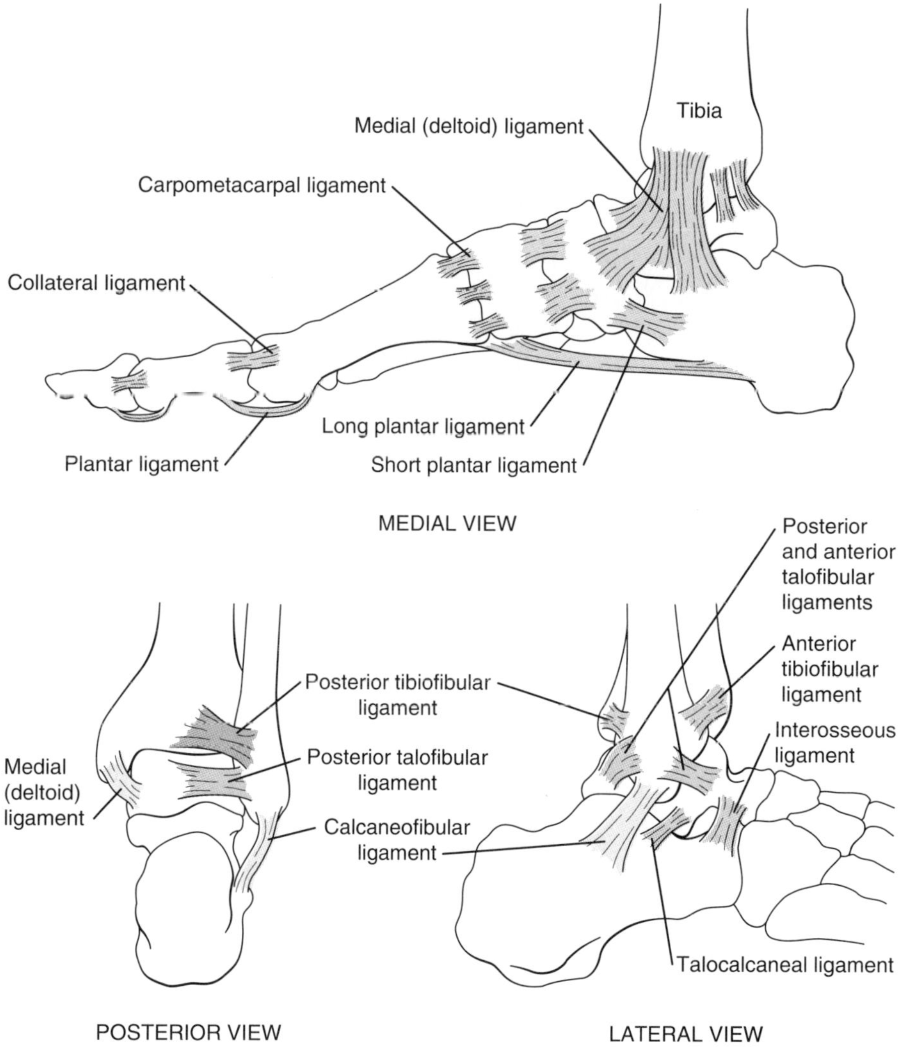

FIGURE 14–2. The ligaments that support the lower leg and ankle.

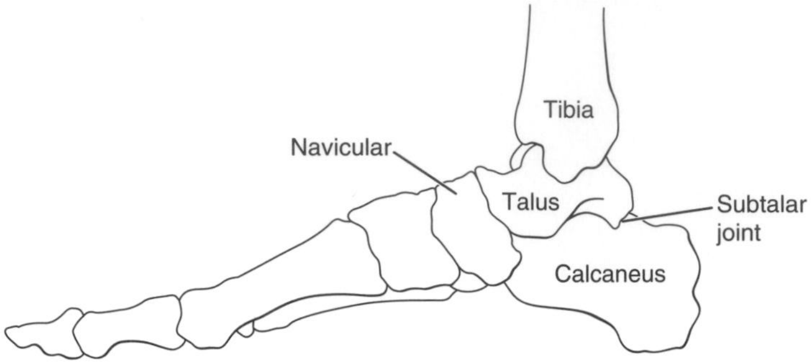

FIGURE 14–3. The subtalar joint (heel) and related bones.

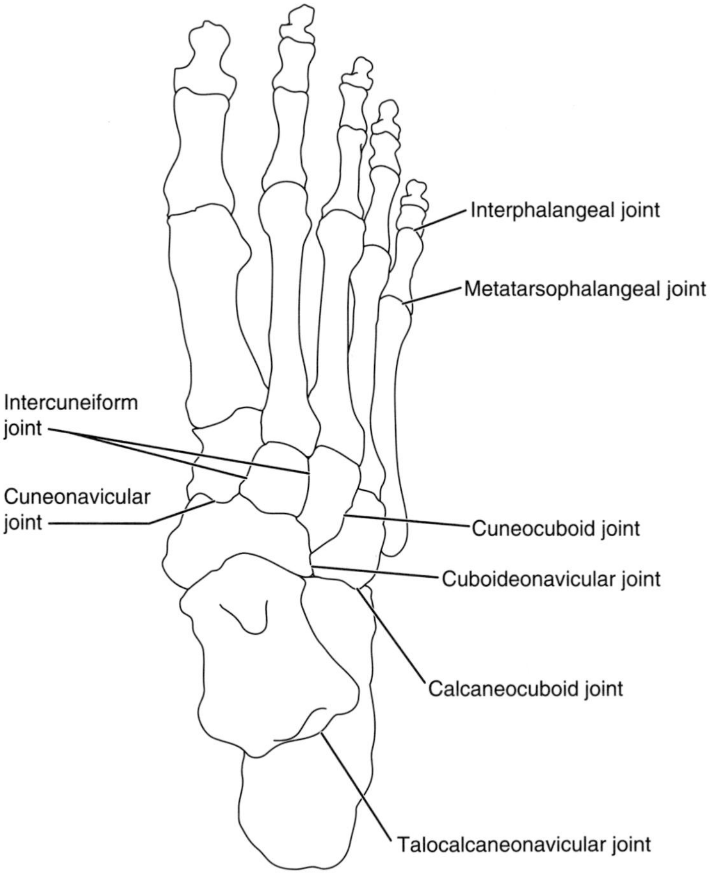

FIGURE 14–4. The joints of the midfoot and forefoot.

ankle permits the following movements[3] (Fig. 14–5):

- dorsiflexion and plantar flexion (Table 14–1)
- inversion and eversion (Table 14–2)

The toes permit the following movements:

- flexion and extension (Table 14–3)

Table 14–4 summarizes the muscles involved in the movements of the ankle and foot.

Measuring the Range of Motion of the Ankle

To measure ankle dorsiflexion and plantar flexion, the examiner places the stationary arm of the goniometer parallel to the lateral midline of the fibula, in line with the lateral malleolus and head of the fibula.[4] The moving arm is placed parallel to the lateral midline of the fifth metatarsal[3] (Fig. 14–6).

Text continued on page 223

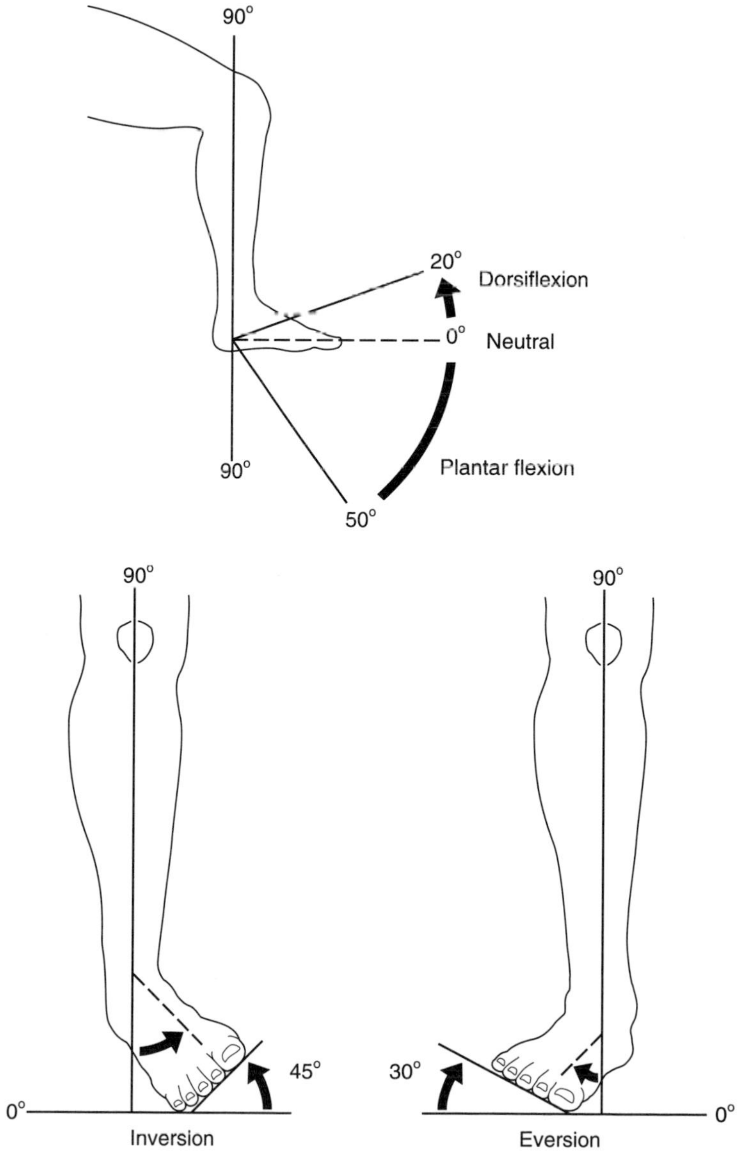

FIGURE 14–5. Movements of the ankle joint showing normal range of motion. (Adapted from Green W, Heckman J. Measurement of Joint Motion. Rosemont, IL: American Academy of Orthopaedic Surgeons, 1994.)

TABLE 14–1. The Muscles Involved in Ankle Plantar Flexion and Dorsiflexion

Muscle	Origin (O)	Insertion (I)	Action
Gastrocnemius 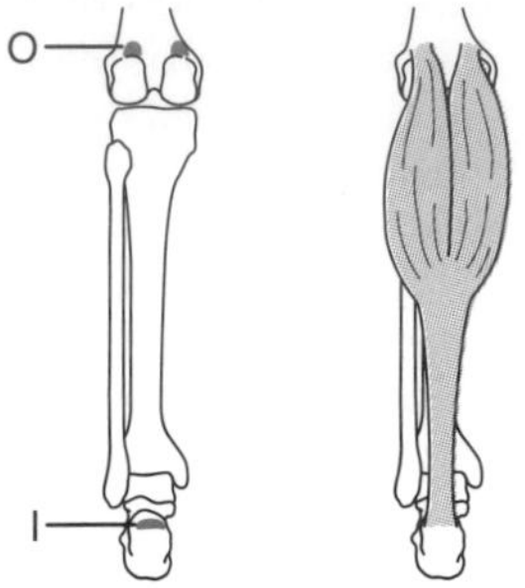 POSTERIOR VIEW	Posterior femoral condyles	Posterior surface of the calcaneus	Ankle plantar flexion Accessory movement: Knee flexion
Soleus 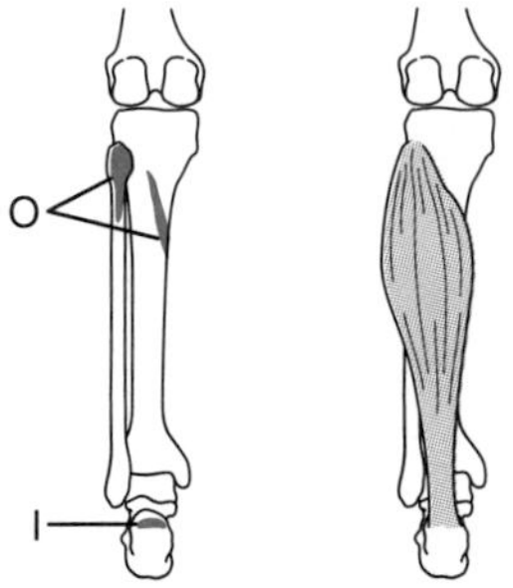 POSTERIOR VIEW	Posterior upper tibia and fibula	Posterior surface of the calcaneus	Ankle plantar flexion
Tibialis anterior 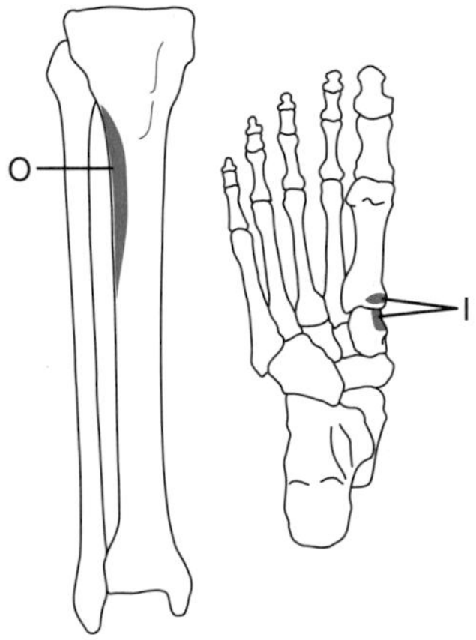 ANTERIOR VIEW AND PLANTAR ASPECT	Upper two-thirds of the outer tibia	Medial and plantar surfaces of the cuneiform bones Base of the first metatarsal	Ankle dorsiflexion Accessory movement: Ankle inversion

TABLE 14–1. The Muscles Involved in Ankle Plantar Flexion and Dorsiflexion *Continued*

Muscle	Origin (O)	Insertion (I)	Action
Extensor digitorum longus 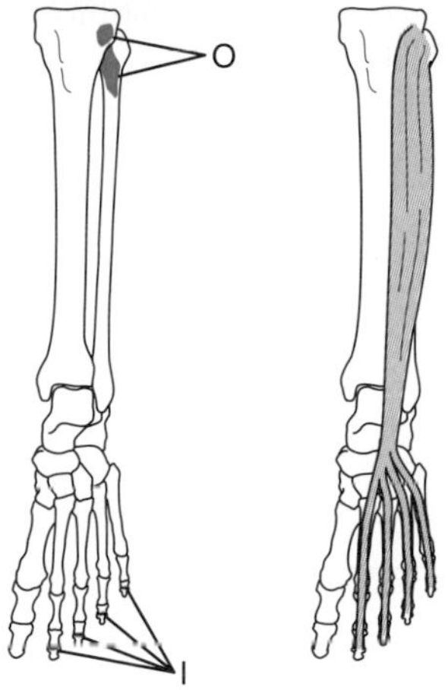	Lateral condyle of the tibia Anterior fibula	Dorsal surfaces of the middle and distal phalanges of the outer four toes	Ankle dorsiflexion Accessory movements: Ankle eversion Toe extension

TABLE 14–2. The Muscles Involved in Ankle Eversion and Inversion

Muscle	Origin (O)	Insertion (I)	Action
Tibialis posterior 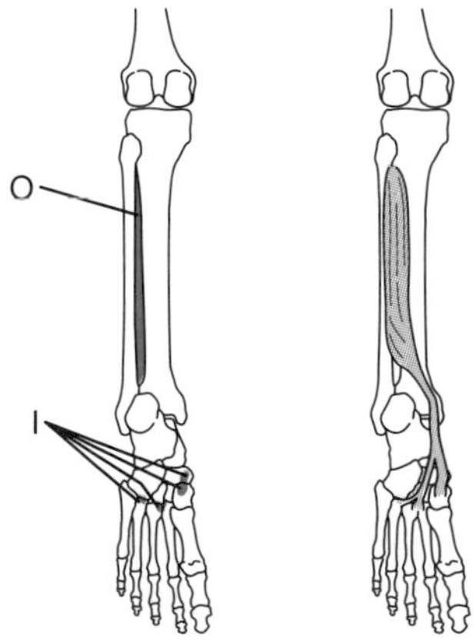	Posterior shaft of the tibia and fibula	Tendon fans out to insert into the navicular, medial cuneiform, and bases of the metatarsals	Ankle inversion Accessory movement: Plantar flexes the foot

Table continued on following page

TABLE 14–2. The Muscles Involved in Ankle Eversion and Inversion *Continued*

Muscle	Origin (O)	Insertion (I)	Action
Peroneus longus 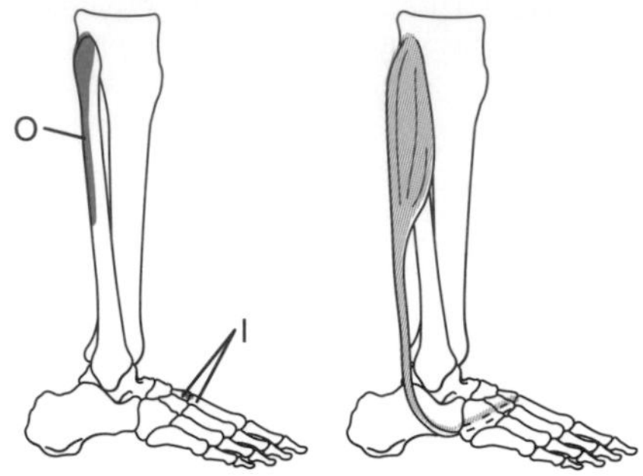 LATERAL VIEW	Upper two-thirds of the outer surface of the fibula	Plantar surface of the medial cuneiform and first metatarsal	Ankle eversion Accessory movement: Plantar flexes the foot
Peroneus brevis 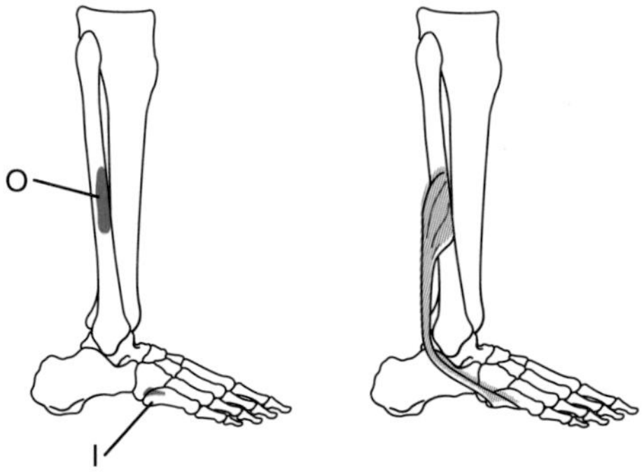 ANTERIOR VIEW	Lower two-thirds of the outer surface of the fibula	Base of the fifth metatarsal Note: The tendon crosses the sole of the foot to insert on the plantar surface, medial border	Ankle eversion Accessory movement: Plantar flexes the foot

TABLE 14–3. The Muscles Involved in Movement of the Toes

Muscle	Origin (O)	Insertion (I)	Action
Extensor hallucis longus 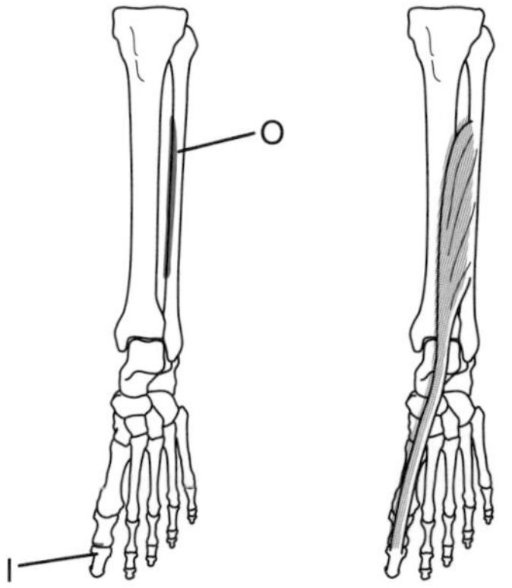 ANTERIOR VIEW	Anterior surface of the fibula	Base of the distal phalanx of the big toe	Extends the big toe Accessory movements: Ankle dorsiflexion Ankle inversion
Flexor digitorum longus 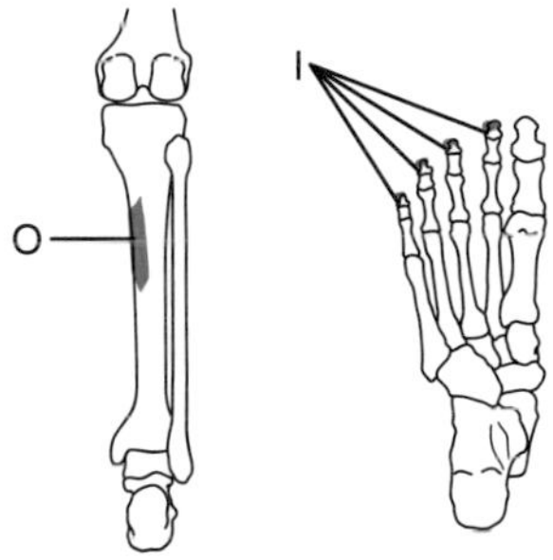 POSTERIOR VIEW AND PLANTAR ASPECT	Posterior tibia	Bases of the distal phalanges of the outer four toes	Flexion of the distal phalanges of the outer four toes Accessory movement: Foot inversion
Flexor hallucis longus 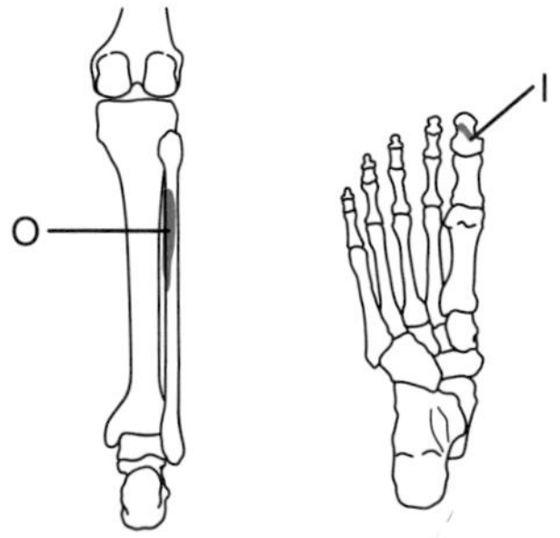 POSTERIOR VIEW AND PLANTAR ASPECT	Lower one-third posterior surface of the fibula	Base of the distal phalanx of the big toe	Flexion of the big toe Accessory movement: Plantar flexes the fore-foot

TABLE 14–4. Summary of the Muscles Involved in the Movements of the Ankle and Foot

Action	Prime Movers	Assistant Movers	Nerve Root Level	Range of Motion
Dorsiflexion	Tibialis anterior Extensor digitorum longus	Peroneus tertius Extensor hallucis longus	L5 to S1	0°–20°
Plantar flexion	Gastrocnemius Soleus	Plantaris Peroneus longus Flexor digitorum longus Flexor hallucis longus Tibialis posterior	L4 to S2	0°–50°
Inversion	Tibialis anterior Tibialis posterior	Flexor digitorum longus Flexor hallucis longus Extensor hallucis longus	L4 to L5	0°–45°
Eversion	Extensor digitorum longus Peroneus tertius Peroneus longus Peroneus brevis		L4 to S1	0°–30°

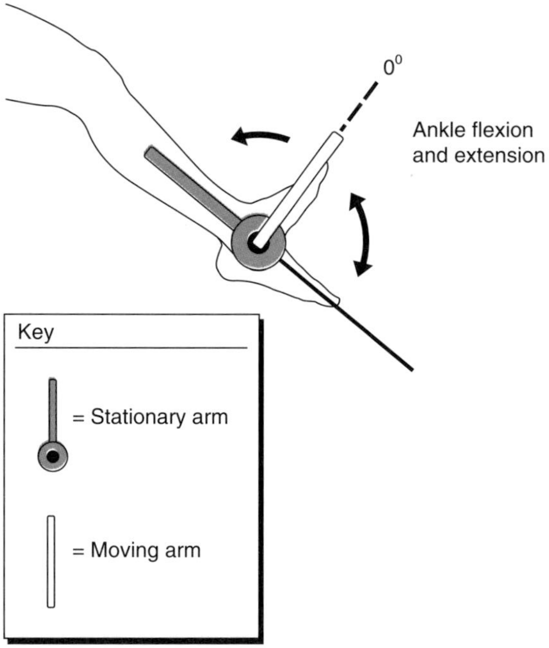

FIGURE 14–6. Measuring the range of motion of the ankle joint.

ANKLE AND FOOT STRETCHES

Calf Stretch (Fig. 14–7)

Prime movers: gastrocnemius, soleus, and hamstrings.

- Stand facing the pool wall, and hold on to the edge of the pool with the elbows straight and the legs together
- Take one step forward with the uninvolved leg, touching the toes against the pool wall, while simultaneously bending the elbows as the trunk moves forward
- Keep the heel of the back foot on the floor
- Push the hips forward and the back heel down, using the edge of the pool for stability to counteract the upward thrust of buoyancy.
- Hold, then return to the original position

Forefoot, Calf Stretch (Fig. 14–8)

Prime movers: gastrocnemius, soleus, flexor digitorum longus, flexor digitorum brevis, and flexor hallucis longus.

- Stand facing the pool wall, and hold on to the edge of the pool with the elbows straight and the legs together
- Take one step forward with the involved leg, placing the heel near the wall and the toes up on the wall, while simultaneously bending the elbows as the trunk moves forward
- Keep the heel of the back foot on the floor
- Push downward on the front heel, using the edge of the pool for stability to counteract the upward thrust of buoyancy
- Hold, then return to the original position

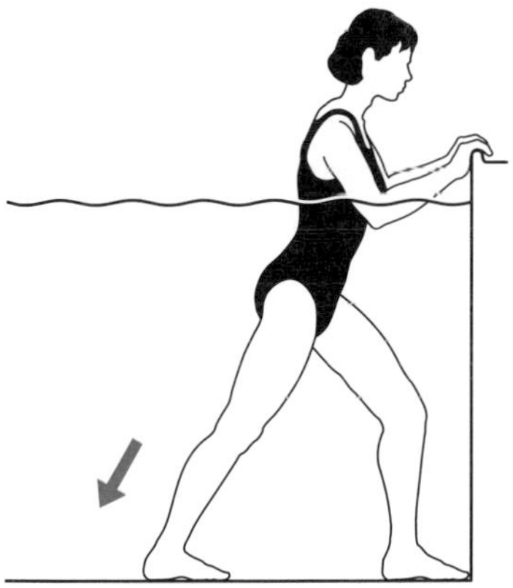

FIGURE 14–7. Calf stretch.

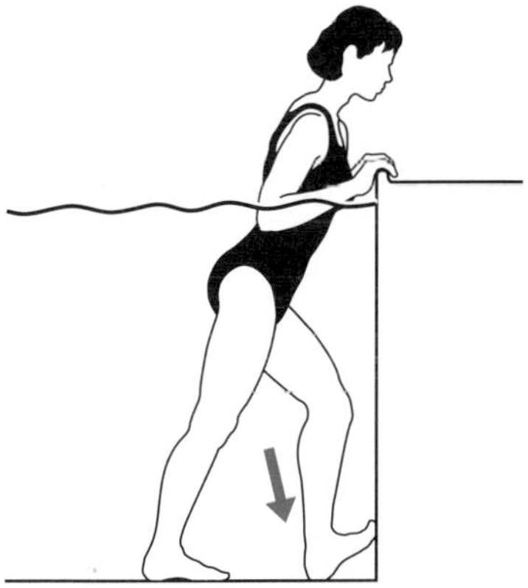

FIGURE 14–8. Forefoot, calf stretch.

Shin Stretch (Fig. 14–9)

Prime movers: tibialis anterior, extensor digitorum longus, extensor digitorum brevis, extensor hallucis longus, extensor hallucis brevis, and lumbricales.

- Stand facing the pool wall, and flex the knee of the involved leg so that the dorsal surface of the toes of the foot are on the pool floor
- Slowly press the dorsal surface of the foot toward the floor
- Hold, then relax

Soleus Stretch (Fig. 14–10)

Prime mover: soleus.

- Stand facing the pool wall, and hold on to the edge of the pool with the elbows straight and the legs together
- Take one step forward with the involved leg, placing the toes against the pool wall
- Keeping the heel of the back foot on the floor, bend the back knee
- Hold, then return to the original position

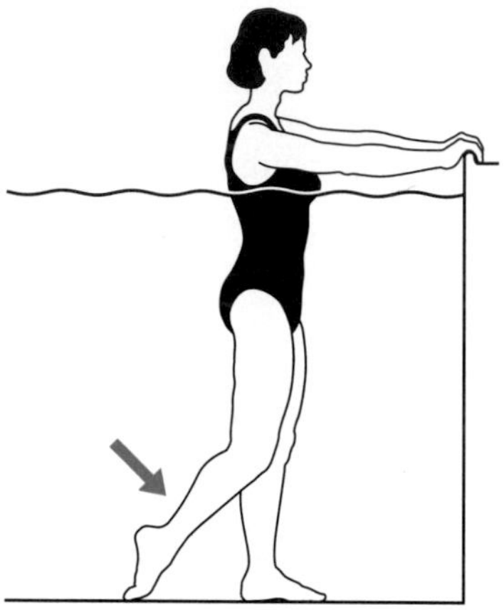

FIGURE 14–9. Shin stretch.

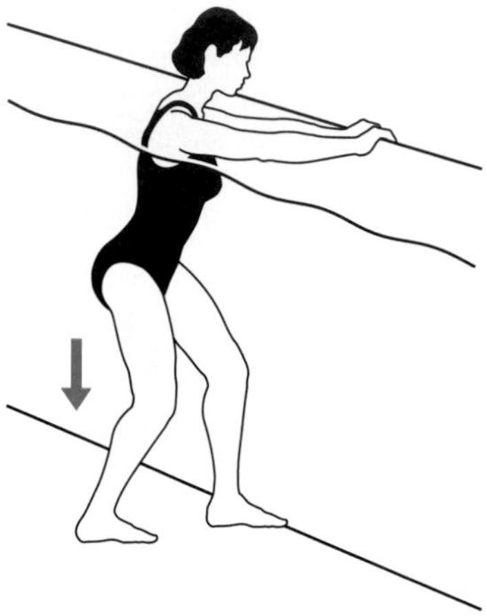

FIGURE 14–10. Soleus stretch.

Plantar Fascia Stretch (Fig. 14–11)

Prime movers: flexor digitorum longus, flexor digitorum brevis, flexor hallucis longus, gastrocnemius, and soleus.

- Stand with the ball of the foot on the stair of the pool ladder or a platform
- Drop the heel below the level of the step until a stretch is felt through the arch of the foot
- Hold, then return to the original position

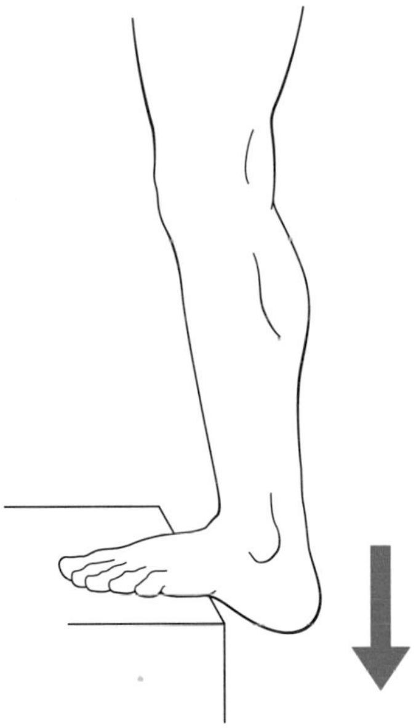

FIGURE 14–11. Plantar fascia stretch.

ANKLE AND FOOT EXERCISES

Ankle Dorsiflexion (Fig. 14–12)

Prime mover: tibialis anterior.

- Stand with the back against the pool wall and the involved leg extended in front of the body
- Slowly lift the toes toward the head (dorsiflexion)
- Hold, then relax

VARIATION: Place an ankle weight on the forefoot to increase the resistancc

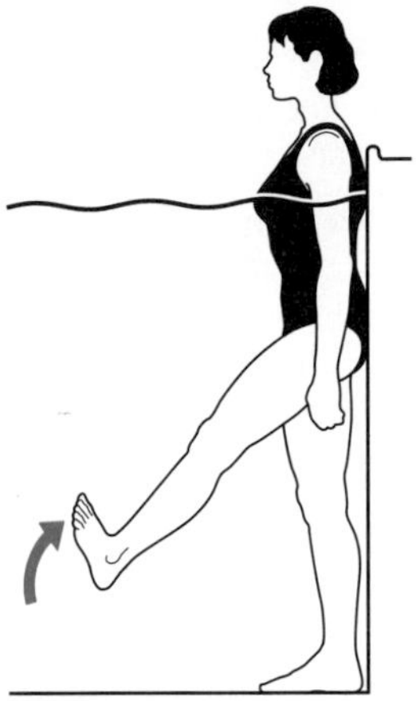

FIGURE 14–12. Ankle dorsiflexion.

Ankle Plantar Flexion (Fig. 14–13)

Prime movers: gastrocnemius and soleus

- Stand with thc back against the pool wall and the involved leg extended in front of the body
- Slowly press the toes toward the bottom of the pool (plantar flexion)
- Hold, then relax

VARIATION: Place an ankle float on the forefoot to increase the resistance

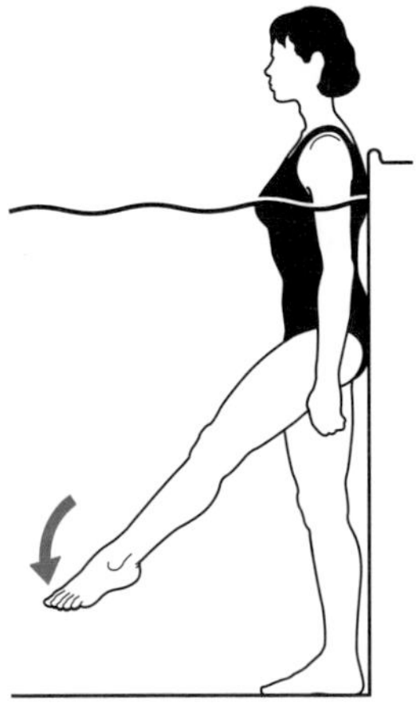

FIGURE 14–13. Ankle plantar flexion.

Ankle Eversion and Inversion (Fig. 14–14)

Prime movers: Peroneus longus, peroneus brevis, tibialis posterior, and tibialis anterior.

- Stand with the back against the pool wall and the involved leg extended in front of the body
- Keeping the leg stationary, turn the outer border of the foot outward (eversion) and then inward (inversion)

VARIATIONS: Place an ankle weight on the forefoot to increase the resistance

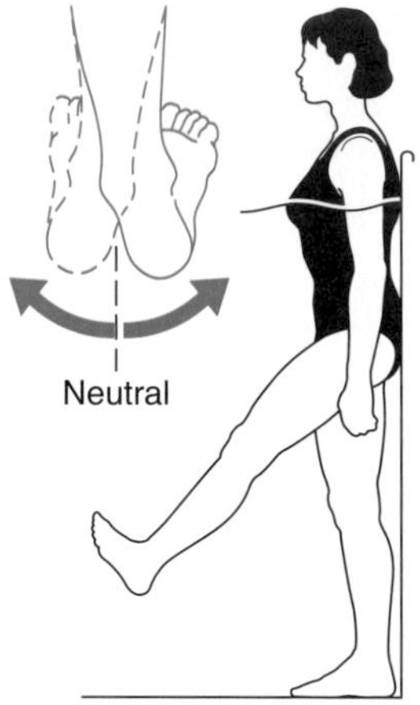

FIGURE 14–14. Ankle eversion and inversion.

Ankle Alphabet (Fig. 14–15)

Prime movers: gastrocnemius, soleus, peronei, tibialis anterior, and tibialis posterior.

- Stand with the back against the pool wall and the involved leg extended in front of the body
- Using the ankle and foot only, trace the letters of the alphabet with the big toe in the water

VARIATION: Place an ankle weight on the forefoot to increase the resistance

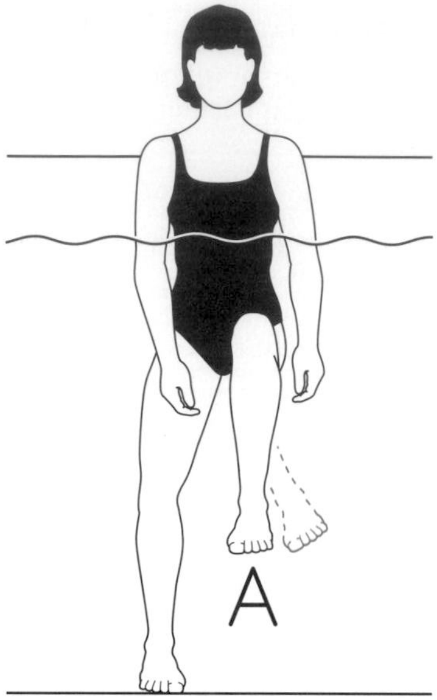

FIGURE 14–15. Ankle alphabet.

Heel Raises (Fig. 14–16)

Prime movers: gastrocnemius and soleus.

- Holding on to the edge of the pool, slowly raise on to the toes
- Hold, then relax
- The deeper the water, the less the resistance

VARIATION: Raise onto the toes of one leg at a time

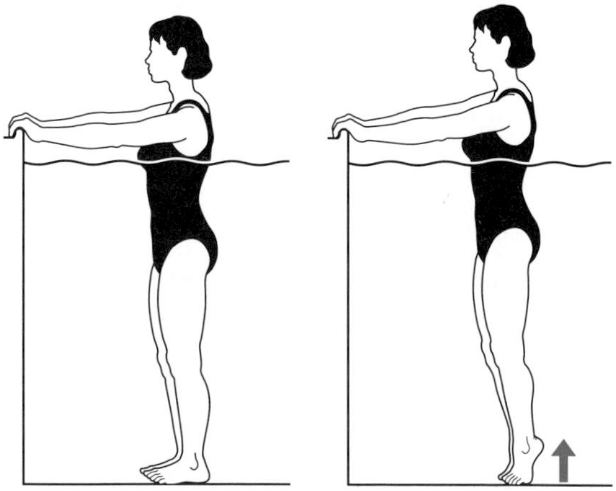

FIGURE 14–16. Heel raises.

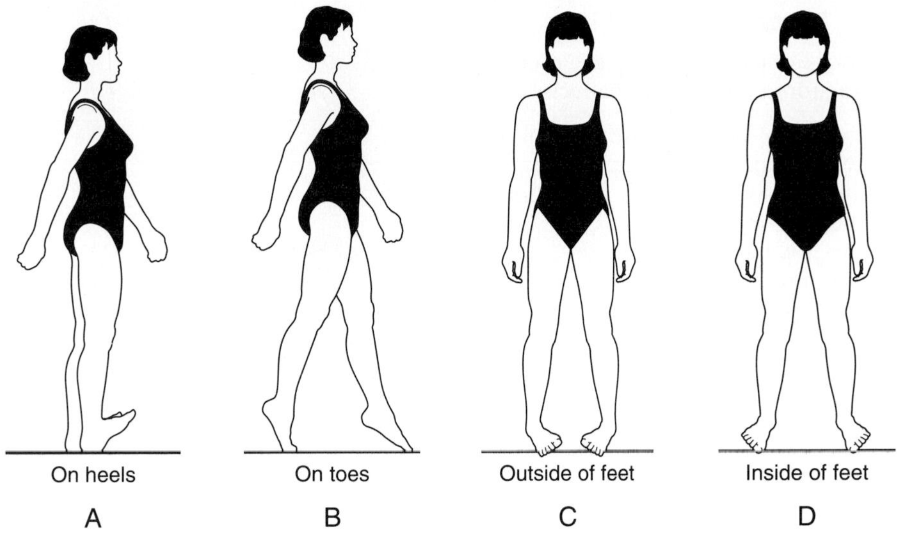

FIGURE 14–17. Ankle walking.

Ankle Walking (Fig. 14–17)

Prime movers: gastrocnemius, soleus, peronei, tibialis anterior, and tibialis posterior. This exercise is performed in four parts:

Part A

Walk on the heels: dorsiflex the forefoot as far as possible and walk forward on the heels

Part B

Walk on the toes: plantar flex the forefoot and walk forward on the toes

Part C

Walk on the outer edge of the feet

Part D

Walk on the inner edge of the feet

Hopping (Fig. 14–18)

Prime movers: quadriceps, hamstrings, gluteus maximus, hip flexors, hip adductors, gastrocnemius, and soleus.

- Stand upright and flex at the hips and knees
- Jump forward, using the arms to assist
- Land on both feet, bending at the knees to absorb the impact
- The deeper the water, the lower the impact forces

VARIATIONS: Hopping forward and backward; hopping on one leg; hopping from side-to-side; hopping on one spot

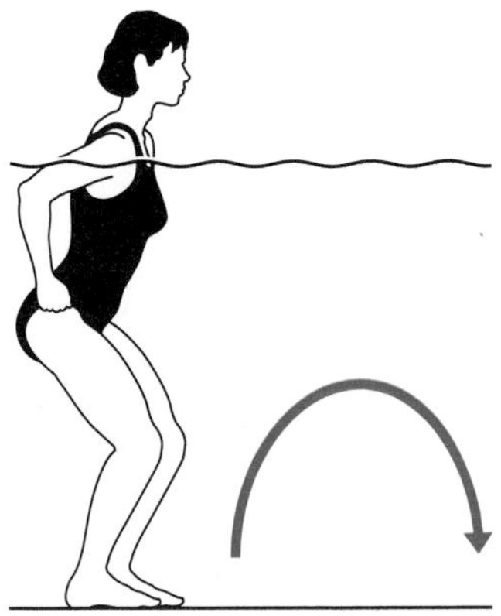

FIGURE 14–18. Hopping.

Toe Flexion and Extension (Fig. 14–19)

Prime movers: extensor hallucis, extensor digitorum, flexor digitorum, and flexor hallucis.

- Stand with the back against the pool wall
- Shift weight to the involved leg
- Curl the toes down toward the bottom of the pool (extension)
- Hold briefly, then relax
- Flex toes upward
- Hold briefly, then relax

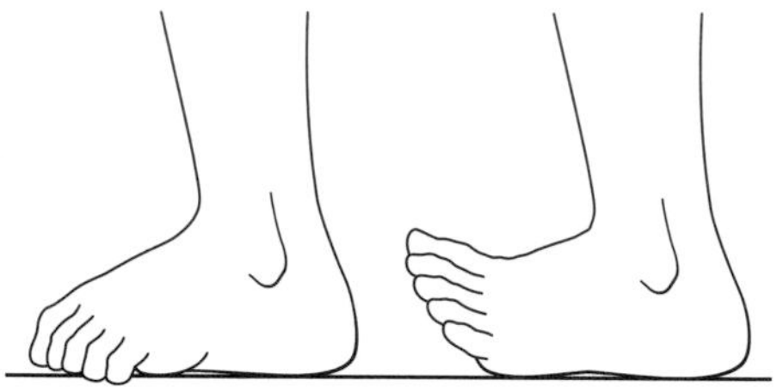

FIGURE 14–19. Toe flexion and extension.

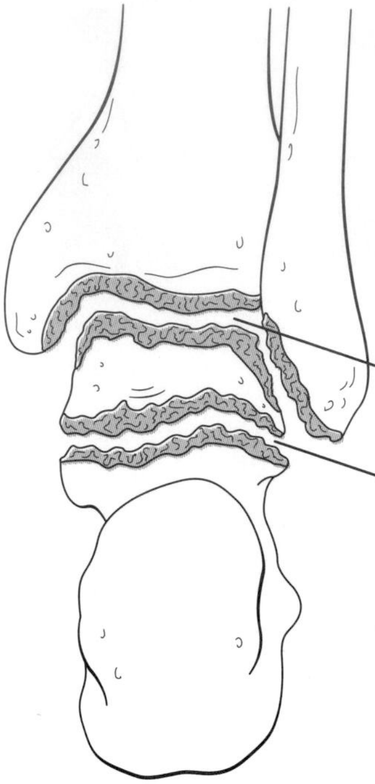

FIGURE 14–20. Ankle arthritis.

COMMON CONDITIONS OF THE ANKLE AND FOOT

Ankle Arthritis

This general term can be used whenever any of the arthritic conditions described in Chapter 7 involve the ankle joint.

Origin

Arthritis of the ankle is relatively common because it is a weight-bearing joint. It is also common for an old ankle fracture that involved the joint to develop into arthritis.

Pathology

Arthritis can affect either the talocrural joint (between the talus and the socket formed by the tibia and the fibula) or the subtalar joint (talocalcaneal joint). These are depicted in Figure 14–20. The various pathologic processes are described in Chapter 7.

Signs and Symptoms

The pain, decreased range of motion, and decreased strength contribute to poor gait. An arthritic ankle may cause a limp that is severe enough to require a walking aid.

Body Parts Affected

- Bones (tibia, fibula, talus, calcaneus)
- Joint surfaces (articular cartilage)
- Soft tissues (joint capsule, muscles, tendons, ligaments)

Exercise Priorities

- Establish a controlled exercise program (be careful that the patient does not overdo it)
- Maximize range of motion
- Strengthen all ankle muscles
- Correct balance and gait abnormalities

Ankle Fracture

Ankle fractures most often involve the tibia and fibula. Less common are fractures of the talus or the calcaneus.

Origin

An ankle eversion injury can result in a fracture of the lateral malleolus. Inversion injuries can also result in fractures, but they are usually small avulsion fractures, in which a piece of the bone breaks off before the ligament tears (Fig. 14–21). Fractures of both the tibia and the fibula are commonly the result of a direct blow, such as would occur in a motor vehicle accident.

Pathology

If there is no displacement, these fractures are splinted or placed in a cast. If there is significant displacement or if the fracture enters the joint, internal fixation is used. With internal fixation, aquatic therapy can begin as soon as the incisions are healed. It is still important, however, to find out if the surgeon has placed any weight-bearing restrictions on the patient.

Signs and Symptoms

Pain, stiffness, and swelling are present to some degree. Although the most important goal of treatment is to increase range of motion, pushing the patient too hard can cause increased pain and swelling, which in the long run may slow the rehabilitation process.

Body Parts Affected

- Bones (tibia, fibula, talus, calcaneus)
- Muscles of the ankle and foot
- Ligaments of the ankle (also may be injured)

Exercise Priorities

- Restore range of motion
- Strengthen ankle muscles
- Restore balance and coordination
- Correct gait abnormalities

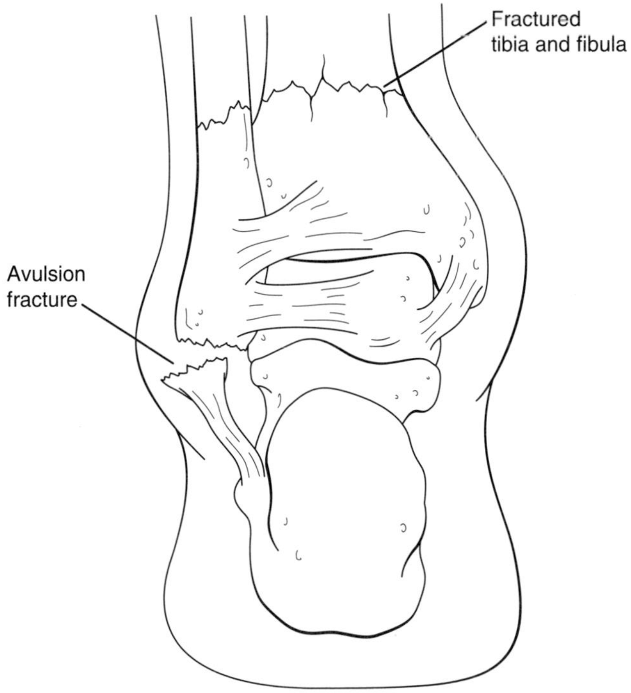

FIGURE 14–21. Ankle fracture.

Ankle Sprain

This well-known injury involves one or more ligaments of the ankle.

Origin

The most common type of ankle sprain is an inversion sprain. This occurs when the ankle is forced into inversion, which stresses the lateral ligaments (Fig. 14–22).

Pathology

The pathology of a sprain is outlined in Chapter 7. The most commonly involved ligaments are the anterior talofibular, calcaneofibular, and posterior talofibular. Of these, the anterior talofibular is sprained most often.

Signs and Symptoms

Although some swelling is always present, pain is usually the factor that limits range of motion. It is often beneficial to treat this injury first with physical therapy modalities. It is also beneficial to use taping to control swelling while the injury is acute. As rehabilitation progresses, it becomes evident that balance, coordination, and ankle muscle strength are also lacking.

Body Parts Affected

- Ankle ligaments (anterior talofibular, calcaneofibular, posterior talofibular)
- Ankle bones (rule out fracture of tibia, fibula, or talus)
- Ankle muscles

Exercise Priorities

- Restore range of motion
- Strengthen ankle muscles
- Improve balance and coordination (to decrease the risk of respraining ankle)

Achilles Tendon Injury

This term refers to an injury to the gastrocnemius muscle–Achilles tendon complex (Fig. 14–23).

Origin

Achilles tendonitis is caused by a repetitive activity such as hiking or cycling. A first-, second-, or third-degree strain of the gastrocnemius muscle or a rupture of the Achilles tendon usually occurs during an activity that involves an explosive pushing off with one foot (eg, raquetball, basketball, skiing).

Pathology

The pathology of a strain is outlined in Chapter 7. If the injury involves a complete tear, it is often repaired surgically. Some doctors may choose to treat it conservatively by securing the ankle in a cast in a plantarflexed position. In either case, recovery takes up to a year.

Signs and Symptoms

A patient with Achilles tendonitis has increased pain during the push-off phase of gait and when the calf is stretched. The patient may also walk with the leg externally rotated to avoid dorsiflexion (which

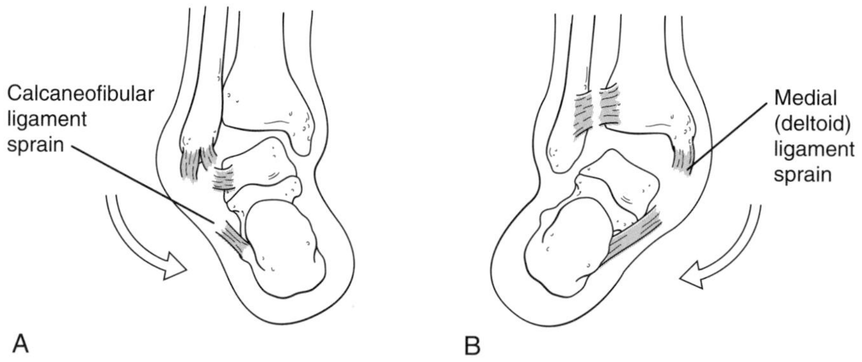

FIGURE 14–22. Ankle sprain (left posterior view). *A,* Inversion. *B,* Eversion.

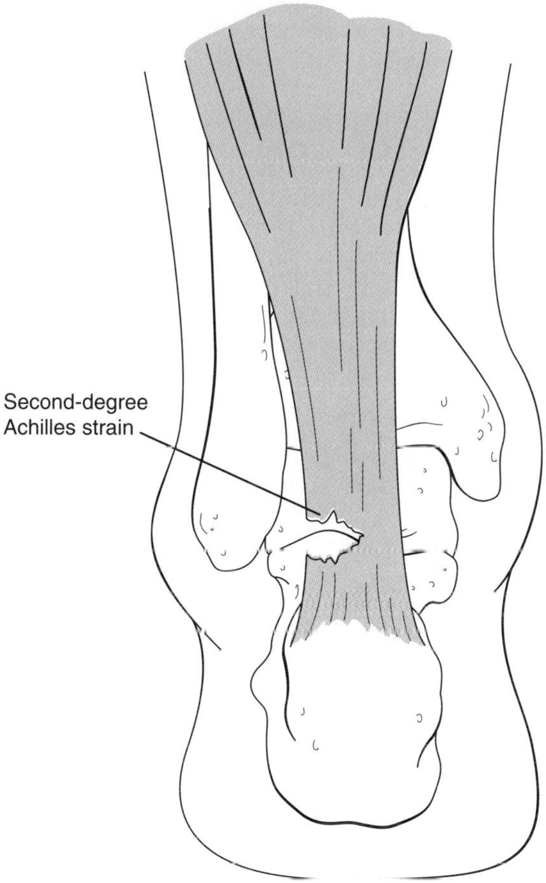

FIGURE 14–23. Achilles tendon strain.

would stretch the Achilles). If the tendonitis becomes chronic, a lump of scar tissue may form on the Achilles tendon. Tears in the gastrocnemius muscle or in the Achilles tendon must be large for the examiner to palpate the defect.

Body Parts Affected

- Muscles (gastrocnemius and soleus)
- Achilles tendon

Exercise Priorities

- Restore range of motion (stretch Achilles tendon)
- Strengthen calf muscles
- Improve balance and coordination

Plantar Fasciitis

Plantar fasciitis is an inflammation of the plantar fascia (Fig. 14–24).

Origin

This is commonly an overuse injury. Improper or worn-out footwear (lacking in arch support) is often a contributing factor. Treatment of the pathology without rectifying the cause may be fruitless.

Pathology

Plantar fasciitis is basically a tendonitis that occurs where the intrinsic muscles of the foot attach to the calcaneus. The pathology of tendonitis discussed in Chapter 7 therefore applies to this condition. If the condition is persistent, a heel spur may develop at the point at which the plantar fascia attaches to the calcaneus.

Signs and Symptoms

The only objective finding with this condition is point tenderness at the insertion of the plantar fas-

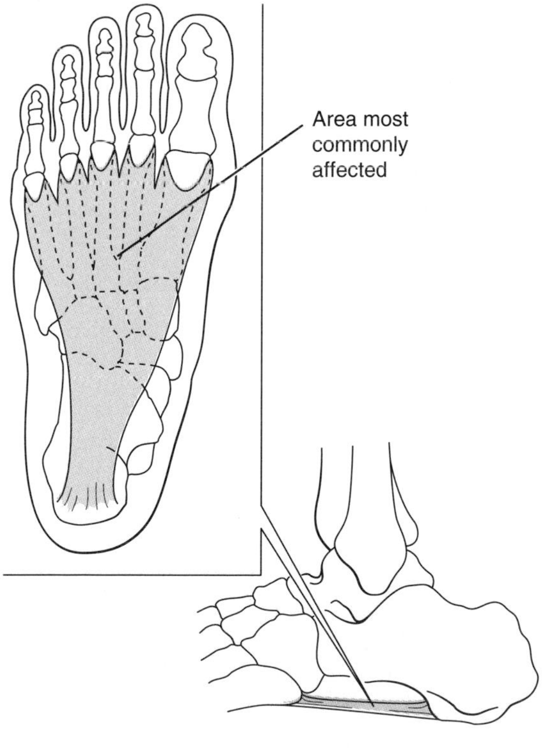

FIGURE 14–24. Plantar fasciitis.

cia, which is exacerbated by weight bearing. Range of motion is usually full, and stretching does not always reproduce the pain.

Body Parts Affected

- Plantar fascia
- Intrinsic muscles of the foot
- Gastrocnemius-soleus muscle complex

Exercise Priorities

- Stretch plantar fascia and gastrocnemius-soleus complex
- Strengthen intrinsic foot muscles
- Improve balance and coordination

Shin Splints

The common term "shin splints" covers several conditions that cause anterior lower leg pain (Fig. 14–25).

Origin

Shin splints have a variety of causes:

- running on hard or uneven terrain
- muscle imbalance between dorsiflexors and plantar flexors
- heels of running shoes too high or too low
- patient overweight
- poor flexibility in lower leg

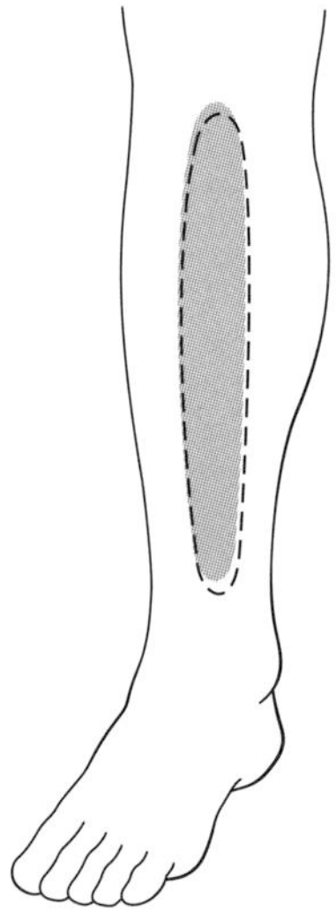

FIGURE 14–25. Typical area of shin splint pain.

- anatomic predisposition (ie, pronated foot or short Achilles tendon)
- overuse

Pathology

As previously mentioned, the term shin splints is used for several different conditions. The most straightforward of these is tendonitis of the anterior compartment muscles. Stress fractures are also common causes of shin pain. Periostitis (muscle being pulled away from its insertion) and inflammation of the interosseous membrane (between the tibia and fibula) are additional types of shin splints.

Signs and Symptoms

All of these conditions result in pain. The pain often increases with running but may decrease, in some cases after a good warm-up. Decreased ankle range of motion also may accompany the pain.

Body Parts Affected

- Bones (tibia, fibula, bones of the foot)
- Muscles and tendons of the lower leg
- Interosseous membrane

Exercise Priorities

- Restore full range of motion
- Restore muscle balance between doriflexors and plantar flexors
- Improve balance and coordination

THE AQUATIC EXERCISE THERAPY PROTOCOL FOR CONDITIONS OF THE ANKLE AND FOOT

Phase One

Warm-up

Perform each exercise for 2 minutes.

- Forward Walking (see Fig. 5–21)
- Backward Walking (see Fig. 5–22)
- Side Stepping (see Fig. 5–23)

Stretch

Perform six repetitions of each exercise, holding for 10 seconds.

- Calf Stretch (see Fig. 14–7)
- Soleus Stretch (see Fig. 14–10)
- Hamstring Stretch (see Fig. 13–10)
- Passive Quadriceps Stretch (see Fig. 13–6)
- Shin Stretch (see Fig. 14–9

Strengthen

Perform one set of 8 to 12 repetitions.

- Ankle Dorsiflexion (see Fig. 14–12)
- Ankle Plantar Flexion (see Fig. 14–13)
- Ankle Eversion and Inversion (see Fig. 14–14)
- Ankle Alphabet (see Fig. 14–15)
- Toe Flexion and Extension (see Fig. 14–19)

Phase Two

Warm-up

Perform each exercise for 2 minutes.

- Forward Walking (see Fig. 5–21)
- Backward Walking (see Fig. 5–22)
- Crossover Stepping (see Fig. 5–24)
- Bicycle (see Fig. 5–31)

Stretch

Perform five repetitions of each exercise, holding 20 seconds.

- Calf Stretch (see Fig. 14–7)
- Soleus Stretch (see Fig. 14–10)
- Lunge Stretch (see Fig. 13–9)
- Plantar Fascia Stretch (see Fig. 14–11)
- Shin Stretch (see Fig. 14–9)

Strengthen

Perform two sets of 8 to 12 repetitions.

- Ankle Dorsiflexion (see Fig. 14–12)
- Ankle Plantar Flexion (see Fig. 14–13)
- Ankle Eversion and Inversion (see Fig. 14–14)
- Side Stepping (see Fig. 5–23)
- Stork Stand (see Fig. 11–8)
- Heel Raises (see Fig. 14–16)

Phase Three

Warm-up

Perform each exercise for 2 minutes.

- Marching (see Fig. 5–28)
- Backward Walking (see Fig. 5–22)
- Crossover Stepping (see Fig. 5–24)
- Bicycle (see Fig. 5–31)

Stretch

Perform five repetitions of each exercise, holding 30 seconds.

- Calf Stretch (see Fig. 14–7)
- Soleus Stretch (see Fig. 14–10)
- Shin Stretch (see Fig. 14–9)
- Forefoot, Calf Stretch (see Fig. 14–8)

Strengthen

Perform three sets of 8 to 12 repetitions.

- Side Stepping (see Fig. 5–23)
- Stork Stand (see Fig. 11–8)
- Heel Raises (see Fig. 14–16)
- Four-Corner Pivot (see Fig. 11–11)
- Leg Balance Exercises (see Fig. 11–9)
- Ankle Walking (see Fig. 14–17)

Phase Four

Warm-up

Perform each exercise for 2 minutes.

- Marching (see Fig. 5–28)
- Backward Walking (see Fig. 5–22)
- Crossover Stepping (see Fig. 5–24)
- Leg Exchange (see Fig. 5–29)
- Jogging (see Fig. 5–30)

Stretch

Perform five repetitions of each exercise, holding 30 seconds.

- Calf Stretch (see Fig. 14–7)
- Soleus Stretch (see Fig. 14–10)
- Shin Stretch (see Fig. 14–9)
- Forefoot, Calf Stretch (see Fig. 14–8)

Strengthen

Perform four sets of 8 to 12 repetitions.

- Side Stepping (see Fig. 5–23)
- Stork Stand (see Fig. 11–8)
- Heel Raises (see Fig. 14–16)
- Four-Corner Pivot (see Fig. 11–11)
- Leg Balance Exercises (see Fig. 11–9)
- Ankle Walking (see Fig. 14–17)

REFERENCES

1. Magee D. Orthopedic Physical Assessment. Philadelphia: W.B. Saunders, 1987.
2. Gould J, Davis G. Orthopedic and Sports Physical Therapy. St. Louis: CV Mosby Company, 1985.
3. Green W, Heckman J. Measurement of Joint Motion. Rosemont, IL: American Academy of Orthopaedic Surgeons, 1994.
4. Arnheim D. Modern Principles of Athletic Training. St. Louis: Times Mirror/Mosby College Publishing, 1985.

Aquatic Rehabilitation of the Spine

CHAPTER 15

THE STRUCTURE AND FUNCTION OF THE SPINE

The spinal column consists of 33 vertebrae that extend from the occipital condyles of the neck to the base of the coccyx. The column can be divided into five regions: the cervical spine (7 vertebrae); the thoracic spine (12 vertebrae); the lumbar spine (5 vertebrae); the sacrum (5 fused vertebrae); and the coccyx (4 variably fused vertebrae). These divisions are shown in Figure 15–1.

Each vertebra is an individual movable segment, and the vertebrae are lined up one on top of the other. The vertebrae have certain anatomic characteristics in common: the vertebral body; two pedicles and two laminae, which enclose the vertebral

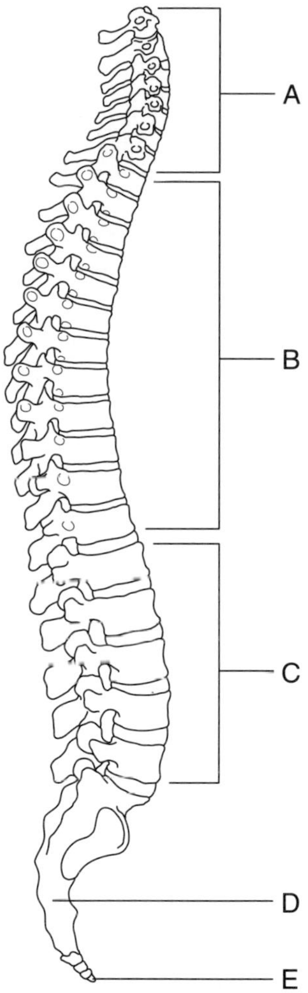

FIGURE 15–1. Regions of the spinal column: A, Cervical spine; B, thoracic spine; C, lumbar spine; D, sacrum; E, coccyx.

foramen; the spinous process; two transverse processes; and four articular processes, two articulating with the vertebra above and two with the vertebra below[1] (Fig. 15–2). The structure and shape of the vertebral features influence the range of motion permitted in each region of the spine.[2] For example, the superior and inferior articular processes of adjacent vertebrae in the cervical region are relatively flat, so that region of the spine can move freely. In the thoracic region, however, the intervertebral articulations permit somewhat less freedom of movement because of the length of the overlapping vertebral spines (that is, the plane of the facets). The design of the lumbar articulations restricts spinal rotation but allows relatively free movement in the two other planes.

Each pair of vertebrae is separated by an intervertebral disc. Each disc acts as a shock absorber for the spinal column to permit compression and distortion and thereby allow some degree of movement in all directions. Each disc has a "gelatinous" central mass called the nucleus, which is contained

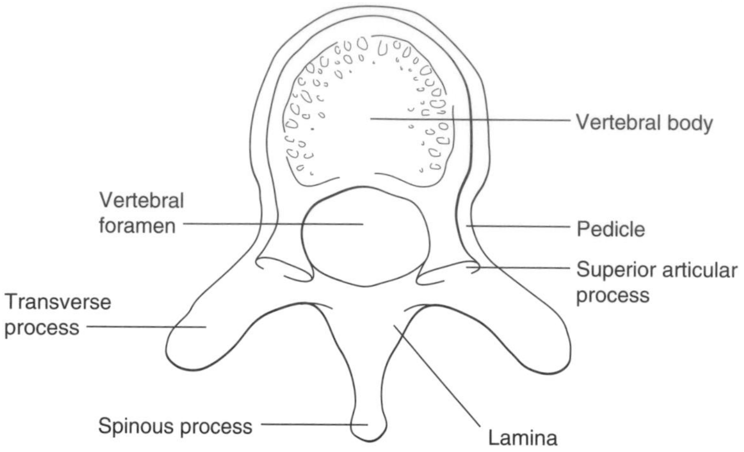

FIGURE 15–2. Features of a typical vertebra.

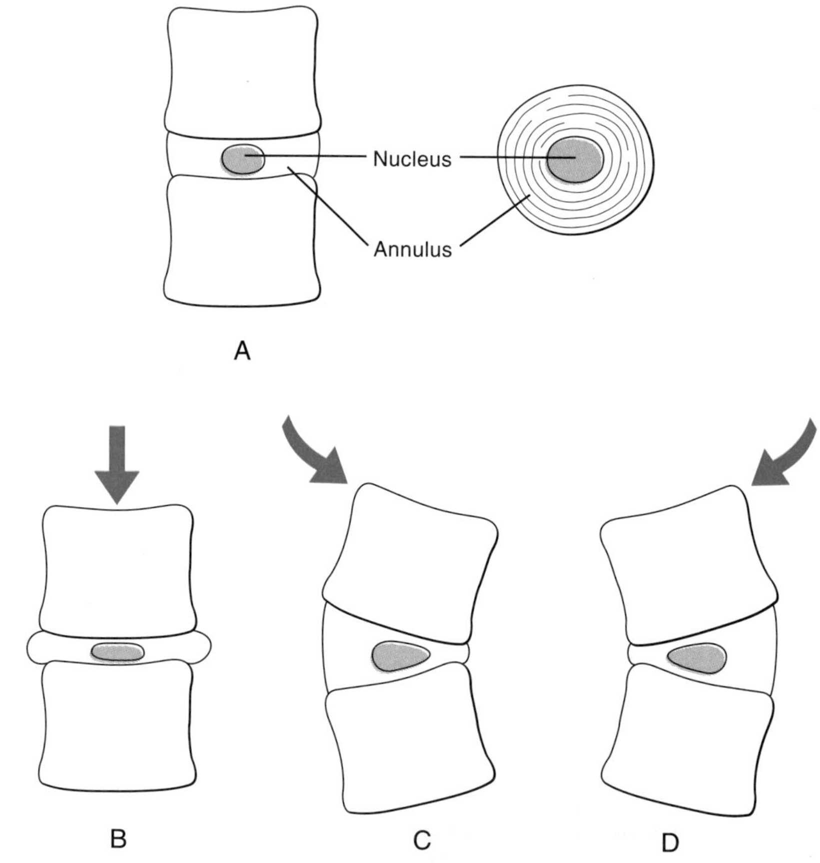

FIGURE 15–3. External forces cause pressure on the disc, deforming the nucleus. *A,* Normal disc space with nucleus intact. *B,* Compression. *C,* Extension. *D,* Flexion.

within elastic fibers, the annulus. External forces acting on the spine deform the nuclei of the discs. How the intervertebral disc reacts to pressure depends on the type and severity of the force (Fig. 15–3). A healthy disc returns quickly to its normal position after the force is removed.

Intervertebral disc lesions most commonly occur at levels at which there is a change from mobility to stability in the spine. The most vulnerable sites seem to be at L5-S1 and L4-L5 in the lumbar region and at C5-C6 and C6-C7 in the cervical spine.[3] The most common lesions are disc protrusion and extrusion (Fig. 15–4). As a disc ages, there is a loss in fluidity of the nucleus, so this type of injury is most common in younger individuals, usually between the ages of 20 and 55 years.

Strong ligaments run along the length of the spinal column, the anterior longitudinal ligament in front and the posterior longitudinal ligament behind the vertebral bodies. A series of elastic ligaments,

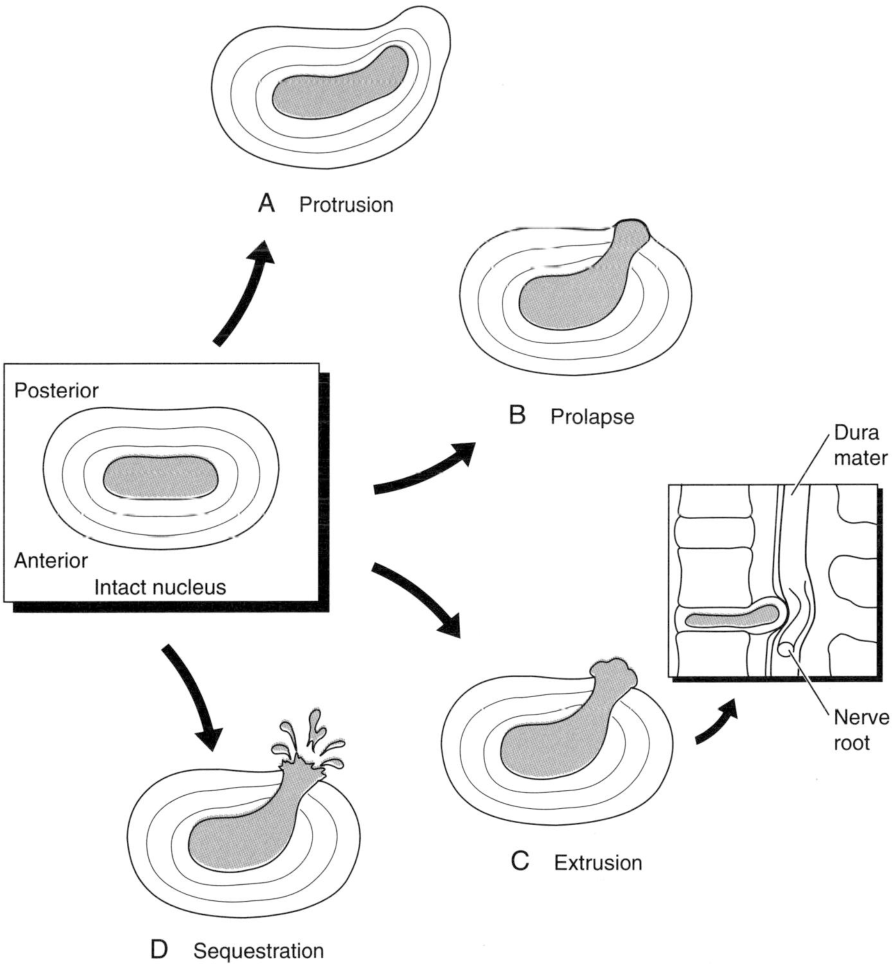

FIGURE 15–4. Types of disc herniation. *A,* Protrusion—annular fibers weaken and nuclear fluid bulges into the annulus. *B,* Prolapse—nuclear fluid bulges into the annulus, but it is still contained by the outermost fibers. *C,* Extrusion—nuclear fluid enters into the epidural space (disc herniation). *D,* Sequestration—nuclear fluid bursts and is free to move around epidural space. (Adapted from Magee D. Orthopedic Physical Assessment. Philadelphia: W.B. Saunders, 1987.)

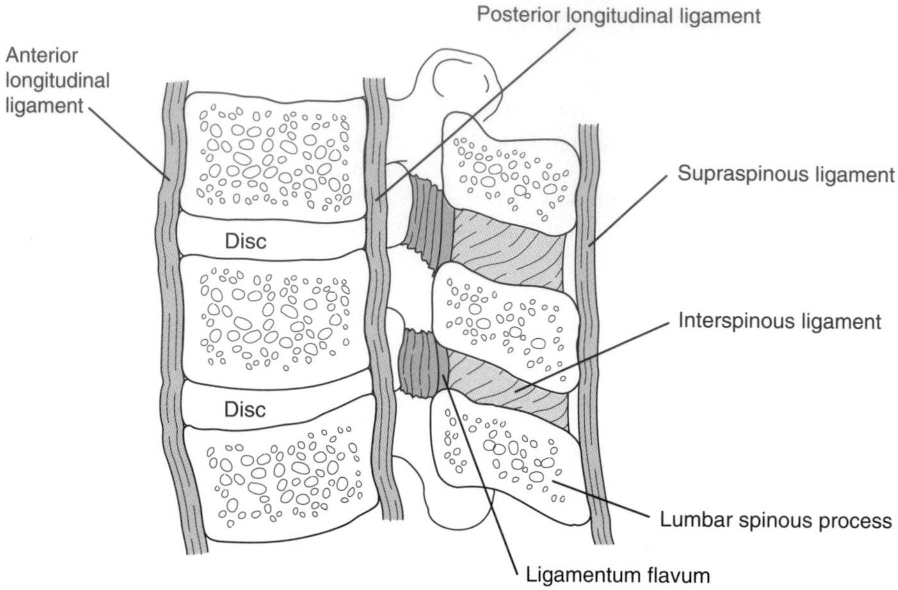

FIGURE 15–5. Spinal ligaments of the lumbar region.

the ligamenta flava, connect the laminae of the vertebrae and help restore the erect posture after flexion (Fig. 15–5).

The Anatomic Parts

CERVICAL SPINE. The cervical spine consists of seven vertebrae, numbered C1 through C7. The first two vertebrae, the atlas and the axis, are uniquely designed and function together to provide the majority of movement in this region (Fig. 15–6).

The atlanto-occipital joint occurs between the atlas of the vertebral column and the occipital condyles of the skull; it is the most superior joint. The atlas has no vertebral body or spinous processes and is designed to support the skull on the vertebral column (Fig. 15–7). This joint allows neck flexion and extension and some side flexion.

The atlantoaxial joint occurs between the atlas and the axis. The axis is the second cervical vertebra and is designed to allow rotation of the skull. The odontoid process looks like a small spike that fits into the atlas and acts as a pivot point (see Fig. 15–7).

The remaining cervical vertebrae are of more typical vertebral design and help to maintain the cervical curve. The greatest amount of neck flexion and extension occurs at C4-C5 and C5-C6.[4]

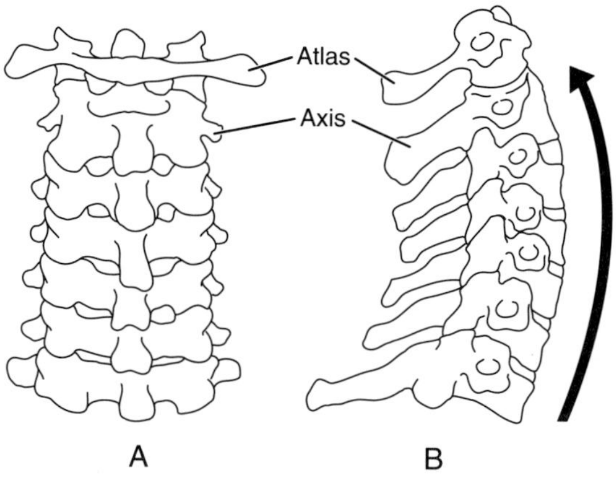

FIGURE 15–6. The cervical spine. *A,* Posterior view. *B,* Lateral view.

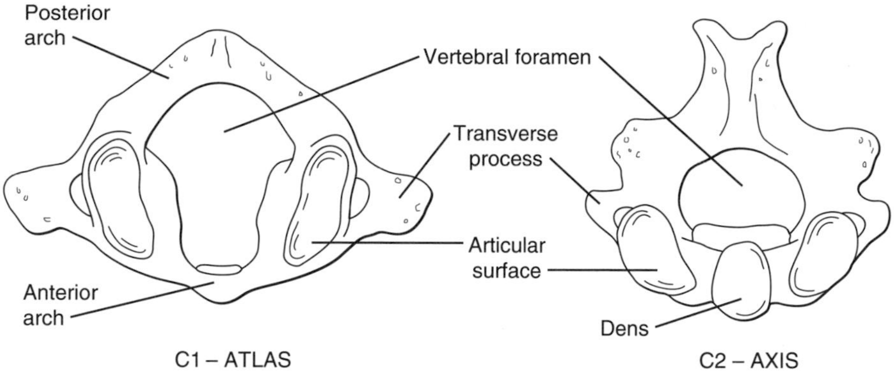

FIGURE 15–7. Structures of the atlas and the axis.

THORACIC SPINE. The thoracic spine consists of 12 vertebrae (Fig. 15–8). The costovertebral joints are synovial joints that occur between the vertebral bodies and the ribs. The costotransverse joints are synovial joints that occur between ribs 1 through 10 and the corresponding transverse processes of the vertebrae. The two floating ribs, ribs 11 and 12, do not attach directly to the spine (Fig. 15–9). Both costovertebral and costotransverse joints add stability to this area. The vertebrae of this region are very similar. The spinous processes are long and thin, angling downward at various levels. As a result, this region is quite rigid. The 12 ribs form the thorax or chest and function to protect the vital organs.

LUMBAR SPINE. The lumbar spine consists of five vertebrae. In erect posture, these vertebrae form a normal curve (lordosis). The vertebrae are large and strong and provide stability to the lower back (Fig. 15–10). In this region, the shape of the facet joints limits the amount of flexion, extension, lateral flexion, and rotation produced at each level. Most trunk flexion occurs at L5-S1, 15% to 70% occurs at L4-L5, and the remaining vertebrae provide 5% to 10% of trunk flexion.[5] Extension is the closed pack position of the lumbar region (the position in

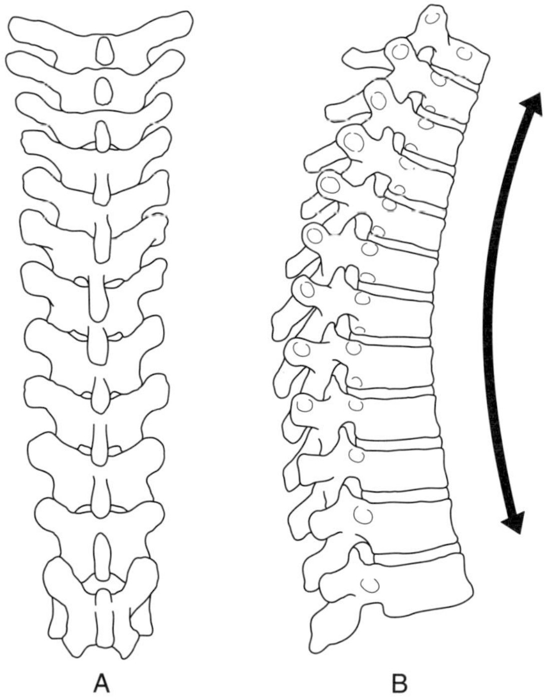

FIGURE 15–8. The thoracic spine. *A*, Posterior view. *B*, Lateral view.

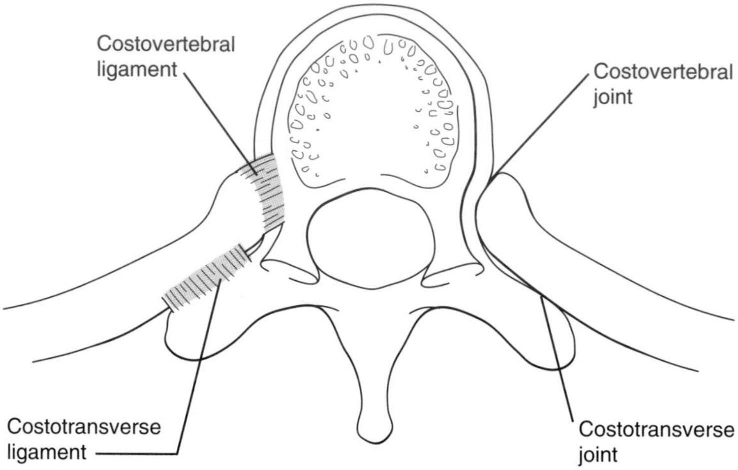

FIGURE 15–9. Joints of the thoracic spine.

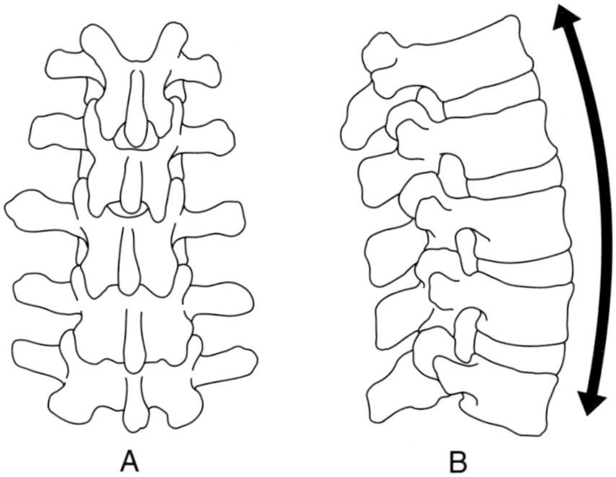

FIGURE 15–10. The lumbar spine. *A,* Posterior view. *B,* Lateral view.

which the facet joints are most compacted).[6] Rotation is minimal in the lumbar spine.

The lumbar spine is often the location of chronic or mechanical low back pain, vertebral degeneration, and numerous surgical procedures. Incorrect mechanics is perhaps the most common cause of pain, spasm, tension, and scoliosis.

The Muscles and Their Actions

A muscle must cross a joint in order to act directly on that joint. The way in which a muscle crosses a joint affects the action. The joints of the neck permit the following movements (Fig. 15–11):

- flexion and extension (Table 15–1)
- lateral flexion (Table 15–1)
- rotation (Table 15–2)

The joints of the trunk permit the following movements (Fig. 15–12):

- flexion and extension (Tables 15–3 and 15–4)
- lateral flexion
- rotation

The action of latissimus dorsi is outlined in Table 8–1.

Text continued on page 250

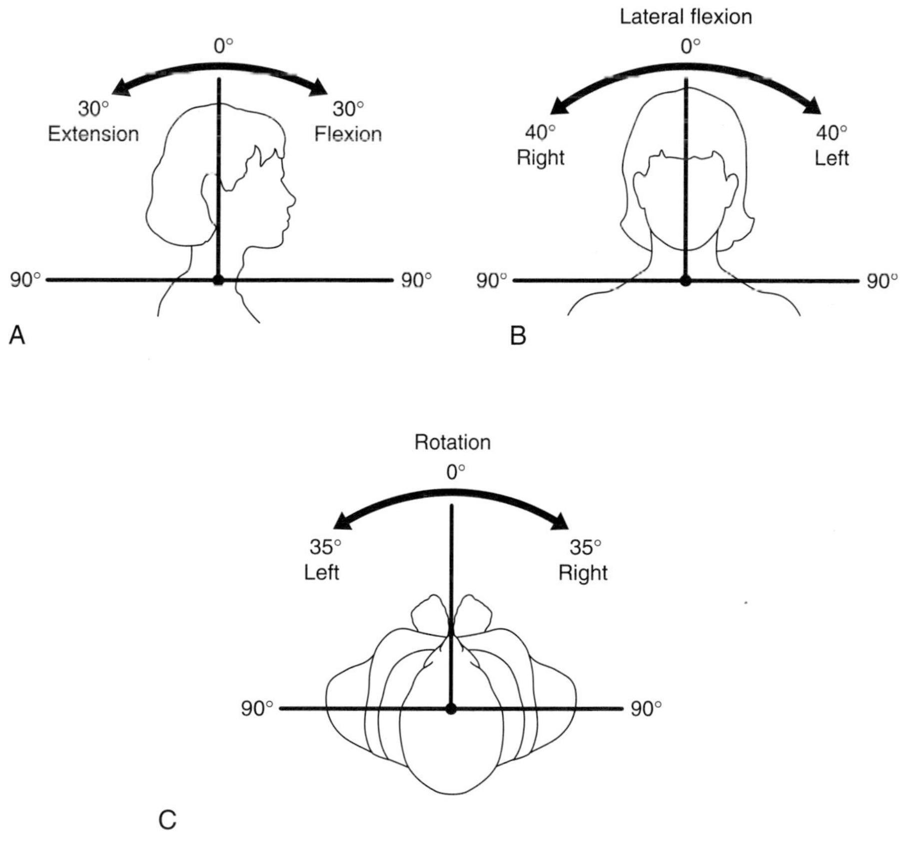

FIGURE 15–11. Movements of the cervical spine showing normal range of motion. *A,* Flexion and extension. *B,* Lateral flexion. *C,* Rotation.

TABLE 15–1. The Muscles Involved in Neck Flexion, Extension, and Lateral Flexion

Muscle	Origin (O)	Insertion (I)	Action
Sternocleidomastoid 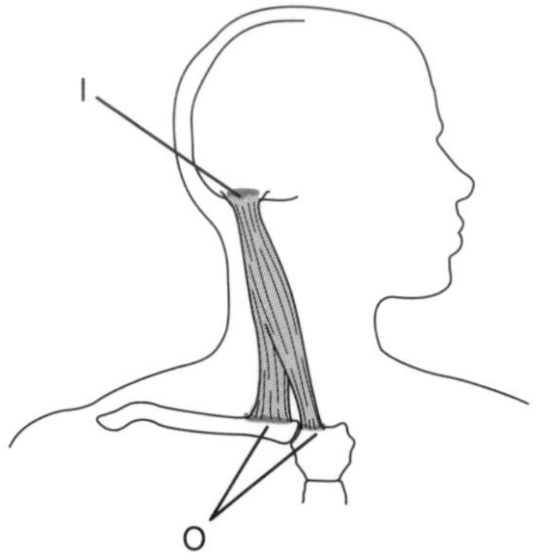 	Manubrium and medial third of the clavicle	Mastoid process of the temporal bone	Neck flexion Accessory movements: Neck extension Neck rotation Flexes upper vertebral column
Trapezius (superior fibers) 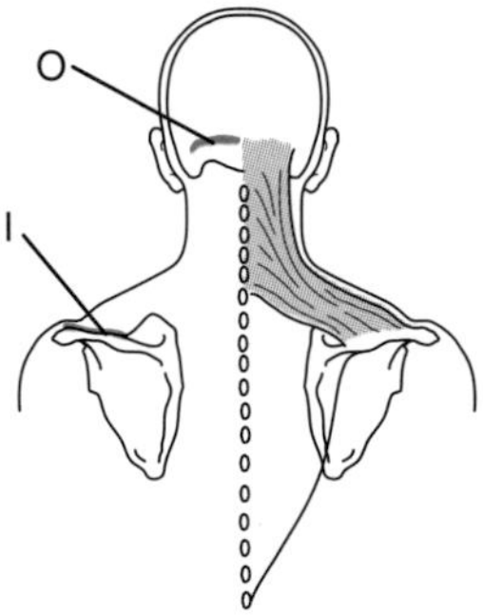 	Base of the skull Ligament of the neck	Lateral third of the clavicle (posterior border)	Neck extension Accessory movement: Scapular elevation
Splenius 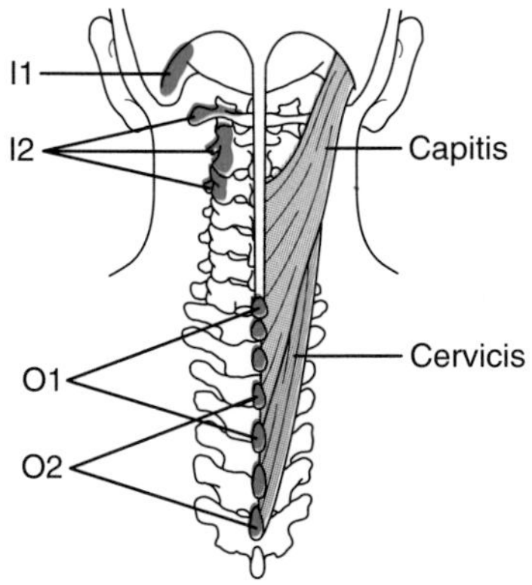 	Splenius capitis Ligamentum nuchae (lower half) Spinous processes (C7, T1-T4) Splenius cervicis Spinous process (T3-T6)	Occipital bone Mastoid process of the temporal bone Transverse processes, posterior tubercles (C1, C2, and C3)	Neck extension (and hyperextension) Accessory movements: Neck rotation Lateral flexion

TABLE 15–1. The Muscles Involved in Neck Flexion, Extension, and Lateral Flexion *Continued*

Muscle	Origin (O)	Insertion (I)	Action
Erector spinae: semispinalis 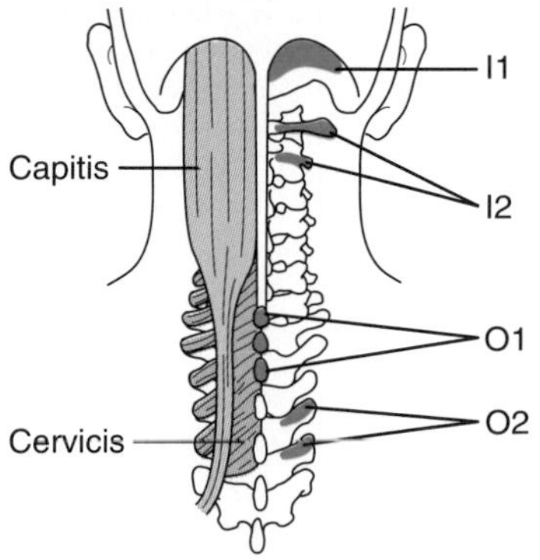	Semispinalis capitis Transverse processes (C7, T1-T7) Articular processes of C4, C5, and C6 Semispinalis cervicis Transverse processes of the upper five or six thoracic vertebrae	Occipital bone (between the superior and inferior nuchal lines) Spinous processes of axis to C5	Neck extension (and hyperextension) Accessory movement: Lateral flexion
Erector spinae 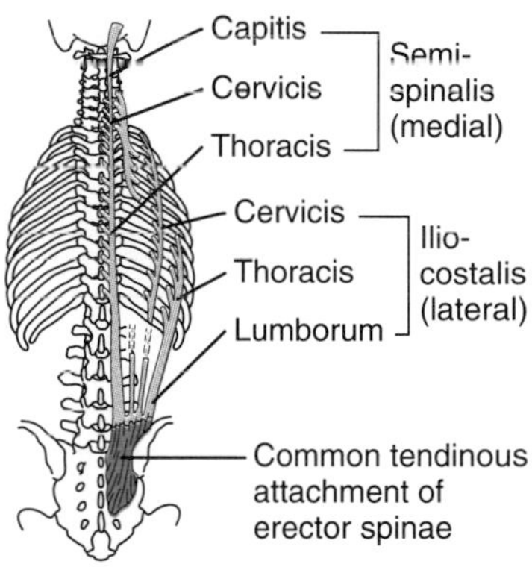	Transverse processes of the lower thoracic, upper thoracic, and C7 vertebrae Sacrum, iliac crest, angles of the lower and middle ribs	Spinous processes of the upper thoracic and cervical vertebrae and base of the skull Transverse processes of the lower cervical vertebrae and angles of the ribs	Extends the neck and trunk (capitis) Accessory movement: Lateral flexion Extends the trunk Accessory movement: Side bending to one side
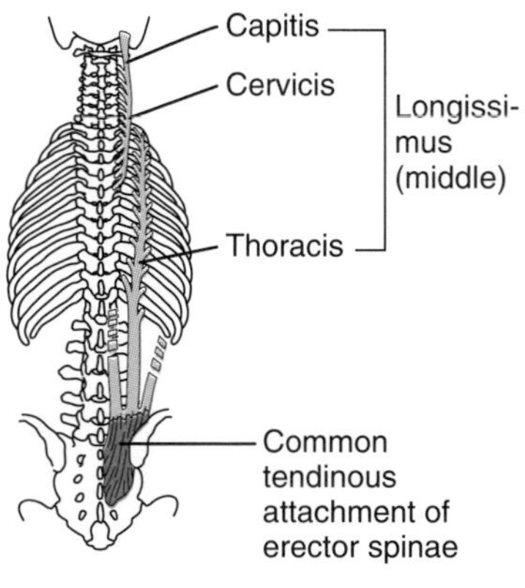	Transverse processes of the lower cervical, thoracic, and lumbar vertebrae	Inferior borders of the ribs, transverse processes of the vertebrae above, and base of the skull	Extends neck (capitis) Accessory movements: Rotates head (capitis) Extends trunk

TABLE 15–2. The Muscles Involved in Neck Rotation

Muscle	Origin (O)	Insertion (I)	Action
Rotators (deep to multifidus) 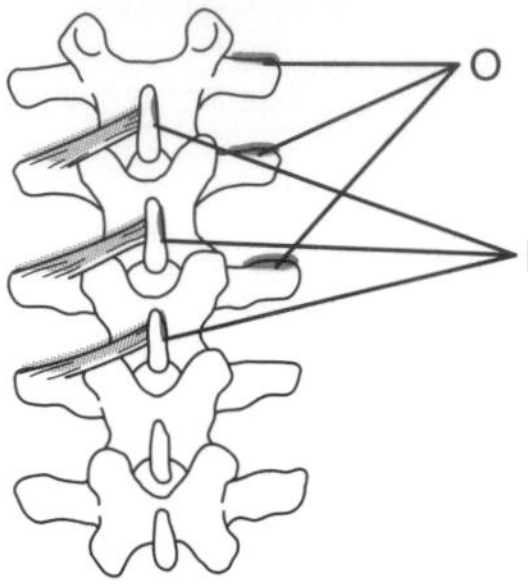	Transverse processes of the vertebrae	Bases of the spinous processes and laminae of the vertebrae above origin	Small rotational movements of the vertebral column Accessory movements: Extension and hyperextension of the spine when both sides act together
Multifidus 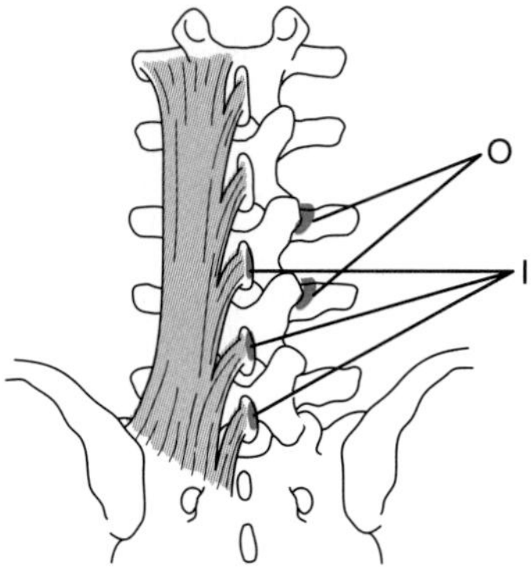	Posterior sacrum Dorsal end of the iliac crest Transverse processes of the lumbar and thoracic vertebrae Articular processes (C4-C7)	Spinous processes of all the vertebrae except the atlas	Rotation Accessory movements: Lateral flexion Extension and hyperextension of the spine

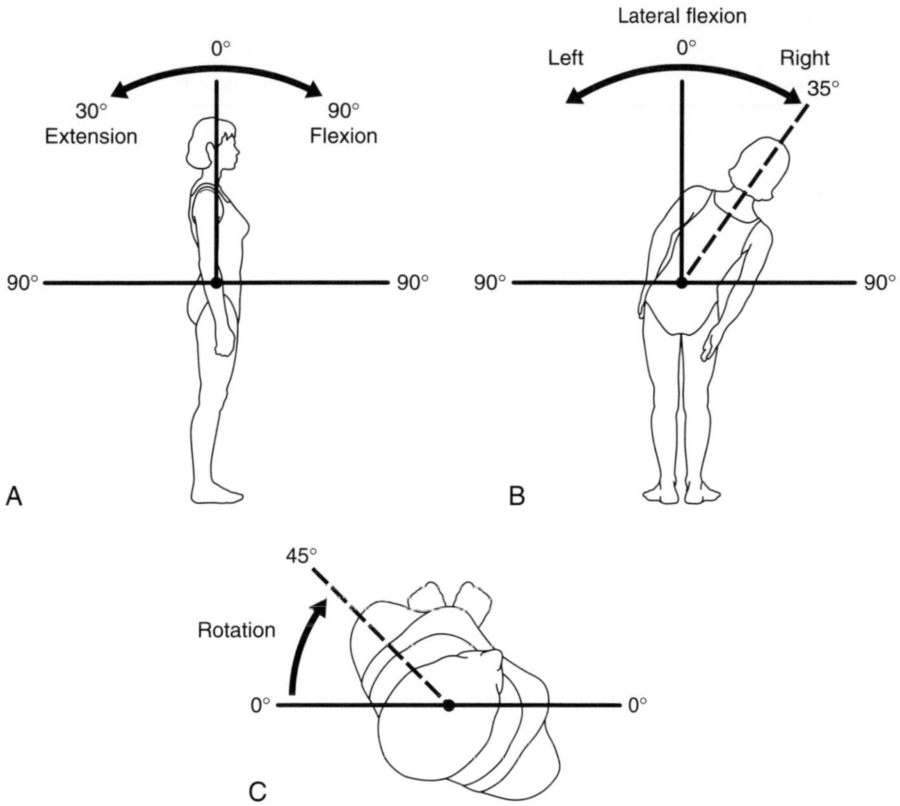

FIGURE 15–12. Movements of the lumbar and thoracic spine showing normal range of motion. *A*, Flexion and extension. *B*, Lateral flexion. *C*, Rotation.

TABLE 15–3. The Muscles Involved in Trunk Forward Flexion

Muscle	Origin (O)	Insertion (I)	Action
Rectus abdominis 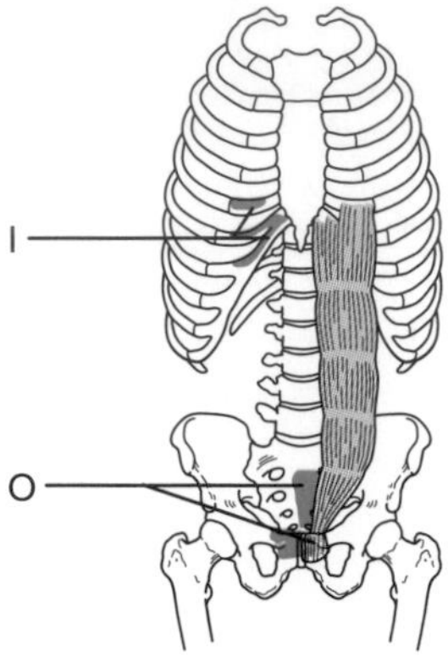	Pubic crest	Costal cartilages of ribs 5 to 7	Trunk flexion Accessory movement: Lateral flexion of the trunk to one side
External abdominal oblique 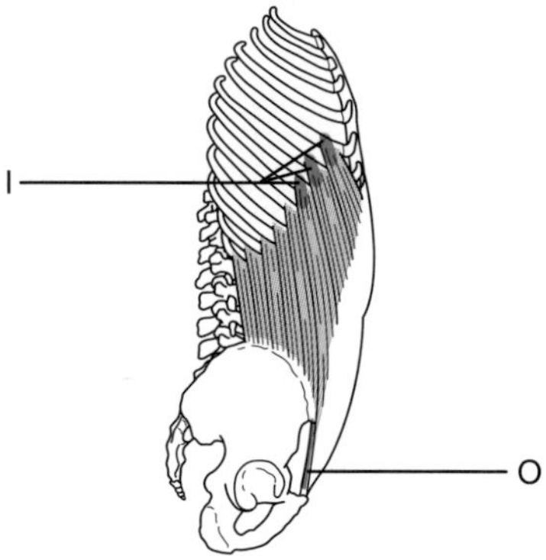	Inguinal ligament, linea alba, pubis, iliac crest	Outer surface of the lower eight ribs	Trunk flexion Accessory movement: Rotates the trunk to the same side
Internal abdominal oblique 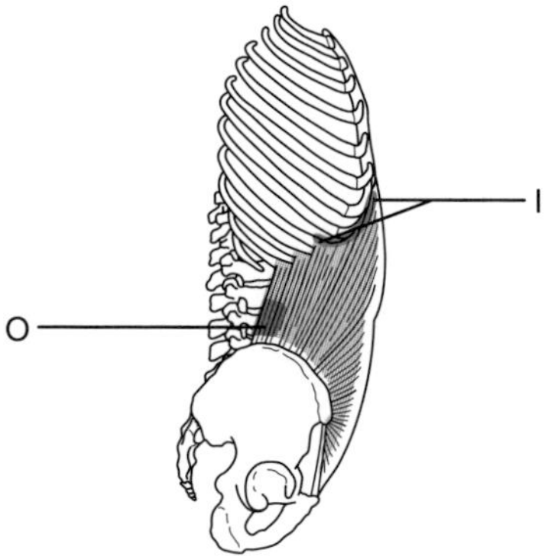	Inguinal ligament, iliac crest, lumbar fascia	Costal cartilages of ribs 8 to 10 Xiphoid process and linea alba	Trunk flexion Accessory movement: Rotates the trunk to the same side

TABLE 15–3. The Muscles Involved in Trunk Forward Flexion *Continued*

Muscle	Origin (O)	Insertion (I)	Action
Transverse abdominal oblique 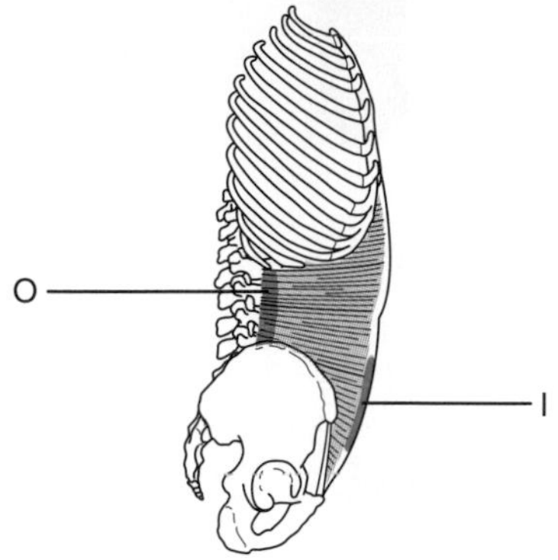	Inguinal ligament, iliac crest, costal cartilage of ribs 6 to 12 Lumbar fascia	Xiphoid process, linea alba, pubis	Compresses abdomen Trunk flexion Accessory movement: Assists forced expiration
Psoas major (See hip flexion)			

TABLE 15–4. The Muscles Involved in Trunk Extension

Muscle	Origin (O)	Insertion (I)	Action
Quadratus lumborum 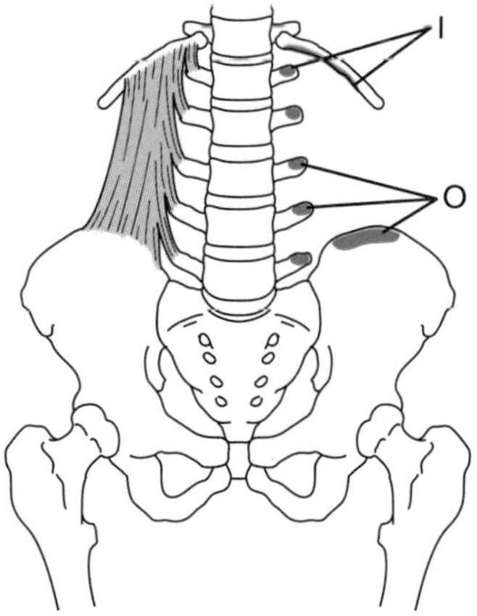	Iliac crest and lower lumbar vertebrae	Upper lumbar vertebrae and rib 12	Trunk extension (lower back) Accessory movement: Lateral flexion to one side
Other muscles involved in trunk extension: **Erector spinae** **Latissimus dorsi** **Interspinales**			

STRETCHES FOR THE SPINE

Neck Stretches

Neck Side Stretch (Fig. 15–13)

Prime movers: trapezius, semispinalis capitis, splenius capitis, splenius cervicis, and levator scapulae.

- Grasp the arm of the involved side above the wrist
- Pull the arm downward and across the body with the other hand
- Gently tilt the head away from the shoulder being pulled
- Hold, then relax

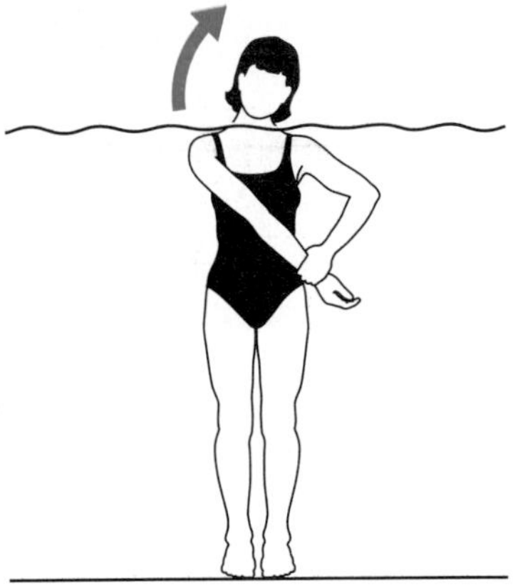

FIGURE 15–13. Neck side stretch.

Upper Trapezius Stretch (Fig. 15–14)

Prime movers: trapezius, semispinalis capitis, splenius capitis, splenius cervicis, and levator scapulae.

- Reach over the top of the head with the (uninvolved) left arm, putting the left middle finger over the right ear
- Put the right hand behind the back
- Gently pull the head toward the left shoulder looking straight ahead
- Hold, then relax

PROGRESSION: After the neck has been side-flexed, rotate the head to look up toward the ceiling

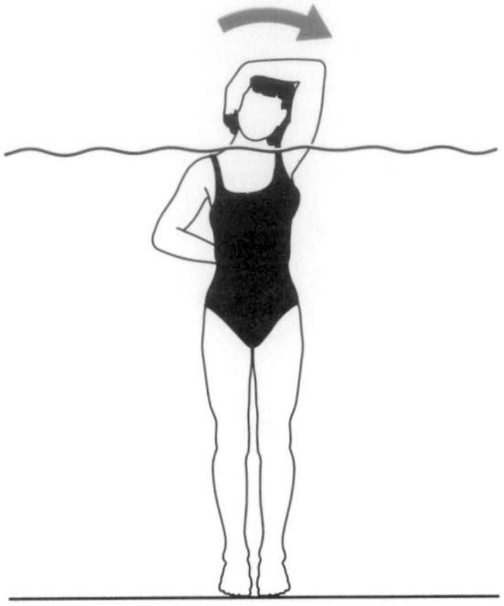

FIGURE 15–14. Upper trapezius stretch.

Neck Flexion Stretch (Fig. 15–15)

Prime movers: trapezius, semispinalis capitis, splenius capitis, splenius cervicis, and levator scapulae.

- Tuck the chin toward the chest
- Maintain a flat thoracic spine
- Hold, then relax

VARIATION: Place the hands on the head
PROGRESSION: Place the hands on the back of the head to increase the stretch

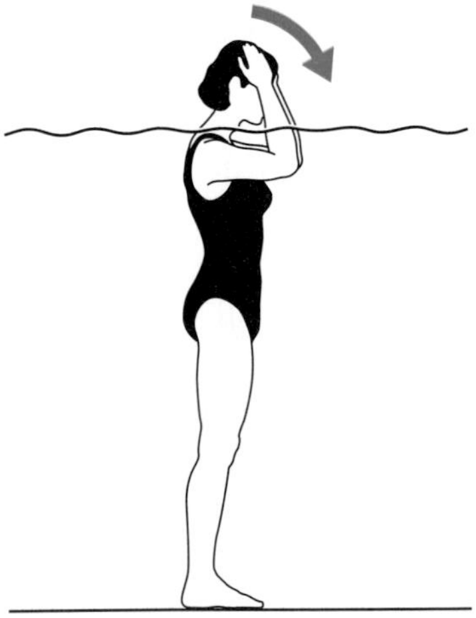

FIGURE 15–15. Neck flexion stretch.

Trapezius Stretch (Fig. 15–16)

Prime movers: trapezius, semispinalis capitis, splenius capitis, splenius cervicis, levator scapulae, and rhomboids.

- Interlock the fingers and extend the arms forward, pressing the palms away from the body
- Protract the shoulders while tucking the chin toward the chest
- Hold, then relax

VARIATION: Alter the angle of the arms with respect to the body, to vary the stretch

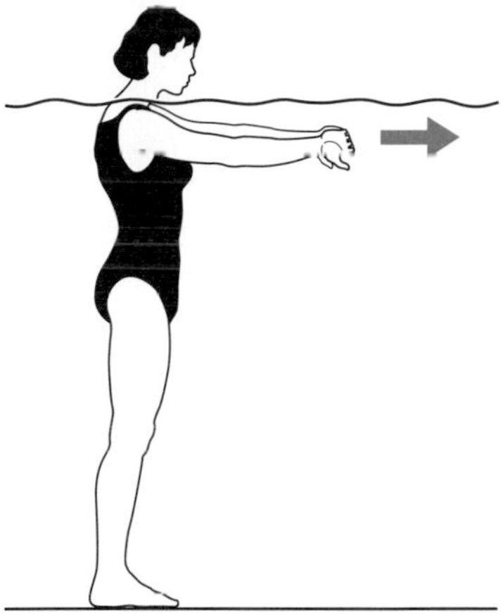

FIGURE 15–16. Trapezius stretch.

Levator Scapulae Stretch (Fig. 15–17)

Prime movers: trapezius and levator scapulae.

- Reach over the top of the head with the (uninvolved) left arm, putting the left middle finger over the right ear
- Reach as far as possible behind the back with the right hand;
- Gently pull the head toward the left shoulder flexing the neck slightly to face downward
- Hold, then relax

PROGRESSION: After the neck has been side-flexed, rotate the head to look down at the floor

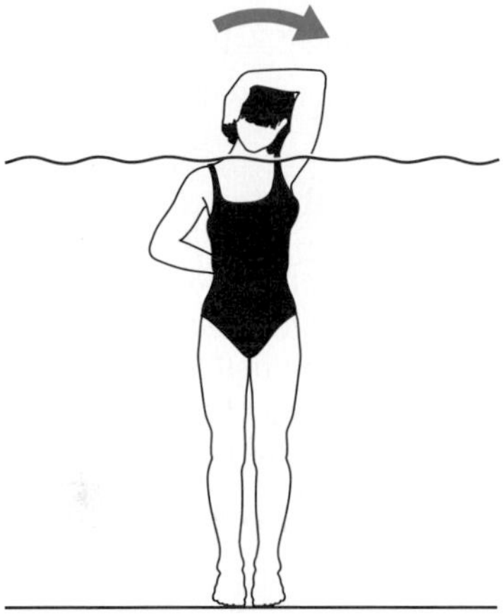

FIGURE 15–17. Levator scapulae stretch.

Trunk Stretches—Flexion

Back Stretch (Fig. 15–18)

Prime movers: quadratus lumborum, erector spinae, sacrospinalis, latissimus dorsi, and gluteus maximus.

- Hang vertically in a flotation tube
- Bring both knees toward the chest and grab under the knees with the hands
- Flex the spine forward. Hold, then relax

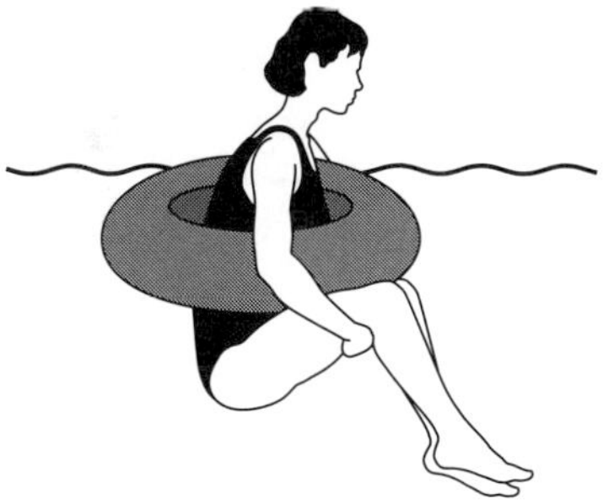

FIGURE 15–18. Back stretch.

Knee Lift Stretch (Fig. 15–19)

Prime movers: quadratus lumborum and gluteus maximus.

- Stand with the feet together, the arms at the sides, and the back against the pool wall
- Lift the involved knee and grasp under the knee with both hands
- Pull the knee up toward the chest, keeping the opposite leg straight
- Hold, then relax

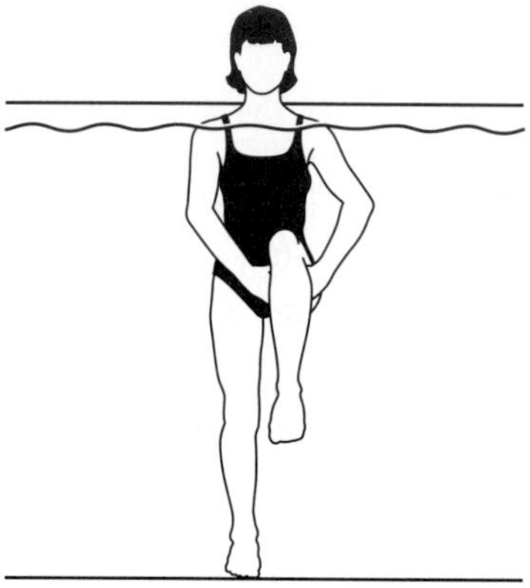

FIGURE 15–19. Knee lift stretch.

Trunk Stretches—Extension

Spine Extension Stretch (Fig. 15–20)

Prime movers: rectus abdominis, internal obliques, external obliques, transverse abdominals, and psoas major.

- Stand with the back against the pool wall and place the arms on the edge of the wall
- Take one small step forward while keeping the arms on the edge of the pool wall
- Gently press the pelvis forward while lifting the chest and arching lumbar spine
- Do not hyperextend the neck
- Use caution if shoulder problems are present

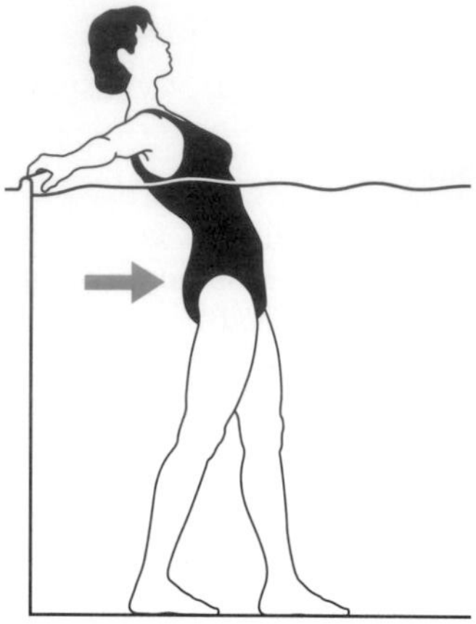

FIGURE 15–20. Spine extension stretch.

Active Spine Flexion and Extension (Fig. 15–21)

Prime movers: rectus abdominis, internal obliques, external obliques, transverse abdominals, psoas major when extending, and sacrospinalis when flexing.

- Stand with the feet shoulder-width apart facing the pool wall
- Hold on to the edge of the pool with both hands at arm's length
- Keeping the arms straight, press the hips forward while gently lifting the chest upward; hold
- Press the hips backward while flexing the spine
- Hold, then relax

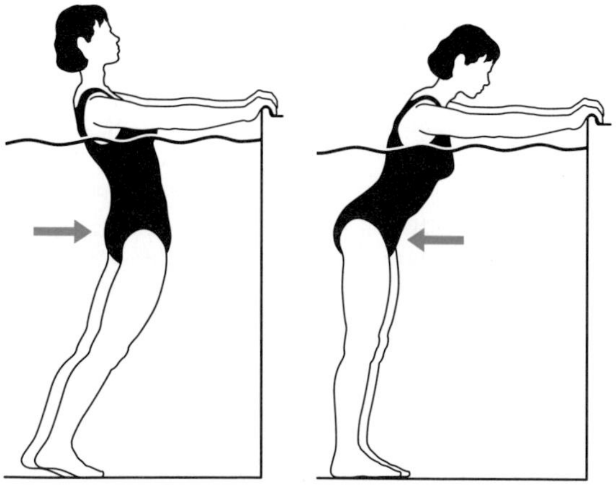

FIGURE 15–21. Active spine flexion and extension.

Press-ups (Fig. 15–22)

Prime movers: rectus abdominis, internal obliques, external obliques, transverse abdominals, and psoas major.

- Lie prone across the parallel bars, maintaining a neutral neck position with the elbows bent
- Slowly straighten the elbows while arching the lower back; hold, then relax
- Make sure the fronts of the thighs remain on the bar throughout the exercise, and do not hyperextend the neck

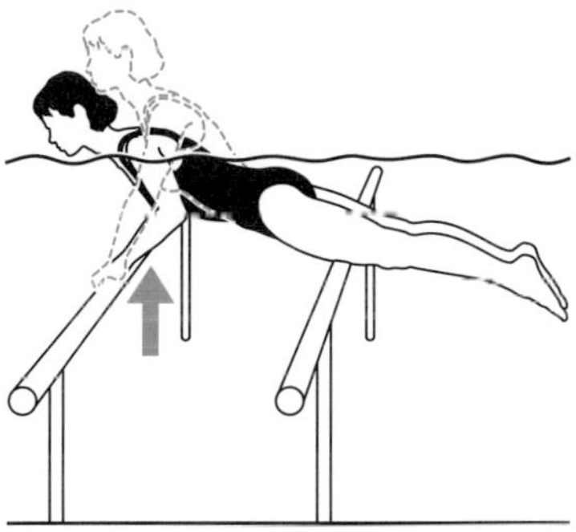

FIGURE 15–22. Press ups.

Thoracic Extension (Fig. 15–23)

Prime mover: sacrospinalis.

- Place the lumbar spine flat against the pool wall
- The pool wall or deck should be at thoracic level (the exact level can be varied)
- Slowly extend the spine, using the corner or edge of the pool as a fulcrum
- Do not hyperextend the neck

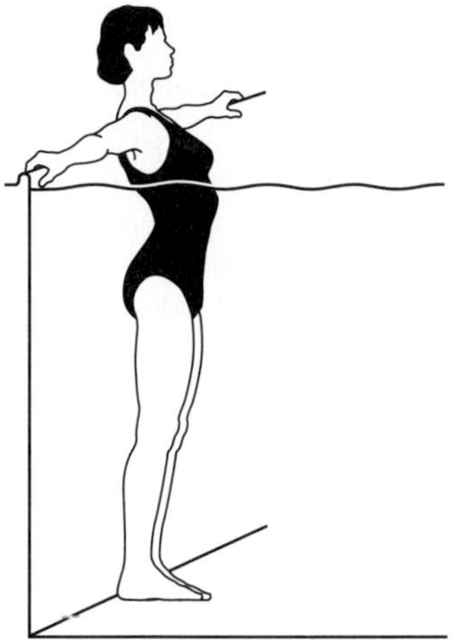

FIGURE 15–23. Thoracic extension.

Trunk Stretches—Lateral Flexion

Cross-Body Stretch (Fig. 15–24)

Prime movers: latissimus dorsi, quadratus lumborum, internal obliques, external obliques, sacrospinalis, psoas major, and teres major.

- Stand with the feet shoulder-width apart and the knees slightly flexed
- Put one hand on the hip
- Lift the involved arm above the head, pressing the palm up and across the midline of the body
- Hold, then relax

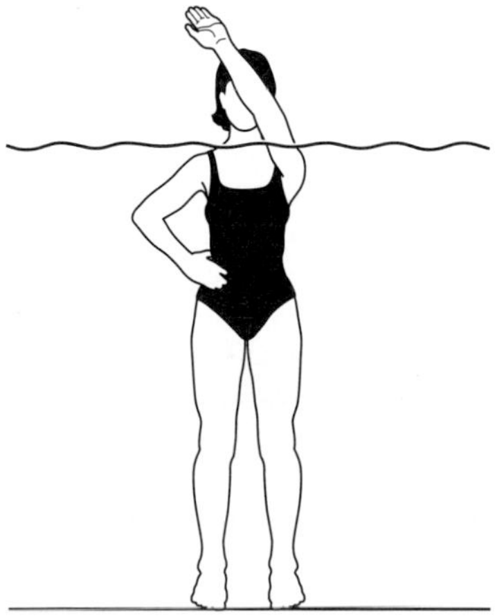

FIGURE 15–24. Cross-body stretch.

Standing Side Stretch (Fig. 15–25)

Prime movers: sacrospinalis, quadratus lumborum.

- Stand sideways with the feet together, arm's length away from the wall; hold on to the wall with the hand of the involved side and place the other hand on the hip
- Press the hip toward the pool wall, keeping the arm straight; feel a stretch on the side closer to the wall
- Hold, then relax

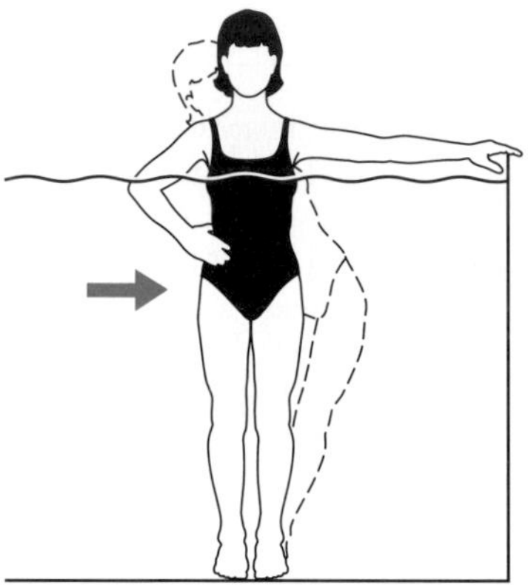

FIGURE 15–25. Standing side stretch.

Piriformis Stretches

Standing Piriformis Stretch (Fig. 15–26).

- Stand with the back against the pool wall
- Flex the (involved) left hip and place the left hand on the outside of the knee
- Press the bent leg toward the right hip
- While maintaining this position of the knee, place the right hand on the left ankle
- Gently pull the ankle in the same direction as the stretch, causing slight external rotation of the left hip
- Hold, then relax

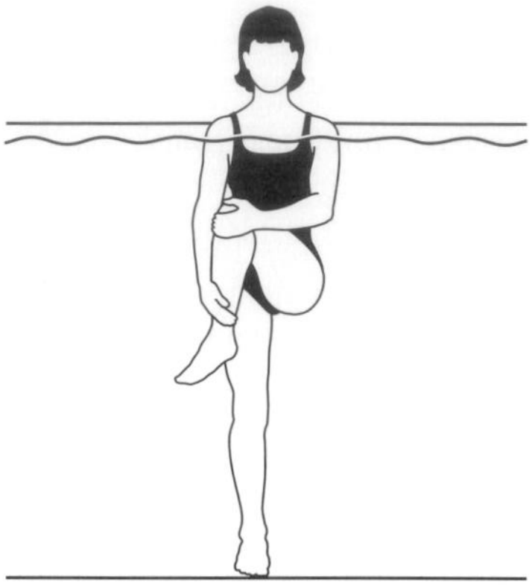

FIGURE 15–26. Standing piriformis stretch.

Seated Piriformis Stretch (Fig. 15–27).

- In a seated position, place the lateral aspect of the (involved) right foot on the left thigh
- Lean forward with the chest while pressing down the right knee
- Hold, then relax

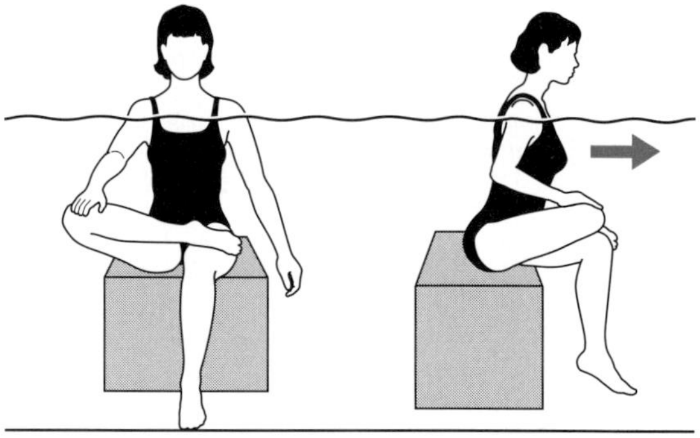

FIGURE 15–27. Seated piriformis stretch.

STRENGTHENING EXERCISES FOR THE SPINE

Neck Exercises

Patients who have rheumatoid arthritis of the cervical spine *must* avoid neck flexion, extension, and circumduction because of atlantoaxial instability. The instability observed between C1 and C2 is often a result of ligamentous laxity as well as structural changes to the vertebrae. These patients *must* have the permission of their doctor or physiotherapist before performing neck range of motion exercises.

For optimal results, patients should perform neck exercises underwater with a snorkel and a mask.

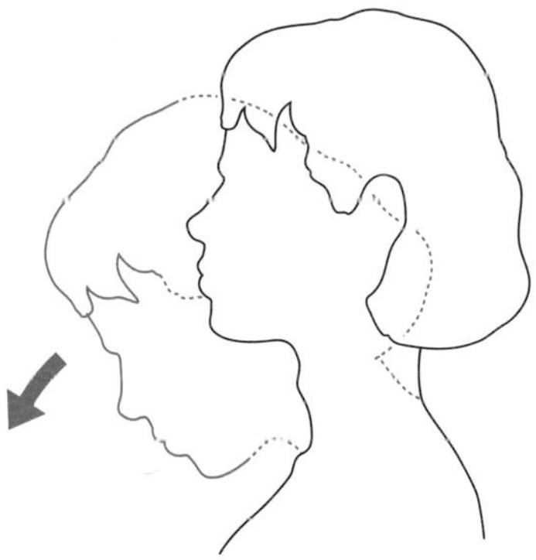

FIGURE 15–28. Neck flexion.

Neck Flexion (Fig. 15–28)

Prime movers: sacrospinalis, trapezius, sternocleidomastoids, and scalenes.

- Slowly lower the chin to the chest; hold
- Raise the head until facing forward

Neck Extension (Fig. 15–29)

Prime movers: splenius, semispinalis capitis, longissimus capitis, sternocleidomastoid, and trapezius.

- Slowly extend the neck backward; hold
- Return the head to an upright position

CAUTION: This exercise is necessary for the complete rehabilitation of the neck range of motion; however, prolonged or excessive hyperextension *must* be avoided.

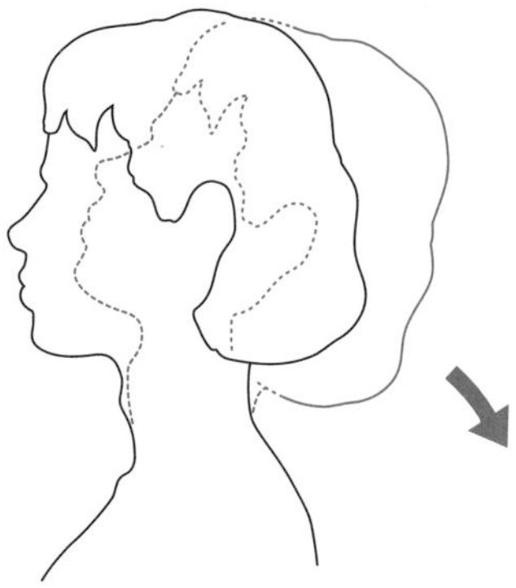

FIGURE 15–29. Neck extension.

Neck Lateral Flexion (Fig. 15–30)

Prime movers: splenius, sacrospinalis, semispinalis cervicis, trapezius, sternocleidomastoid, and scalenes.

- Slowly tilt the head so the left ear (on the involved side) is as far as possible away from the left shoulder; hold
- Return the head to an upright position

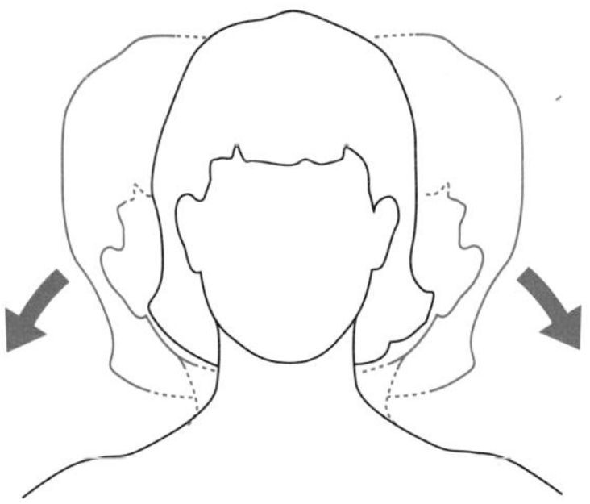

FIGURE 15–30. Neck lateral flexion.

Neck Rotation (Fig. 15–31)

Prime movers: sternocleidomastoid, longissimus capitis, multifidi, rotators, sacrospinalis, and splenius.

- Turn the head to look over the left shoulder; hold
- Return the head to face forward
- Turn the head to look over the right shoulder; hold
- Return the head to face forward
- Keep the movements slow and controlled, and avoid lateral flexion while rotating

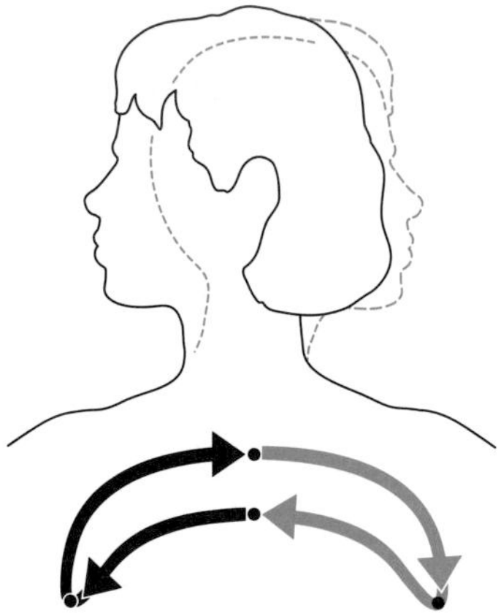

FIGURE 15–31. Neck rotation.

Neck Retraction (Fig. 15–32)

Prime movers: trapezius, splenius, scalenes, sternocleidomastoid, and sacrospinalis.

- Pull the head straight back, keeping the jaw and eyes level
- Return to the neutral position

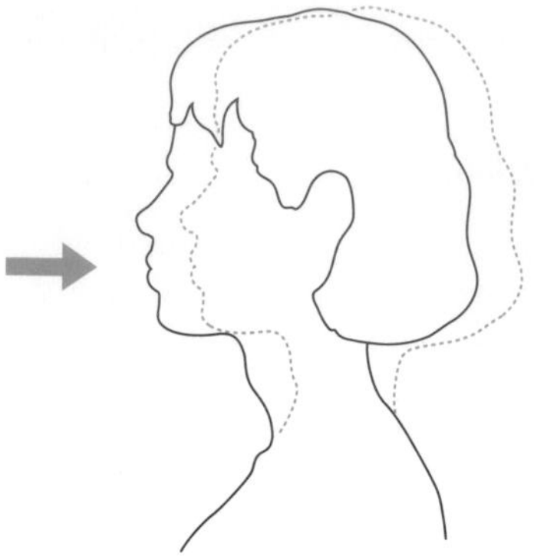

FIGURE 15–32. Neck retraction.

Trunk Exercises—Flexion

Pelvic Tilt (Fig. 15–33)

Prime movers: transverse abdominals, rectus abdominis, internal obliques, and external obliques.

- Stand with the back against the pool wall, feet shoulder-width apart, and knees over the toes
- Contact the lower abdominals, pulling the pubic bone forward and up toward the navel (posterior tilt)
- Hold, then relax (anterior tilt)

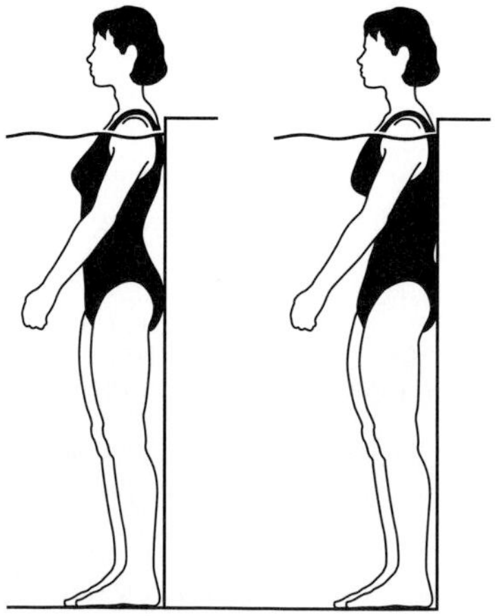

FIGURE 15–33. Pelvic tilt.

Pelvic Curl (Fig. 15–34)

Prime movers: rectus abdominis, internal obliques, external obliques, iliopsoas, and rectus femoris.

- Place the back against the pool wall and hold on to the edge of the pool with both hands
- Slowly lift the legs off the pool floor until the knees are at 90° and the lumbar spine is flat against the pool wall
- Keeping the knees and hips in this fixed position, slowly lift the pelvis or tailbone off the pool wall by tightening the abdominal muscles
- Release the contraction and allow the pelvis to make contact with the pool wall

VARIATION: This exercise can also be done in deep water, holding onto flotation bells

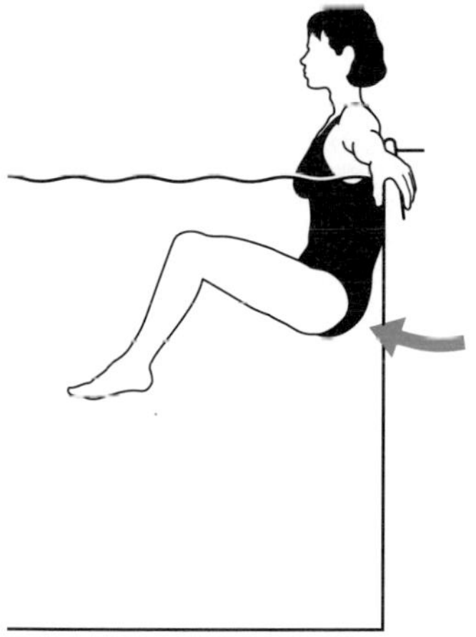

FIGURE 15–34. Pelvic curl.

Standing Crunches (Fig. 15–35)

Prime movers: rectus abdominis, internal obliques, external obliques, and transversus abdominis.

- Stand upright with the pelvis tilted back (see Fig. 15–33)
- Hold a ball or flotation device snugly against the chest
- Gently contract the abdominal muscles to flex the spine
- Hold the contraction for four counts, and then relax for four counts; maintain pelvic tilt throughout

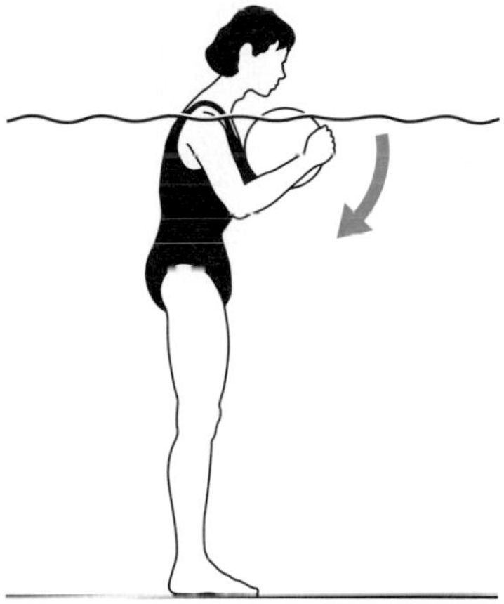

FIGURE 15–35. Standing crunches.

Knees to Chest (Fig. 15–36)

Acute, in Tube

Prime movers: hip flexors, rectus abdominis, and rectus femoris.

- Lie supine in a flotation tube with a smaller tube around the ankles (the patient must be stabilized by the instructor or in a corner of the pool)
- Slowly flex the hips and knees, bringing the knees up toward the chest
- Gently flex the spine
- Hold, then straighten the legs

Advanced, with Floats

Prime movers: rectus abdominis, internal obliques, external obliques, psoas major, rectus femoris, pectoralis, deltoids, trapezius, latissimus dorsi, and triceps.

- Hold flotation bells in the hands or place them under the arms
- Keeping the abdominals tight, extend the legs in front of the body
- Slowly flex the knees and hips toward the chest, then extend the legs again

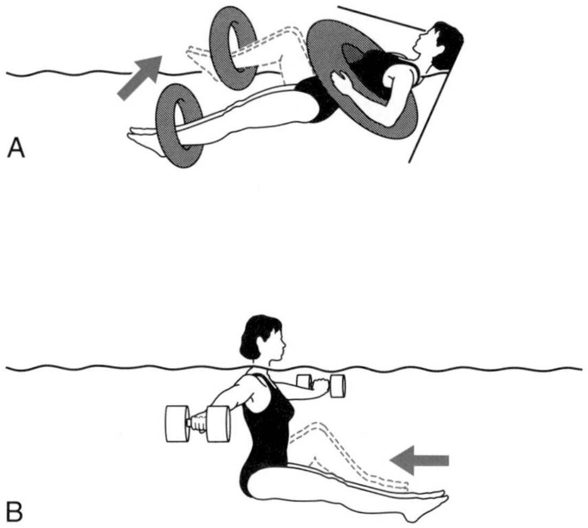

FIGURE 15–36. Knees to chest. *A*, Acute, in tube. *B*, Advanced, with floats.

Sit-ups in Parallel Bars (Fig. 15–37)

Prime movers: rectus abdominis, internal obliques, external obliques, psoas major, and rectus femoris.

- Sit on one parallel bar and hook the toes under the other
- Hold a ring or flotation device extended in front of the body at the surface of the water
- Sit up by contracting the abdominal muscles, keeping the float in front of the body

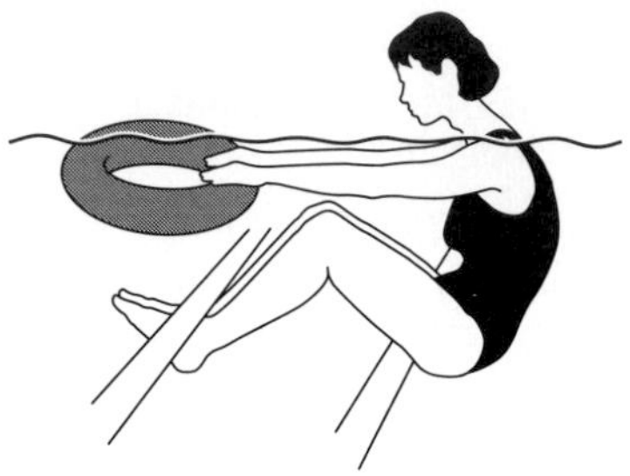

FIGURE 15–37. Sit-ups in parallel bars.

Resistive Band Crunches (Fig. 15–38)

Prime movers: rectus abdominis, internal obliques, and external obliques.

- Secure a stretch band to the pool ladder or any other stable attachment
- Stand with the feet shoulder-width apart (or kneel) facing the ladder, and hold the stretch band with stable (unmoving) flexed arms
- Slowly contract the abdominals to flex the spine, pulling on the band
- Hold, then relax

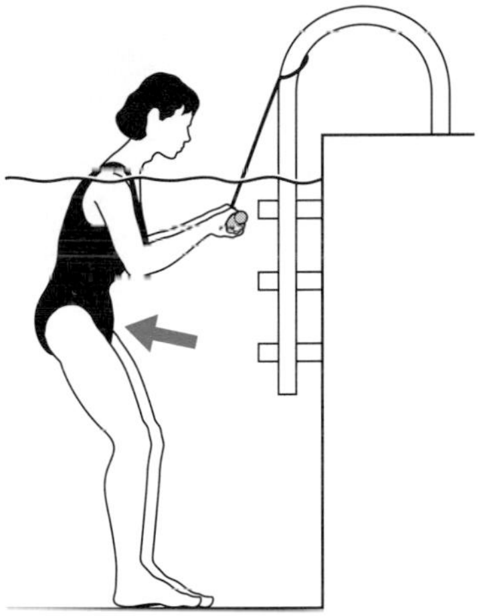

FIGURE 15–38. Resistive band crunches.

Double Leg Lifts (Fig. 15–39)

Prime movers: rectus abdominis and psoas major.

- Assume a vertical position in deep water with the legs together, holding on to flotation devices
- Lift both legs at the same time to approximately 90°; hold, then lower legs.

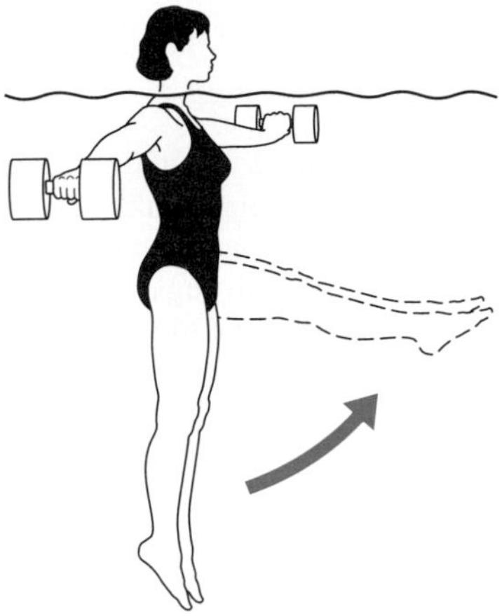

FIGURE 15–39. Double leg lifts.

Trunk Exercises—Extension

Passive Back Extension (Fig. 15–40)

Prime movers: sacrospinalis.

- Hang in a flotation tube with the feet just touching the pool floor
- Keep the legs straight while pressing hips toward the pool floor and gently arching the back
- Hold, then relax

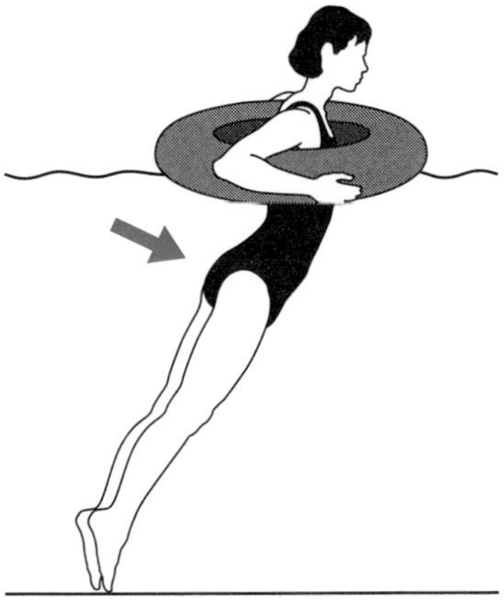

FIGURE 15–40. Passive back extension.

Resistive Back Extension (Fig. 15–41)

Prime movers: sacrospinalis.

- Lie supine in a large flotation tube with floats on both ankles, or with both feet in a small flotation tube
- Gently press both legs toward the bottom of the pool as the hips come up
- Keep the abdominals tight
- Hold the contraction, then relax

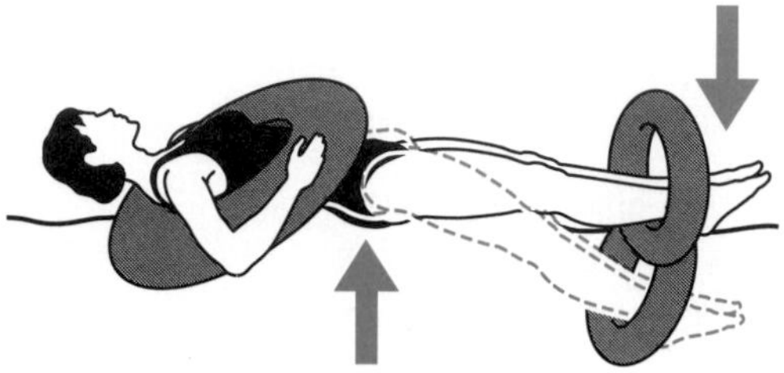

FIGURE 15–41. Resistive back extension.

Standing Back Press[7] (Fig. 15–42)

Prime movers: sacrospinalis.

- Stand with the feet shoulder-width apart and square to the pool wall, holding on to the pool wall
- Slowly look up at the ceiling without hyperextending the neck
- Allow the upper torso to fall away from the pool wall; hold, then relax

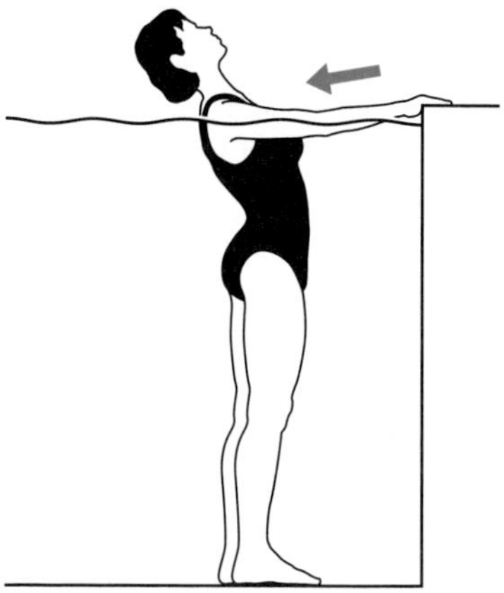

FIGURE 15–42. Standing back press.

Trunk Exercises—Rotation

Standing Cross-Crunches (Fig. 15–43)

Prime movers: rectus abdominis, internal obliques, and external obliques.

- Stand upright with the pelvis tilted back
- Hold a ball or flotation device snugly against the chest
- Gently contract the abdominals, rotating the trunk 10° to one side before flexing the spine
- Hold the contraction for four counts, then relax for four counts

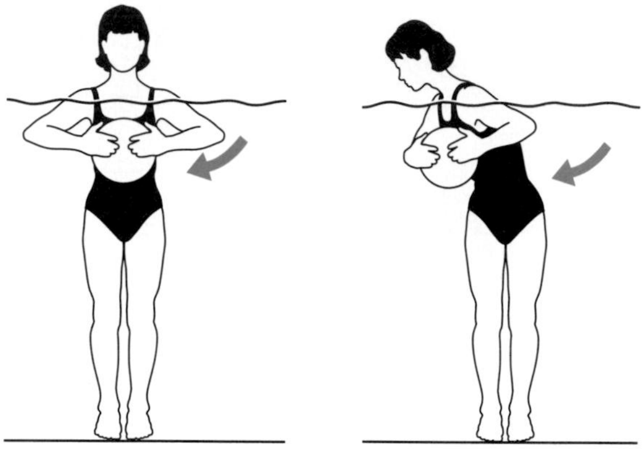

FIGURE 15–43. Standing cross-crunches.

Resistive Band Cross-Crunches[7] (Fig. 15–44)

Prime movers: rectus abdominis, internal obliques, and external obliques.

- Secure a stretch band to the pool ladder or any other stable attachment
- Stand with the feet shoulder-width apart (or kneel) facing the ladder, and hold the stretch band with stable (unmoving) flexed arms
- Contract the abdominals slowly to flex the trunk forward and rotate it slightly to one side
- Hold, then relax

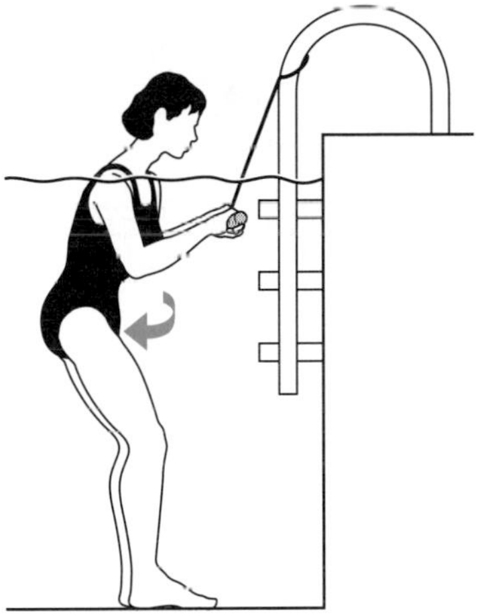

FIGURE 15–44. Resistive band cross-crunches.

Standing Trunk Rotation (Fig. 15–45)

Prime movers: internal obliques and external obliques.

- Stand with the feet shoulder-width apart and the knees slightly bent
- Place the arms on a kickboard that is floating on the surface of the water
- Slowly rotate the trunk to the uninvolved side
- Return to neutral

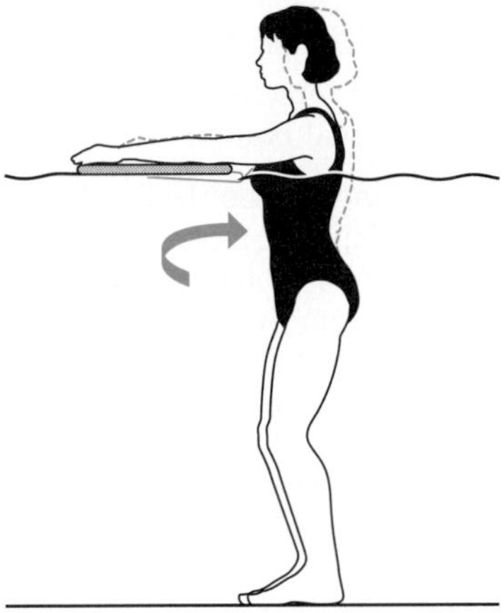

FIGURE 15–45. Standing trunk rotation.

Resistive Trunk Rotation (Fig. 15–46)

Prime movers: internal obliques and external obliques.

- Stand with the feet shoulder-width apart and the knees slightly bent
- Hold resistive paddle or a kickboard vertically in front of the chest with the arms extended
- Slowly rotate the trunk to the uninvolved side
- Return to neutral

PROGRESSION: Increase the surface area of resistance

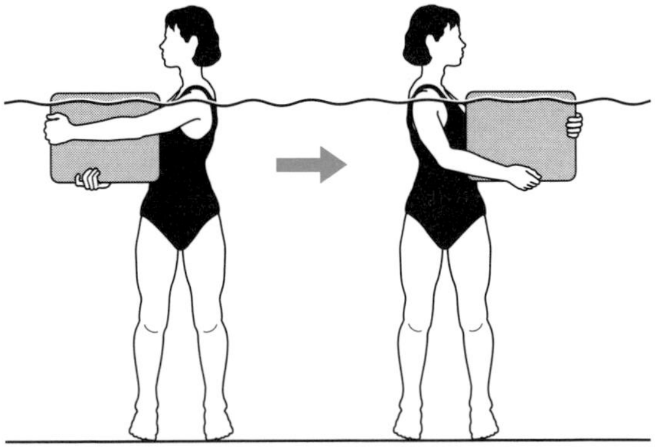

FIGURE 15–46. Resistive trunk rotation.

Crossover Sit-ups in Parallel Bars (Fig. 15–47)

Prime movers: rectus abdominis, internal obliques, and external obliques.

- Sit on one parallel bar and hook the toes under the other
- Hold a small flotation tube in the left hand in front of the body and approximately 45° to the left (uninvolved) side, on the surface of the water
- Contract the abdominal muscles, bringing the right hand across the midline of the body to touch the tube, moving the flotation device along the surface of the water

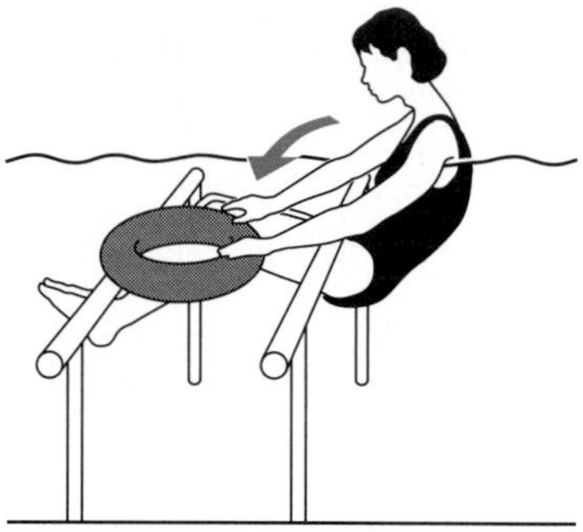

FIGURE 15–47. Crossover sit-up in parallel bars.

Bent Knee Twists (Fig. 15–48)

Prime movers: internal obliques, external obliques, and rectus abdominis.

- Assume a vertical position in deep water, using a flotation tube
- Gently flex the hips and knees
- Use the oblique muscles to rotate or swivel the hips to the left and then to the right

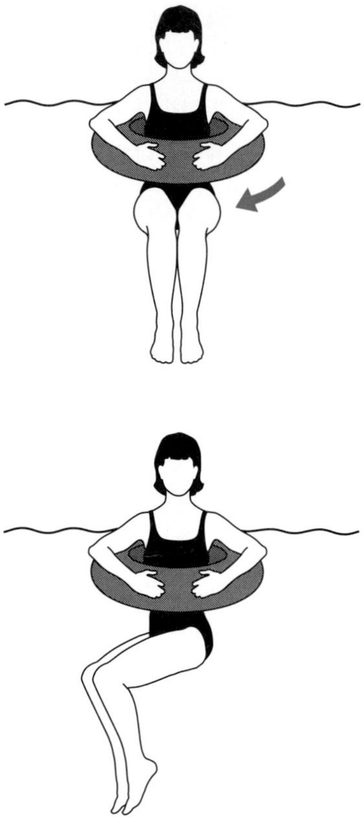

Bent knee twists.

Standing Cross-Crunches with Bent Knee (Fig. 15–49)

Prime movers: rectus abdominis, internal obliques, and external obliques.

- Place the back against the pool wall with the left hand on the edge of the wall and the right hand behind the head
- Flex the left hip and knee to 90°
- Slowly bring the right elbow toward the left hip, crossing the midline of the body

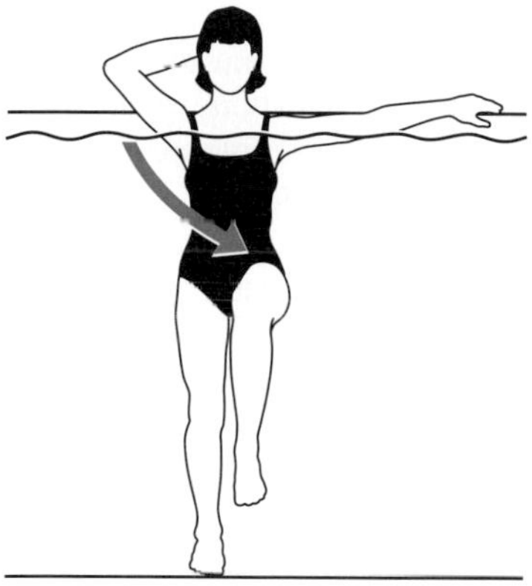

FIGURE 15–49. Standing cross-crunches with bent knee.

Trunk Exercises—Lateral Flexion

Thigh Side Bends (Fig. 15–50)

Prime movers: sacrospinalis, quadratus lumborum, internal obliques, and external obliques.

- Stand with the feet shoulder-width apart and the hands at the sides
- Slowly slide the palm of the hand on the uninvolved side down the side of the leg to the knee, laterally flexing the spine
- Return to original position

PROGRESSION: Hold flotation bells in the hands close to the body

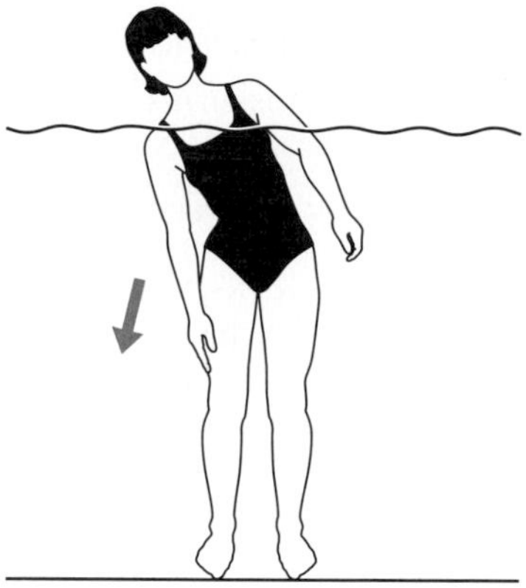

FIGURE 15–50. Thigh side bends.

Suspended Lateral Flexion[7] (Fig. 15–51)

Prime movers: sacrospinalis, quadratus lumborum, internal obliques, and external obliques.

- Use a flotation tube or bells to float with the knees and hips flexed to 90°
- Contract the abdominals laterally, bringing the left ribs slightly closer to the left hip

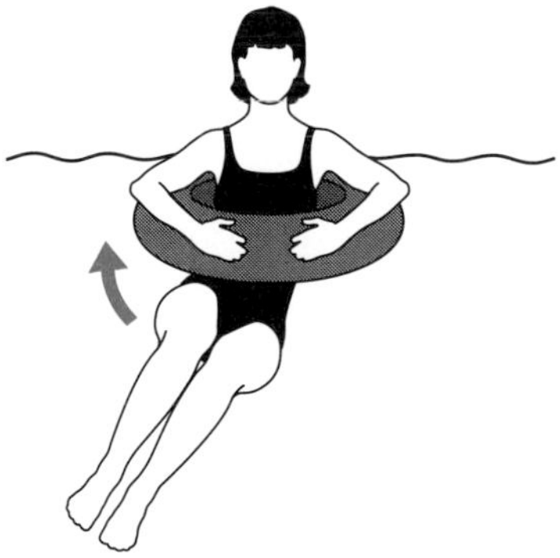

FIGURE 15–51. Suspended lateral flexion.

Resistive Band Lateral Flexion[7] (Fig. 15–52)

Prime movers: sacrospinalis, quadratus lumborum, internal obliques, and external obliques.

- Secure the stretch band to the pool ladder or any other stable attachment
- Stand with the feet shoulder-width apart (or kneel) with the left (uninvolved) side next to the pool wall, holding the stretch band close to the shoulder with both hands
- Laterally contract away from the band, bringing the right ribs closer to the right hip
- Return to original position

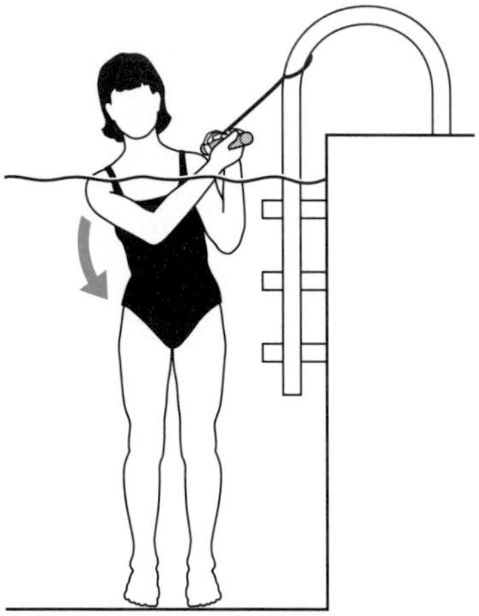

FIGURE 15–52. Resistive band lateral flexion.

Side Flexion in Tube (Fig. 15–53)

Prime movers: rectus abdominis, internal obliques, external obliques, hip abductors, hip adductors, quadratus lumborum, and sacrospinalis.

- Float supine in a flotation tube with floats on both ankles or with both feet in a small flotation tube (the patient must be stabilized by the instructor or in a corner of the pool)
- Place the legs firmly together and keep the knees slightly bent
- Slowly move the legs to the involved side by contracting the internal and external oblique muscles
- Keep the upper body fixed and the pelvis tilted back; isolate the movement to the lower back

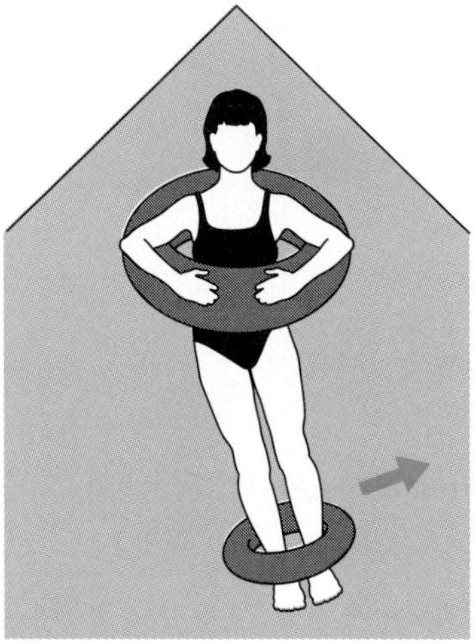

FIGURE 15–53. Side flexion in tube.

Trunk Exercises—Active Trunk Flexion and Extension

Tuck and Roll (Fig. 15–54)

Prime movers: rectus abdominis, quadriceps, gluteus, iliopsoas, sacrospinalis, and hamstring.

- Hang vertically in a flotation tube or in the parallel bars
- Bring the knees to the chest and hold; then roll back, extend the legs to the front, and hold
- Bring the knees to the chest, roll forward, and extend the legs behind
- Bring the knees to the chest, then relax and return to the original position

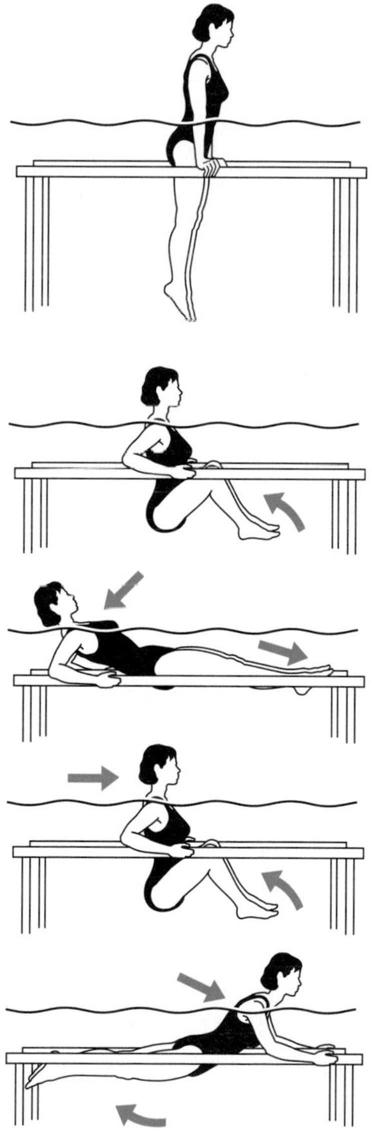

FIGURE 15–54. Tuck and roll.

Thoracic Spine Exercises

Push-offs (Fig. 15–55)

Prime movers: pectoralis, rhomboids, triceps, anterior deltoids, and posterior deltoids.

- Stand with the feet shoulder-width apart facing the pool wall; hold on to the edge of the pool wall with both hands at arm's length
- Keeping the body straight (no arch in the back), lean forward by bending the arms until the chest touches or is close to the pool wall
- Do not move the feet; keep the heels on the floor
- Push off with both hands to the starting position
- All movements should flow smoothly and continuously

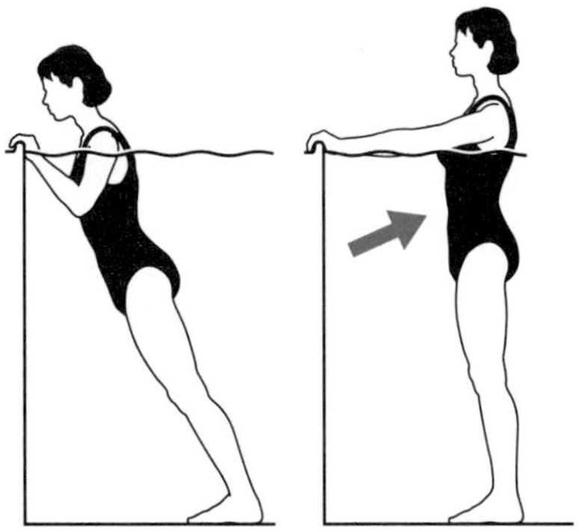

FIGURE 15–55. Push-offs.

Bent Arm Pull-backs (Fig. 15–56)

Prime movers: infraspinatus, teres minor, deltoids, trapezius, and rhomboids.

- Stand upright with the elbows bent at shoulder level and the forearms parallel to the water surface
- Slowly press the elbows back, moving the shoulder blades closer to each other
- Slowly reach forward as far as possible; relax

PROGRESSION: To increase resistance, use spa bells or floats

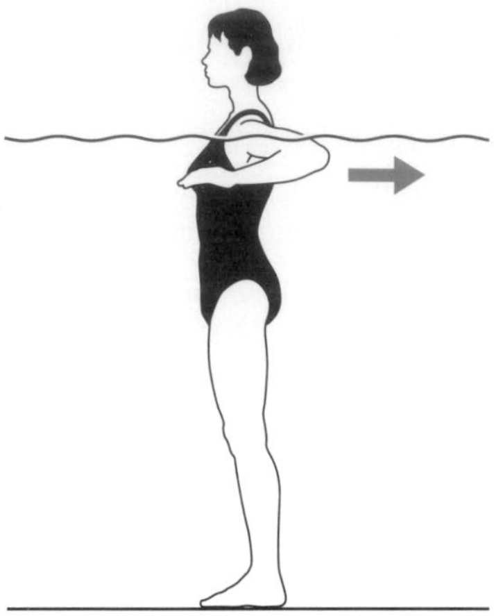

FIGURE 15–56. Bent arm pull-backs.

Scapular Retraction (Fig. 15–57)

Prime movers: deltoid, pectoralis, coracobrachialis, infraspinatus, teres minor, rhomboids, and trapezius.

- Stand upright with the elbows slightly bent, arms slightly below shoulder level in forward flexion
- Slowly press the arms back, moving the shoulder blades closer together
- Return to starting position and relax

PROGRESSION: To increase the resistance, use hand paddles

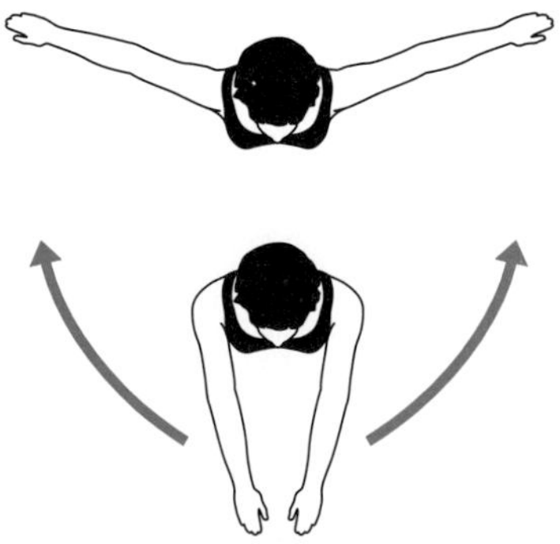

FIGURE 15–57. Scapular retraction.

Lateral Pull-downs (Fig. 15–58)

Prime movers: latissimus dorsi, teres major, and triceps.

- Using flotation bells, stand with the feet shoulder-width apart, the knees slightly bent, and the arms in front of the body
- Maintain elbow flexion throughout the exercise, and do not twist or rotate the trunk
- Slowly pull the arms down toward the sides
- Return to the starting position and relax

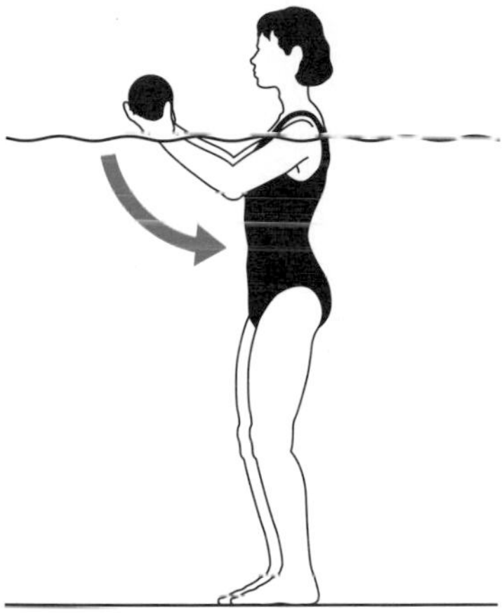

FIGURE 15–58. Lateral pull-downs.

COMMON CONDITIONS OF THE SPINE

Conditions of the Cervical Spine

Cervical Arthritis

There are two types of joints in the cervical spine that are commonly affected by arthritis: the intervertebral joint and the facet joint. If the intervertebral joint is involved, the condition is often referred to as degenerative disc disease. The various types of arthritis are presented in Chapter 7.

Origin

Arthritis of the cervical spine is often due to a previous injury. The injury may have involved a traumatic incident, such as a fracture or whiplash injury. Old disc lesions that have caused a decrease in disc height also can lead to arthritis. The most common cause, however, is simply wear and tear. This is usually a result of years of poor posture or activities that have harmed the spine.

Pathology

A degeneration of the disc results in a decrease in disc height. This allows the anterior and posterior longitudinal ligaments to slacken, forming small pockets where the vertebral body and disc meet. If these pockets calcify, bone spurs result (Fig. 15–59). These spurs encroach on the spinal canal, causing pain and decreased range of motion. Decreased disc height also results in narrowing of the facet joint space. This contributes to the pain and stiffness and can also lead to the formation of osteophytes in the facet joints.

Signs and Symptoms

As with any arthritic condition, pain and stiffness are the chief complaints. Crepitus may or may not be present. Acute exacerbations may involve headaches or pain that radiates down the arm.

Body Parts Affected

- Vertebrae
- Paraspinal muscles
- Spinal ligaments
- Nerves
- Discs
- Facet joints

Exercise Priorities

- Maximize range of motion (stretch all tight neck and shoulder girdle muscles)
- Correct postural misalignment
- Strengthen neck and shoulder muscles

Acute Cervical Sprain or Strain

This condition presents as neck pain that follows an acute injury to the soft tissues of the cervical spine.

Origin

This condition can be caused by a repetitive strain injury, which may result from poor working posture. The most common cause, however, is a traumatic injury such as whiplash. This typically involves both a hyperflexion and a hyperextension

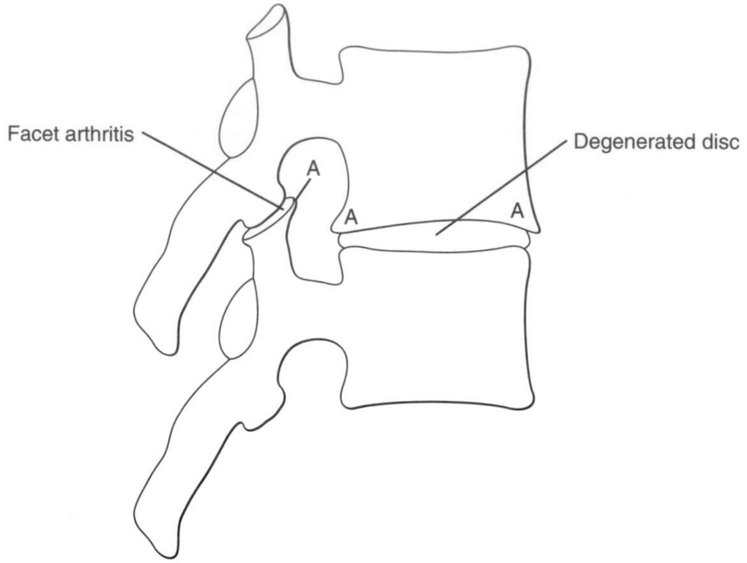

FIGURE 15–59. Arthritic changes in the spine. A = osteophytes.

injury to the neck (Fig. 15–60). The muscles and ligaments of the area are violently overstretched, and the discs, the facet joints, or the vertebrae themselves may also be injured.

Pathology

Chapter 7 describes the pathology of soft-tissue injuries. X-ray studies must always be taken to rule out fractures. It is also important to determine whether any of the arm pain is caused by a disc injury. Because the neck is a very pain-sensitive structure, care must always be taken not to cause more pain.

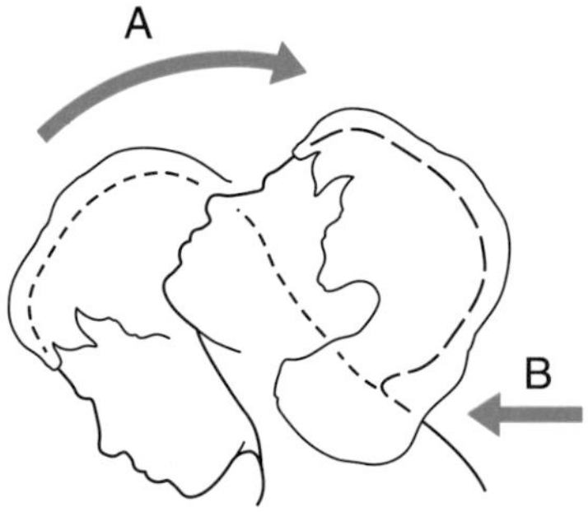

FIGURE 15–60. Mechanism of a whiplash injury. *A*, Hyperextension is followed by *B*, hyperflexion.

Signs and Symptoms

Pain and stiffness are the most common symptoms. Headaches and referred pain down the arm are also common.

Body Parts Affected

- Vertebrae
- Paraspinal muscles
- Spinal ligaments
- Nerves
- Discs
- Facet joints

Exercise Priorities

- Gently increase range of motion to decrease pain and muscle spasm
- Restore neck range of motion
- Maintain thoracic spine and shoulder mobility and strength
- Correct postural misalignment

Cervical Disc Bulge

The terms "disc bulge" or "disc protrusion" are far more accurate than the term "slipped disc." As depicted in Figure 15–61, the nucleus of the disc protrudes, causing the bulge.

Origin

This condition usually results from a traumatic injury such as a jarring or twisting stress. It can also be caused by wear and tear or chronic poor posture.

Pathology

In the typical disc bulge, a part of the nucleus protrudes through a tear in the annulus. A small bulge puts pressure on the posterior longitudinal ligament, resulting in acute neck pain. A large bulge can put pressure on a nerve root, causing radicular signs and symptoms. A central bulge can press on the spinal cord itself. Any of these types of bulges can lead to arthritis because they result in a decrease in disc height.

Signs and Symptoms

An acute bulge results in neck pain that is exacerbated by coughing. Pressure on a nerve root may cause pain or paraesthesia along that nerve. There may also be weakness in a muscle innervated by that particular nerve and a decrease in the corresponding reflex.

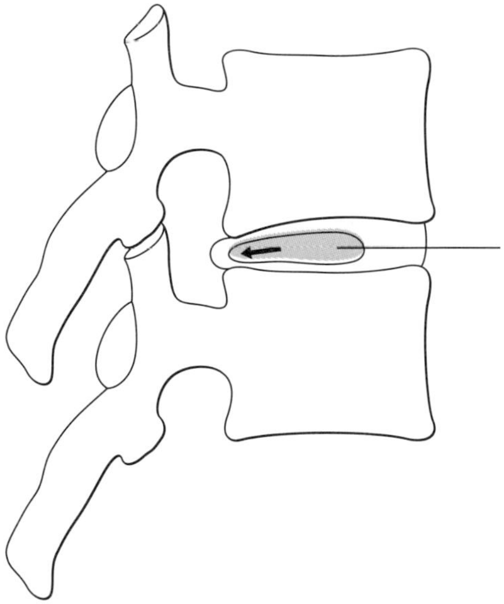

FIGURE 15–61. Cervical or thoracic disc bulge.

Body Parts Affected

- Vertebrae
- Paraspinal muscles
- Spinal ligaments
- Nerves
- Discs
- Facet joints

Exercise Priorities

- Perform neck extension exercises
- Begin with side flexion away from the painful side
- Add remaining range of motion exercises as pain subsides
- Correct postural misalignment

Chronic Neck Pain

This term generally refers to any neck pain that has persisted for longer than 3 months and is not caused by a disc protrusion.

Origin

Chronic neck pain often starts with a traumatic incident. It may, however, be caused by repetitive strain or poor posture, such as an increased cervical lordosis (Fig. 15–62).

Pathology

The pain experienced with this condition can be muscular or ligamentous in origin. X-ray studies may or may not show degeneration, so they are not useful in predicting whether chronic pain will develop. Because there is no specific pathology, it is not surprising that passive modalities provide only temporary relief.

Signs and Symptoms

Pain and stiffness are always present to some degree. Pain is not a good indicator of whether rehabilitation is being successful, because it can fluctuate for no apparent reason. Objective signs, such as range of motion, are better indicators of a patient's progress. These measurements can be used as evidence that a patient is improving even if the pain has not changed.

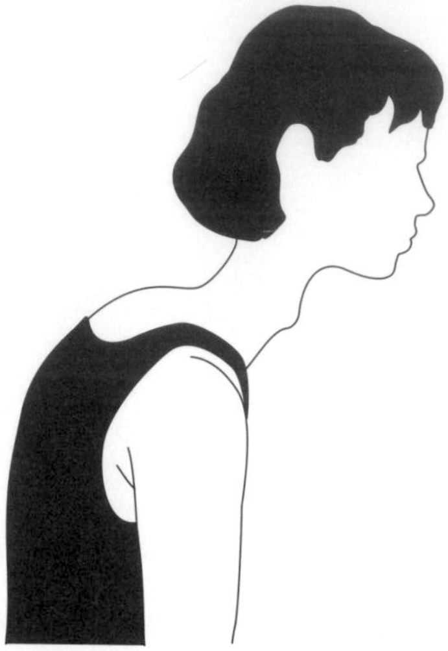

FIGURE 15–62. Increased cervical lordosis and kyphotic thoracic spine.

Body Parts Affected

- Vertebrae
- Paraspinal muscles
- Spinal ligaments
- Nerves
- Discs
- Facet joints

Exercise Priorities

- Maximize range of motion (stretch all tight neck and shoulder girdle muscles)
- Correct postural misalignment
- Strengthen neck and shoulder muscles

Conditions of the Thoracic Spine

Thoracic Arthritis

As with other parts of the spine, thoracic arthritis may involve the intervertebral joints or the facet joints. The various types of arthritis are discussed in Chapter 7.

Origin

The most common cause of arthritis in the thoracic spine is poor posture that has existed for several years. Wear and tear can also result from a previous injury, disease (such as osteochondritis), or a disc lesion.

Pathology

The pathology of thoracic arthritis is similar to that of cervical arthritis. Disc degeneration can lead to osteophyte formation in both intervertebral and facet joints. This leads to the classic symptoms of spinal arthritis.

Signs and Symptoms

Pain and stiffness are the primary complaints. During an acute exacerbation, movement may be guarded because of pain. After the pain subsides, the patient is usually left with some degree of stiffness.

Body Parts Affected

- Vertebrae
- Paraspinal muscles
- Spinal ligaments
- Nerves
- Discs
- Facet joints

Exercise Priorities

- Maximize range of motion (stretch all tight neck and shoulder girdle muscles)
- Correct postural misalignment (emphasize shoulder retraction and good neck posture)

Acute Thoracic Sprain or Strain

Thoracic soft-tissue injuries present as sprains and strains (see Chapter 7).

Origin

Because the thoracic spine is a transition area between the cervical and lumbar regions, thoracic conditions can be related to either neck or low back injuries. Upper thoracic problems often accompany neck and shoulder injuries. Lower thoracic injuries can essentially be treated as lumbar strains.

Pathology

The general pathology of sprains and strains also applies to the thoracic spine. Figure 15–63 depicts a thoracic muscle tear. As with other areas of the spine, secondary muscle spasm may be more of a problem than the primary injury.

Signs and Symptoms

Pain and decreased range of motion are the most common signs of this condition, and they may actu-

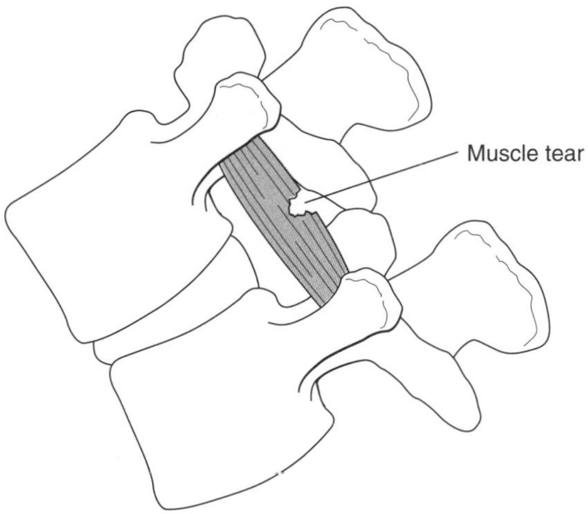

FIGURE 15–63. Acute thoracic muscle tear.

ally increase during the 48 hours after the initial injury. This occurs as the secondary muscle spasm increases.

Body Parts Affected

- Vertebrae
- Paraspinal muscles
- Spinal ligaments
- Nerves
- Discs
- Facet joints

Exercise Priorities

- Increase range of motion (use gentle stretching to prevent movement loss)
- Correct postural misalignment (to prevent further strain of injured tissues)

Thoracic Disc Protrusion

The thoracic spine is the least common area for a disc protrusion to occur.

Origin

This injury may occur as a result of a fall on the buttocks. It can also occur during a twisting stress to the thoracic spine. It may, however, simply be associated with degenerative changes of this area of the spine.

Pathology

Disc bulges anywhere in the spine have essentially the same pathology. The characteristics of a cervical disc bulge also apply to the thoracic spine.

Signs and Symptoms

The position and size of the bulge determine the symptoms. Often, the patient experiences shooting pain from the back through the body. This pain increases when the patient coughs. The patient may also experience numbness in one or both legs. Upper motor neuron signs (such as clonus) indicate a severe problem that warrants immediate medical attention.

Body Parts Affected

- Discs
- Vertebrae
- Spinal ligaments
- Nerves
- Paraspinal muscles

Exercise Priorities

- Establish extension exercises to reduce disc bulge
- Establish range of motion exercises to regain maximum range of motion
- Correct postural misalignment
- Trunk strengthening exercises

Chronic Thoracic Pain

As with the other regions of the spine, chronic pain refers to any pain that has persisted for longer than 3 months and that is not caused by a disc protrusion.

Origin

Chronic pain may start with a traumatic incident or a repetitive strain injury. It may also result from poor posture (see Fig. 15–62).

Pathology

Clinical tests, such as X-ray studies, may or may not point to a specific diagnosis. Even if there is a specific pathology, there is often no "quick fix" to the problem. Consequently, exercise is the basis of the patient's therapy.

Signs and Symptoms

As with any chronically painful joint, pain is not a good sign to observe when trying to plan the patient's treatment. Objective signs, such as range of motion, are better indicators of a patient's progress. Often pain fluctuates even though range of motion does not change.

Body Parts Affected

- Vertebrae
- Paraspinal muscles
- Spinal ligaments
- Nerves
- Discs
- Facet joints

Exercise Priorities

- Maximize range of motion (stretch all tight neck and shoulder girdle muscles)
- Correct postural misalignment (emphasize shoulder retraction and good neck posture)

Conditions of the Lumbar Spine

Lumbar Arthritis

The various types of arthritis are discussed in Chapter 7. Lumbar arthritis can involve the intervertebral joints or the facet joints.

Origin

Arthritis of the spine can be the result of a previous injury. Disc lesions can also lead to arthritis because they cause a decrease in disc height. Arthritis may also result simply from years of wear and tear.

Pathology

Arthritis of the lumbar spine can involve several components. Degenerative disc disease involves a loss of disc height. The disc material bulges, becomes calcified, and forms a spur (see Fig. 15–59). This results in a decreased foramen size and a narrowing of the spinal canal. This narrowing of the canal, also known as spinal stenosis, leads to painful cramping of nerves and vessels passing through the canal. Facet arthritis involves inflammation of the facet joints.

Signs and Symptoms

Spinal stenosis is characterized by increased pain with extension and walking; flexion exercises decrease the pain. Degenerative disc disease usually causes an aching type of pain that varies with activity. The pain may become sharp during acute exacerbations. The loss of range of motion varies from person to person.

Body Parts Affected

- Vertebrae
- Paraspinal muscles
- Spinal ligaments
- Nerves
- Discs
- Facet joints

Exercise Priorities

- Maximize range of motion (stretch all tight low back and lower extremity muscles)
- Strengthen trunk muscles
- Correct postural misalignment

Acute Low Back Pain

Low back pain can be considered acute if it has not been present for an extended period of time. Although it is a matter of opinion, pain that has lasted for more than 3 months is usually referred to as chronic pain rather than acute pain.

Origin

This condition is often caused by a traumatic incident, such as a "twist and lift" stress. It may also be the result of a repetitive strain injury. In either case, poor posture can be a contributing factor. Postsurgical pain can also be considered acute.

Pathology

The pathology of sprains and strains described in Chapter 7 applies also to the low back (Fig. 15–64). The secondary muscle spasm of adjacent muscles that occurs after these injuries is often worse than the original injury. Discectomies and laminectomies are techniques for surgical removal of a piece of disc or bone material to relieve pressure on a nerve root. Ideally, the operation relieves the leg signs and symptoms, but the patient must still undergo a long rehabilitation process.

Signs and Symptoms

Acute low back pain is characterized by sharp pain and decreased mobility. Generally, pain increases with activity and lessens with rest. However, mobility must be restored as soon as possible to prevent the problem from becoming chronic.

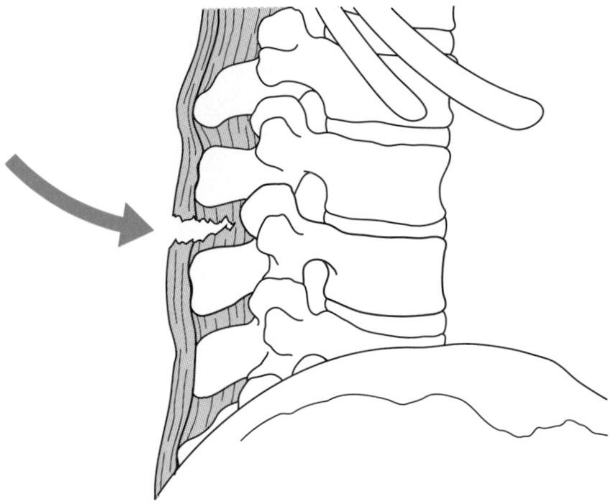

FIGURE 15–64. Acute low back sprain of interspinous ligament.

Body Parts Affected

- Vertebrae
- Paraspinal muscles
- Spinal ligaments
- Nerves
- Discs
- Facet joints

Exercise Priorities

- Maximize range of motion (stretch all tight low back and lower extremity muscles)
- Strengthen trunk muscles
- Correct postural misalignment

Disc Protrusion

The terms disc protrusion, herniation, and bulge refer to the condition wherein part of the nucleus of the disc protrudes through a weakened or torn area of the annulus.

Origin

The most common mechanism is a "twist and lift" injury. The load lifted need not be extremely heavy to cause this injury. Often a disc herniates because the lift is performed when the spine is not prepared to withstand the stress at that particular moment.

Pathology

The protrusion of the disc exerts pressure on the longitudinal ligament, which can cause severe low back pain. If the bulge is large enough, it puts pressure on a nerve root. This can result in numbness, tingling, or weakness in the muscles supplied by that nerve root.

Signs and Symptoms

Numbness, tingling, and weakness are common signs, and they may be present even in the absence of any significant amount of back pain. The pain is increased with coughing and with a straight leg raise test. Flexion exercises also increase pain, but extension exercises relieve it. This occurs because, as depicted in Figure 15–65, lumbar extension causes the nucleus of the disc to move anteriorly, away from the disc bulge.

Body Parts Affected

- Vertebrae
- Paraspinal muscles
- Spinal ligaments
- Nerves
- Discs
- Facet joints

Exercise Priorities

- Establish passive extension exercises
- Correct postural misalignment (including any lateral shifting)

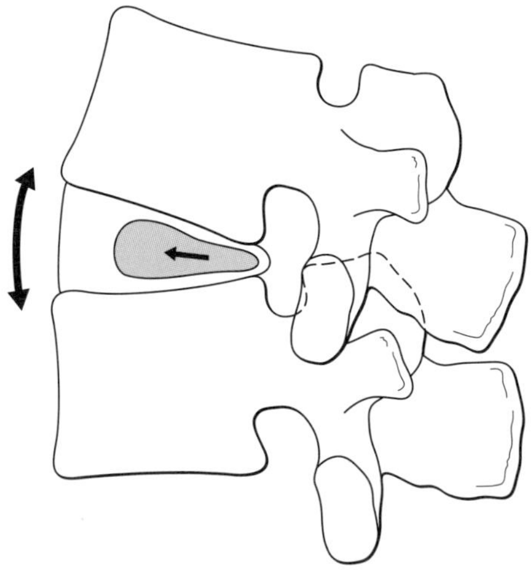

FIGURE 15–65. The effect of lumbar extension on the nucleus of the disc.

- Establish abdominal and extensor muscle strengthening exercises
- Add flexion exercises after pain has subsided

Chronic Low Back Pain

Chronic low back pain is one of the most commonly treated conditions. As with other conditions, the term "chronic" means that is has been present for more than 3 months.

Origin

This condition can start with any acute injury. Often patients have poor posture and are deconditioned. However, there may not be any apparent reason why an acute problem turns into a chronic one.

Pathology

As with other parts of the spine, clinical tests may or may not correlate with the amount of pain and disability experienced by the patient. The injury may begin with a muscle or ligament tear. Some degree of arthritis is often present. There is not usually an acute inflammatory process.

Signs and Symptoms

Decreased range of motion of the lumbar spine and lower extremities is a typical sign of chronic low back pain. Pain usually increases if the patient attempts to maintain a static position or increases his or her activity level. Pain may decrease with rest, but this does not mean that rest is the treatment of choice. As with other chronic orthopedic conditions, exercise should always be the basis of treatment.

Body Parts Affected

- Vertebrae
- Paraspinal muscles
- Spinal ligaments
- Nerves
- Discs
- Facet joints

Exercise Priorities

- Maximize range of motion
- Strengthen trunk muscles
- Correct postural misalignment
- Institute a general conditioning program

Compression Fractures

A compression fracture of the spine is a crush injury to one or more vertebral bodies (Fig. 15–66).

Origin

This condition often occurs as the result of a traumatic injury, such as a motor vehicle accident or a fall. It may also occur spontaneously if the bone has been weakened by osteoporosis.

Pathology

The various types of fractures are outlined in Chapter 7. Like other fractures, compression fractures normally take 6 to 8 weeks to heal. They do not need to be immobilized during the healing process. Conservative treatment usually calls for rest and physical therapy (often commencing within 2 weeks of the injury). The spinal cord and nerve roots are not often affected, but the patient may be predisposed to future arthritic changes in the spine.

Signs and Symptoms

Localized pain is the most common complaint. Pain increases with activities that involve spinal flexion, such as sitting, because flexion causes compression of the fractured vertebral body.

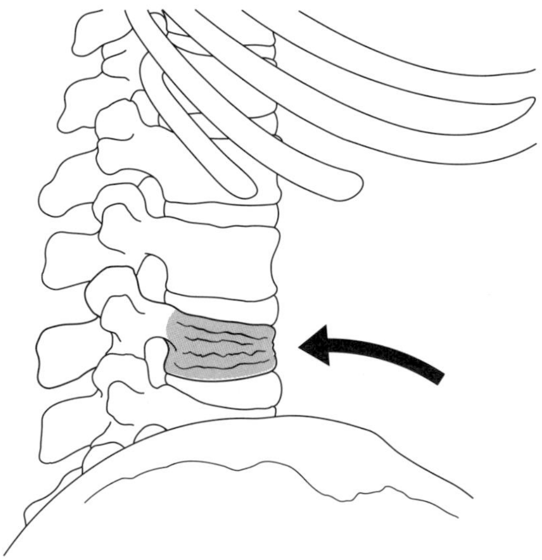

FIGURE 15–66. Compression fracture.

Body Parts Affected

- Vertebrae
- Paraspinal muscles
- Spinal ligaments
- Nerves
- Discs
- Facet joints

Exercise Priorities

- Establish passive spine extension (this opens the front of the spine, allowing more room for the vertebral body)
- Stretch tight low back and lower extremity muscles
- Increase general spine range of motion
- Establish trunk strengthening exercises
- Correct postural misalignment

Spinal Fusion

A spinal fusion is a surgical procedure that involves fusing two adjacent vertebrae using a bone graft (Fig. 15–67).

Origin

This procedure is usually seen as a last resort. It is performed only for severe joint degeneration (as in advanced arthritis or a severe fracture) when activities of daily living are not possible.

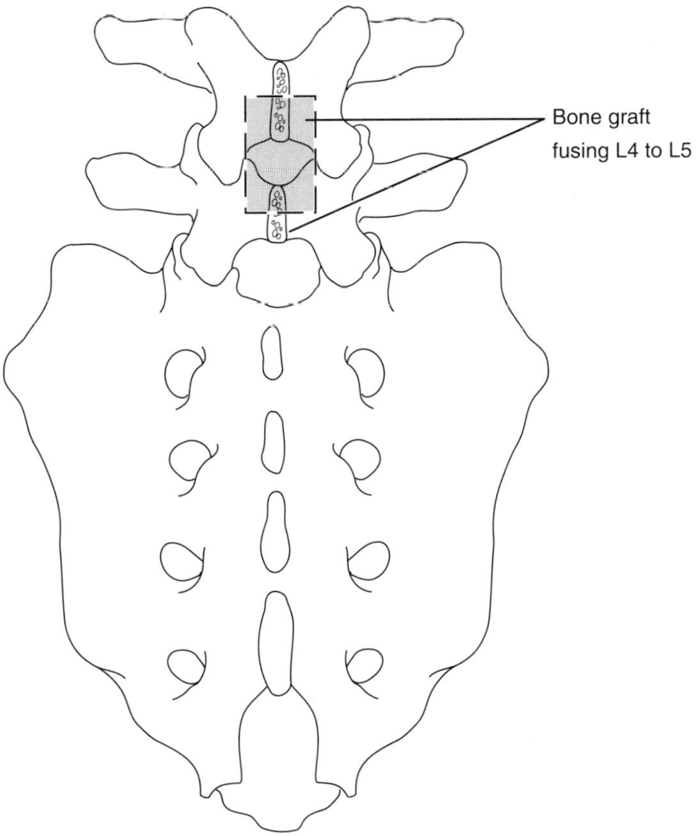

FIGURE 15–67. Spinal fusion. (Redrawn from Magee D. Orthopedic Physical Assessment. Philadelphia: W.B. Saunders, 1987.)

Pathology

As with a fracture, it takes a bone graft 6 to 8 weeks to heal. The bone for the graft is usually taken from the ilium. After the fusion has healed, there can be no movement at that particular level. Attention must then be directed to the spinal levels just above and below the fused level. These levels will now experience increased wear and tear, which predisposes them to disc bulges and arthritis.

Signs and Symptoms

Ideally, pain decreases after this surgery. The extent of pain relief varies from person to person. Generalized decreased range of motion and decreased strength are very common.

Body Parts Affected

- Vertebrae
- Paraspinal muscles
- Spinal ligaments
- Nerves
- Discs
- Facet joints

Exercise Priorities

- Increase range of motion
- Increase trunk muscle strength
- Correct postural misalignment

Spondylolisthesis

This condition involves the forward displacement of one vertebra on another as a result of an instability at that level (Fig. 15–68).

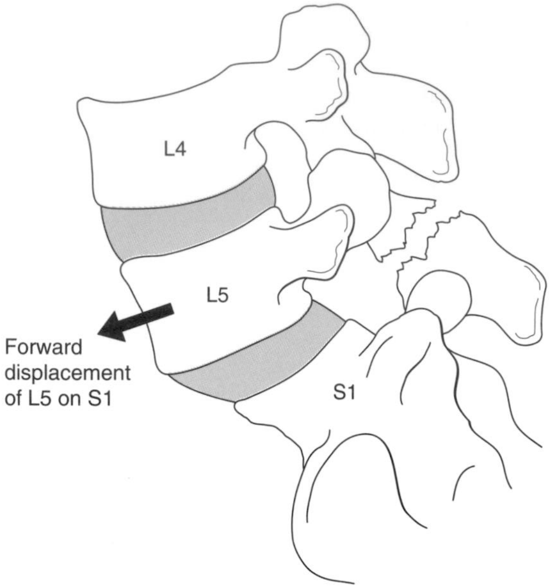

FIGURE 15–68. Spondylolisthesis.

Origin

This condition usually represents a congenital defect. It can also result from a major trauma that causes a poorly united fracture.

Pathology

Under normal circumstances, forward slip of a vertebra is prevented because the facet joints of that vertebra approximate those of the adjacent vertebrae. The term spondylolisthesis refers to a defect in this mechanism.

Signs and Symptoms

This is one of the few conditions characterized by hypermobility. There is often a palpable step defect at the level of the instability when the patient's spine is fully extended.

Body Parts Affected

- Vertebrae
- Paraspinal muscles
- Spinal ligaments
- Nerves
- Discs
- Facet joints

Exercise Priorities

- Strengthen trunk muscles
- Stretch any tight muscles that may increase stress on the hypermobile segment
- Correct postural malalignment (patient must learn to use trunk muscles to maintain spinal stability)

THE AQUATIC EXERCISE THERAPY PROTOCOL FOR CONDITIONS OF THE SPINE

Cervical Spine Flexion Protocol

For maximum benefit, neck range of motion stretches and exercises should be performed underwater, using a snorkel and mask.

Phase One

Warm-up

Perform each exercise for 2 minutes, emphasizing correct postural alignment.

- Forward Walking (see Fig. 5–21)
- Backward Walking (see Fig. 5–22)
- Side Stepping (see Fig. 5–23)
- Bent Arm Pull (see Fig. 5–12)

Stretch

Perform six repetitions of each exercise, holding 10 seconds.

- Neck Flexion (see Fig. 15–28)
- Neck Lateral Flexion (see Fig. 15–30)
- Neck Rotation (see Fig. 15–31)
- Neck Retraction (see Fig. 15–32)

Strengthen

Perform one set of 8 to 12 repetitions.

- Combination Arm Movements (see Fig. 5–20)
- Push-offs (see Fig. 15–55)

Phase Two

Warm-up

Perform each exercise for 2 minutes, emphasizing correct postural alignment.

- Forward Walking (see Fig. 5–21)
- Backward Walking (see Fig. 5–22)
- Side Stepping (see Fig. 5–23)
- Bent Arm Pull (see Fig. 5–12)
- Neck Flexion (see Fig. 15–28)
- Neck Lateral Flexion (see Fig. 15–30)
- Neck Rotation (see Fig. 15–31)
- Neck Retraction (see Fig. 15–32)

Stretch

Perform five repetitions of each exercise holding 20 seconds.

- Neck Side Stretch (see Fig. 15–13)
- Neck Flexion Stretch (see Fig. 15–15)
- Upper Trapezius Stretch (see Fig. 15–14)
- Levator Scapulae Stretch (see Fig. 15–17)

Strengthen

Perform two sets of 8 to 12 repetitions.

- Combination Arm Movements (see Fig. 5–20)
- Push-offs (see Fig. 15–55)
- Pelvic Tilt (see Fig. 15–33)

Phase Three

Warm-up

Perform each exercise for 2 minutes.

- Forward Walking (see Fig. 5–21)
- Backward Walking (see Fig. 5–22)
- Side Stepping (see Fig. 5–23)
- Bent Arm Pull (see Fig. 5–12)
- Neck Flexion (see Fig. 5–28)
- Neck Lateral Flexion (see Fig. 15–30)
- Neck Rotation (see Fig. 15–31)
- Neck Retraction (see Fig. 15–32)

Stretch

Perform five repetitions of each exercise, holding 30 seconds.

- Neck Side Stretch (see Fig. 15–13)
- Neck Flexion Stretch (see Fig. 15–15)
- Upper Trapezius Stretch (see Fig. 15–14)
- Levator Scapulae Stretch (see Fig. 15–17)
- Trapezius Stretch (see Fig. 15–16)
- Thoracic Extension (see Fig. 15–23)

Strengthen

Perform three sets of 8 to 12 repetitions.

- Resistive Shoulder Flexion (see Fig. 8–32)
- Resistive Shoulder Extension (see Fig. 8–33)
- Resistive Shoulder Adduction and Abduction (see Fig. 8–31)
- Resistive Horizontal Abduction and Adduction (see Fig. 8–34)
- Pelvic Tilt (see Fig. 15–33)

Phase Four

Warm-up

Perform each exercise for 2 minutes.

- Forward Walking (see Fig. 5–21)
- Backward Walking (see Fig. 5–22)
- Side Stepping (see Fig. 5–23)
- Bent Arm Pull (see Fig. 5–12)
- Neck Flexion (see Fig. 15–28)

- Neck Lateral Flexion (see Fig. 15–30)
- Neck Rotation (see Fig. 15–31)
- Neck Retraction (see Fig. 15–32)

Stretch

Perform five repetitions of each exercise, holding 45 seconds.

- Neck Side Stretch (see Fig. 15–13)
- Neck Flexion Stretch (see Fig. 15–15)
- Upper Trapezius Stretch (see Fig. 15–14)
- Levator Scapulae Stretch (see Fig. 15–17)
- Trapezius Stretch (see Fig. 15–16)
- Thoracic Extension (see Fig. 15–23)

Strengthen

Perform four sets of 8 to 12 repetitions. Resistive paddles may be used to increase resistance.

- Resistive Shoulder Flexion (see Fig. 8–32)
- Resistive Shoulder Extension (see Fig. 8–33)
- Resistive Shoulder Adduction and Abduction (see Fig. 8–31)
- Resistive Horizontal Abduction and Adduction (see Fig. 8–34)
- Bent Arm Pull-backs (see Fig. 15–56)
- Scapular Retraction (see Fig. 15–57)
- Lateral Pull-downs (see Fig. 15–58)

Cervical Spine Extension Protocol

Phase One

Warm-up

Perform each exercise for 2 minutes, emphasizing correct postural alignment.

- Forward Walking (see Fig. 5–21)
- Backward Walking (see Fig. 5–22)
- Side Stepping (see Fig. 5–23)
- Bent Arm Pull (see Fig. 5–12)

Stretch

Perform six repetitions of each exercise, holding 10 seconds.

- Neck Extension (see Fig. 15–29)
- Neck Lateral Flexion (emphasize stretching away from painful side) (see Fig. 15–30)
- Neck Rotation (emphasize rotation away from painful side) (see Fig. 15–31)
- Neck Retraction (see Fig. 15–32)

Strengthen

Perform one set of 8 to 12 repetitions.

- Combination Arm Movements (see Fig. 5–20)
- Push-offs (see Fig. 15–55)

Phase Two

Warm-up

Perform each exercise for 2 minutes.

- Forward Walking (see Fig. 5–21)
- Backward Walking (see Fig. 5–22)
- Bent Arm Pull (see Fig. 5–12)
- Neck Extension (see Fig. 15–29)
- Neck Lateral Flexion (see Fig. 15–30)
- Neck Rotation (see Fig. 15–31)
- Neck Retraction (see Fig. 15–32)

Stretch

Perform five repetitions of each exercise, holding 20 seconds.

- Neck Side Stretch (see Fig. 15–13)
- Upper Trapezius Stretch (see Fig. 15–14)
- Levator Scapulae Stretch (see Fig. 15–17)

Strengthen

Perform two sets of 8 to 12 repetitions.

- Combination Arm Movements (see Fig. 5–20)
- Push-offs (see Fig. 15–55)
- Pelvic Tilt (see Fig. 15–33)
- Neck Extension (see Fig. 15–29)

Phase Three

Warm-up

Perform each exercise for 2 minutes.

- Forward Walking (see Fig. 5–21)
- Backward Walking (see Fig. 5–22)
- Side Stepping (see Fig. 5–23)
- Bent Arm Pull (see Fig. 5–12)
- Neck Extension (see Fig. 15–29)
- Neck Lateral Flexion (see Fig. 15–30)
- Neck Rotation (see Fig. 15–31)
- Neck Retraction (see Fig. 15–32)

Stretch

Perform five repetitions of each exercise, holding 30 seconds.

- Neck Side Stretch (see Fig. 15–13)

- Neck Flexion Stretch (see Fig. 15–15)
- Upper Trapezius Stretch (see Fig. 15–14)
- Levator Scapulae Stretch (see Fig. 15–17)
- Trapezius Stretch (see Fig. 15–16)
- Thoracic Extension (see Fig. 15–23)

Strengthen

Perform three sets of 8 to 12 repetitions.

- Resistive Shoulder Flexion (see Fig. 8–32)
- Resistive Shoulder Extension (see Fig. 8–33)
- Resistive Shoulder Adduction and Abduction (see Fig. 8–31)
- Resistive Horizontal Abduction and Adduction (see Fig. 8–34)
- Pelvic Tilt (see Fig. 15–33)
- Neck Extension (see Fig. 15–29)

Phase Four

Warm-up

Perform each exercise for 2 minutes.

- Forward Walking (see Fig. 5–21)
- Backward Walking (see Fig. 5–22)
- Side Stepping (see Fig. 5–23)
- Bent Arm Pull (see Fig. 5–12)
- Neck Extension (see Fig. 15–29)
- Neck Lateral Flexion (see Fig. 15–30)
- Neck Rotation (see Fig. 15–31)
- Neck Retraction (see Fig. 15–32)
- Neck Flexion (see Fig. 15–28)

Stretch

Perform five repetitions of each exercise, holding 45 seconds.

- Neck Side Stretch (see Fig. 15–13)
- Neck Flexion Stretch (see Fig. 15–15)
- Upper Trapezius Stretch (see Fig. 15–14)
- Levator Scapulae Stretch (see Fig. 15–17)
- Trapezius Stretch (see Fig. 15–16)
- Thoracic Extension (see Fig. 15–23)

Strengthen

Perform four sets of 8 to 12 repetitions. Resistive paddles may be used to increase resistance.

- Resistive Shoulder Flexion (see Fig. 8–32)
- Resistive Shoulder Extension (see Fig. 8–33)
- Resistive Shoulder Adduction and Abduction (see Fig. 8–31)
- Bent Arm Pull-backs (see Fig. 15–56)
- Scapular Retraction (see Fig. 15–57)
- Lateral Pull-downs (see Fig. 15–58)

Thoracic Spine Flexion Protocol

Phase One

Warm-up

Perform each exercise for 2 minutes, emphasizing correct postural alignment.

- Forward Walking (see Fig. 5–21)
- Backward Walking (see Fig. 5–22)
- Side Stepping (see Fig. 5–23)
- Bent Arm Pull (see Fig. 5–12)

Stretch

Perform six repetitions of each exercise, holding 10 seconds.

- Neck Flexion (see Fig. 15–28)
- Neck Lateral Flexion (see Fig. 15–30)
- Neck Retraction (see Fig. 15–32)
- Pectoral Stretch (see Fig. 8–6)
- Trapezius Stretch (see Fig. 15–16)
- Levator Scapulae Stretch (see Fig. 15–17)

Strengthen

Perform one set of 8 to 12 repetitions.

- Combination Arm Movements (see Fig. 5–20)
- Push-offs (see Fig. 15–55)
- Resistive Horizontal Abduction and Adduction (see Fig. 8–34)
- Pelvic Tilt (see Fig. 15–33)
- Standing Trunk Rotation (see Fig. 15–45)

Phase Two

Warm-up

Perform each exercise for 2 minutes, emphasizing correct postural alignment.

- Forward Walking (see Fig. 5–21)
- Backward Walking (see Fig. 5–22)
- Side Stepping (see Fig. 5–23)
- Bent Arm Pull (see Fig. 5–12)
- Breast Stroke (see Fig. 5–14)

Stretch

Perform five repetitions of each exercise, holding 20 seconds.

- Neck Lateral Flexion (see Fig. 15–30)
- Trapezius Stretch (see Fig. 15–16)
- Levator Scapulae Stretch (see Fig. 15–17)
- Pectoral Stretch (see Fig. 8–6)

- Corner Stretch (see Fig. 8–20)
- Neck Retraction (see Fig. 15–32)

Strengthen

Perform two sets of 8 to 12 repetitions.

- Pelvic Tilt (see Fig. 15–33)
- Resistive Trunk Rotation (see Fig. 15–46)
- Resistive Horizontal Abduction and Adduction (see Fig. 8–34)
- Push-offs (see Fig. 15–55)
- Scapular Retraction (see Fig. 15–57)
- Standing Crunches (see Fig. 15–35)

Phase Three

Warm-up

Perform each exercise for 2 minutes.

- Forward Walking (see Fig. 5–21)
- Backward Walking (see Fig. 5–22)
- Side Stepping (see Fig. 5–23)
- Combination Arm Movements (see Fig. 5–20)

Stretch

Perform five repetitions of each exercise, holding 30 seconds)

- Upper Trapezius Stretch (see Fig. 15–14)
- Trapezius Stretch (see Fig. 15–16)
- Levator Scapulae Stretch (see Fig. 15–17)
- Pectoral Stretch (see Fig. 8–6)
- Corner Stretch (see Fig. 8–20)
- Standing Side Stretch (see Fig. 15–25)

Strengthen

Perform three sets of 8 to 12 repetitions.

- Resistive Trunk Rotation (see Fig. 15–46)
- Resistive Horizontal Abduction and Adduction (see Fig. 8–34)
- Scapular Retraction (see Fig. 15–57)
- Standing Crunches (see Fig. 15–35)
- Resistive Back Extension (see Fig. 15–41)
- Thigh Side Bends (see Fig. 15–50)

Phase Four

Warm-up

Perform each exercise for 2 minutes.

- Forward Walking (see Fig. 5–21)
- Backward Walking (see Fig. 5–22)
- Side Stepping (see Fig. 5–23)
- Combination Arm Movements (see Fig. 5–20)

Stretch

Perform five repetitions of each exercise, holding 45 seconds.

- Upper Trapezius Stretch (see Fig. 15–14)
- Trapezius Stretch (see Fig. 15–16)
- Levator Scapulae Stretch (see Fig. 15–17)
- Corner Stretch (see Fig. 8–20)
- Standing Side Stretch (see Fig. 15–25)
- Thoracic Extension (see Fig. 15–23)

Strengthen

Perform four sets of 8 to 12 repetitions.

- Resistive Trunk Rotation (see Fig. 15–46)
- Resistive Horizontal Abduction and Adduction (see Fig. 8–34)
- Scapular Retraction (see Fig. 15–57)
- Standing Cross-Crunches (see Fig. 15–43)
- Resistive Back Extension (see Fig. 15–41)
- Thigh Side Bends (with bells) (see Fig. 15–50)
- Lateral Pull-downs (see Fig. 15–58)

Thoracic Spine Extension Protocol

Phase One

Warm-up

Perform each exercise for 2 minutes.

- Backward Walking (see Fig. 5–22)
- Side Stepping (see Fig. 5–23)
- Bent Arm Pull (see Fig. 5–12)

Stretch

Perform six repetitions of each exercise, holding 10 seconds.

- Passive Back Extension (see Fig. 15–40)
- Spine Extension Stretch (see Fig. 15–20)
- Neck Extension (see Fig. 15–29)
- Neck Retraction (see Fig. 15–32)
- Upper Trapezius Stretch (see Fig. 15–14)
- Thoracic Extension (see Fig. 15–23)

Strengthen

Perform one set of 8 to 12 repetitions.

- Combination Arm Movements (see Fig. 5–20)
- Resistive Back Extension (see Fig. 15–41)
- Active Spine Flexion and Extension (patient should not flex beyond neutral) (see Fig. 15–21)

- Resistive Horizontal Abduction and Adduction (see Fig. 8–34)

Phase Two

Warm-up

Perform each exercise for 2 minutes.

- Forward Walking (see Fig. 5–21)
- Backward Walking (see Fig. 5–22)
- Side Stepping (see Fig. 5–23)
- Bent Arm Pull (see Fig. 5–12)
- Breast Stroke (see Fig. 5–14)
- Neck Extension (see Fig. 15–29)
- Neck Lateral Flexion (see Fig. 15–30)
- Neck Rotation (see Fig. 15–31)
- Neck Retraction (see Fig. 15–32)

Stretch

Perform five repetitions of each exercise, holding 20 seconds.

- Passive Back Extension (see Fig. 15–40)
- Spine Extension Stretch (see Fig. 15–20)
- Upper Trapezius Stretch (see Fig. 15–14)
- Thoracic Extension (see Fig. 15–23)
- Press-ups (see Fig. 15–22)
- Levator Scapulae Stretch (see Fig. 15–17)

Strengthen

Perform two sets of 8 to 12 repetitions.

- Combination Arm Movements (see Fig. 5–20)
- Resistive Back Extension (see Fig. 15–41)
- Active Spine Flexion and Extension (see Fig. 15–21)
- Standing Back Press (see Fig. 15–42)
- Push-offs (see Fig. 15–55)
- Standing Trunk Rotation (see Fig. 15–45)
- Resistive Horizontal Abduction and Adduction (see Fig. 8–34)

Phase Three

Warm-up

Perform each exercise for 2 minutes.

- Forward Walking (see Fig. 5–21)
- Backward Walking (see Fig. 5–22)
- Side Stepping (see Fig. 5–23)
- Combination Arm Movements (see Fig. 5–20)
- Neck Extension (see Fig. 15–29)
- Neck Lateral Flexion (see Fig. 15–30)
- Neck Rotation (see Fig. 15–31)
- Neck Retraction (see Fig. 15–32)

Stretch

Perform five repetitions of each exercise, holding 30 seconds.

- Spine Extension Stretch (see Fig. 15–20)
- Upper Trapezius Stretch (see Fig. 15–14)
- Thoracic Extension (see Fig. 15–23)
- Press-ups (see Fig. 15–22)
- Cross-Body Stretch (see Fig. 15–24)
- Standing Side Stretch (see Fig. 15–25)
- Thigh Side Bends (see Fig. 15–50)

Strengthen

Perform three sets of 8 to 12 repetitions.

- Active Spine Flexion and Extension (see Fig. 15–21)
- Resistive Horizontal Abduction and Adduction (see Fig. 8–34)
- Resistive Trunk Rotation (see Fig. 15–46)
- Lateral Pull-downs (see Fig. 15–58)
- Pelvic Tilt (see Fig. 15–33)
- Standing Back Press (see Fig. 15–42)
- Scapular Retraction (see Fig. 15–57)

Phase Four

Warm-Up

Perform each exercise for 2 minutes.

- Forward Walking (see Fig. 5–21)
- Backward Walking (see Fig. 5–22)
- Side Stepping (see Fig. 5–23)
- Combination Arm Movements (see Fig. 5–20)
- Neck Flexion (see Fig. 15–28)
- Neck Extension (see Fig. 15–29)
- Neck Lateral Flexion (see Fig. 15–30)
- Neck Rotation (see Fig. 15–31)
- Neck Retraction (see Fig. 15–32)

Stretch

Perform five repetitions of each exercise, holding 45 seconds.

- Upper Trapezius Stretch (see Fig. 15–14)
- Trapezius Stretch (see Fig. 15–16)
- Levator Scapulae Stretch (see Fig. 15–17)
- Thoracic Extension (see Fig. 15–23)
- Standing Side Stretch (see Fig. 15–25)

Strengthen

Perform four sets of 8 to 12 repetitions.

- Resistive Horizontal Abduction and Adduction (see Fig. 8–34)
- Resistive Trunk Rotation (see Fig. 15–46)
- Lateral Pull-downs (see Fig. 15–58)
- Scapular Retraction (see Fig. 15–57)
- Standing Crunches (see Fig. 15–35)
- Thigh Side Bends (with flotation bells) (see Fig. 15–50)

Lumbar Spine Flexion Protocol

Phase One

Warm-up

Perform each exercise for 2 minutes.

- Forward Walking (see Fig. 5–21)
- Backward Walking (see Fig. 5–22)
- Side Stepping (see Fig. 5–23)
- Bicycle (see Fig. 5–31)

Stretch

Perform six repetitions of each exercise, holding 10 seconds.

- Calf Stretch (see Fig. 14–7)
- Hamstring Stretch (see Fig. 13–10)
- Knee Lift Stretch (see Fig. 15–19)
- Seated Piriformis Stretch (see Fig. 15–27)
- Standing Side Stretch (see Fig. 15–25)

Strengthen

Perform one set of 8 to 12 repetitions.

- Knees to Chest (see Fig. 15–36)
- Side Flexion in Tube (see Fig. 15–53)
- Resistive Back Extension (see Fig. 15–41)
- Pelvic Tilt (see Fig. 15–33)
- Standing Trunk Rotation (see Fig. 15–45)
- Active Spine Flexion and Extension (see Fig. 15–21)

Phase Two

Warm-up

Perform each exercise for 2 minutes.

- Forward Walking (see Fig. 5–21)
- Backward Walking (see Fig. 5–22)
- Side Stepping (see Fig. 5–23)
- Bicycle (see Fig. 5–31)
- Hip Flexion (see Fig. 12–11)
- Hip Extension (see Fig. 12–12)
- Hip Abduction and Adduction (see Fig. 12–13)
- Pelvic Movements (see Fig. 5–32)
- Pelvic Tilt (see Fig. 5–33)

Stretch

Perform five repetitions of each exercise, holding 20 seconds.

- Standing Piriformis Stretch (see Fig. 15–26)
- Thigh Side Bends (see Fig. 15–50)
- Groin Stretch (see Fig. 12–9)
- Hamstring Stretch (see Fig. 13–10)
- Back Stretch (see Fig. 15–18)
- Standing Side Stretch (see Fig. 15–25)

Strengthen

Perform sets of 8 to 12 repetitions.

- Knees to Chest (see Fig. 15–36)
- Side Flexion in Tube (see Fig. 15–53)
- Resistive Back Extension (see Fig. 15–41)
- Resistive Trunk Rotation (see Fig. 15–46)
- Standing Crunches (see Fig. 15–35)
- Standing Cross-Crunches (see Fig. 15–43)
- Active Spine Flexion and Extension (see Fig. 15–21)

Phase Three

Warm-up

Perform each exercise for 2 minutes. Resistance may be increased by use of a tray with the walking warm-ups or ankle cuffs with the bicycle warm-up.

- Forward Walking (see Fig. 5–21)
- Backward Walking (see Fig. 5–22)
- Side Stepping (see Fig. 5–23)
- Bicycle (see Fig. 5–31)
- Hip Flexion (see Fig. 12–11)
- Hip Extension (see Fig. 12–12)
- Hip Abduction and Adduction (see Fig. 12–13)
- Pelvic Movements (see Fig. 5–32)
- Pelvic Tilt (see Fig. 5–33)

Stretch

Perform five repetitions of each exercise, holding 30 seconds.

- Standing Piriformis Stretch (see Fig. 15–26)
- Hamstring Stretch (see Fig. 13–10)
- Standing Side Stretch (see Fig. 15–25)

- Back Stretch (see Fig. 15–18)
- Groin Stretch (see Fig. 12–9)
- Cross-Body Stretch (see Fig. 15–24)

Strengthen

Perform three sets of 8 to 12 repetitions.

- Thigh Side Bends (use flotation bells) (see Fig. 15–50)
- Resistive Band Cross-Crunches (see Fig. 15–44)
- Bent Knee Twists (see Fig. 15–48)
- Resistive Band Lateral Flexion (see Fig. 15–52)
- Resistive Trunk Rotation (see Fig. 15–46)
- Standing Cross-Crunches (see Fig. 15–43)
- Sit-ups in Parallel Bars (see Fig. 15–37)

Phase Four

Warm-up

Perform each exercise for 2 minutes. Use tray with walking warm-ups.

- Forward Walking (see Fig. 5–21)
- Backward Walking (see Fig. 5–22)
- Side Stepping (see Fig. 5–23)
- Bicycle (use ankle cuffs for resistance) (see Fig. 5–31)
- Hip Flexion (see Fig. 12–11)
- Hip Extension (see Fig. 12–12)
- Hip Abduction and Adduction (see Fig. 12–13)

Stretch

Perform five repetitions of each exercise, holding 45 seconds.

- Standing Piriformis Stretch (see Fig. 15–26)
- Hamstring Stretch (see Fig. 13–10)
- Standing Side Stretch (see Fig. 15–25)
- Back Stretch (see Fig. 15–18)

Strengthen

Perform four sets of 8 to 12 repetitions.

- Crossover Sit-ups in Parallel Bars (see Fig. 15–47)
- Double Leg Lifts (see Fig. 15–39)
- Pelvic Curl (see Fig. 15–34)
- Deep water exercises for lower extremities (see Figs. 6–12 to 6–29)

Lumbar Spine Extension Protocol

Phase One

Warm-Up

Perform each exercise for 2 minutes.

- Backward Walking (see Fig. 5–22)
- Side Stepping (see Fig. 5–23)

Stretches

Perform 10 repetitions of each exercise, holding 10 seconds.

- Passive Back Extension (see Fig. 15–40)
- Spine Extension Stretch (see Fig. 15–20)

Strengthen

Perform sets of 8 to 12 repetitions.

- Side Flexion in Tube (see Fig. 15–53)
- Resistive Back Extension (see Fig. 15–41)
- Active Spine Flexion and Extension (patient should not flex beyond neutral) (see Fig. 15–21)

Phase Two

Warm-up

Perform each exercise for 2 minutes.

- Backward Walking (see Fig. 5 22)
- Side Stepping (see Fig. 5–23)
- Hip Flexion (see Fig. 12–11)
- Hip Extension (see Fig. 12–12)
- Hip Abduction and Adduction (see Fig. 12–13)
- Forward Walking (slow) (see Fig. 5–21)

Stretch

Perform 10 repetitions of each exercise, holding 10 seconds.

- Passive Back Extension (see Fig. 15–40)
- Spine Extension Stretch (see Fig. 15–20)
- Press-ups (see Fig. 15–22)
- Thoracic Extension (see Fig. 15–23)

Strengthen

Perform two sets of 8 to 12 repetitions.

- Side Flexion in Tube (see Fig. 15–53)
- Resistive Back Extension (see Fig. 15–41)
- Active Spine Flexion and Extension (see Fig. 15–21)
- Standing Back Press (see Fig. 15–42)
- Push-offs (see Fig. 15–55)
- Standing Trunk Rotation (see Fig. 15–45)

Phase Three

Warm-up

Perform each exercise for 2 minutes.

- Forward Walking (see Fig. 5–21)

- Backward Walking (see Fig. 5–22)
- Side Stepping (see Fig. 5–23)
- Hip Flexion (see Fig. 12–11)
- Hip Extension (see Fig. 12–12)
- Hip Abduction and Adduction (see Fig. 12–13)
- Pelvic Movements (see Fig. 5–32)

Stretch

Perform five repetitions of each exercise, holding 20 seconds.

- Spine Extension Stretch (see Fig. 15–20)
- Thoracic Extension (see Fig. 15–23)
- Press-ups (see Fig. 15–22)
- Cross-Body Stretch (see Fig. 15–24)
- Standing Side Stretch (see Fig. 15–25)
- Thigh Side Bends (see Fig. 15–50)

Strengthen

Perform three sets of 8 to 12 repetitions.

- Active Spine Flexion and Extension (see Fig. 15–21)
- Resistive Back Extension (see Fig. 15–41)
- Resistive Trunk Rotation (see Fig. 15–46)
- Lateral Pull-downs (see Fig. 15–58)
- Pelvic Tilt (see Fig. 5–33)
- Standing Back Press (see Fig. 15–42)

Phase Four

Warm-up

Perform each exercise for 2 minutes. Use tray with walking warm-ups.

- Forward Walking (see Fig. 5–21)
- Backward Walking (see Fig. 5–22)
- Side Stepping (see Fig. 5–23)
- Hip Flexion (see Fig. 12–11)
- Hip Extension (see Fig. 12–12)
- Hip Abduction and Adduction (see Fig. 12–13)
- Pelvic Movements (see Fig. 5–32)

Stretch

Perform five repetitions of each exercise, holding 30 seconds.

- Spine Extension Stretch (see Fig. 15–20)
- Standing Side Stretch (see Fig. 15–25)
- Hamstring Stretch (see Fig. 13–10)
- Knee Lift Stretch (see Fig. 15–19)
- Standing Piriformis Stretch (see Fig. 15–26)

Strengthen

Perform three sets of 8 to 12 repetitions.

- Standing Back Press (see Fig. 15–42)
- Resistive Trunk Rotation (see Fig. 15–46)
- Pelvic Tilt (see Fig. 5–33)
- Active Spine Flexion and Extension (see Fig. 15–21)
- Standing Crunches (see Fig. 15–35)
- Standing Cross-Crunches (see Fig. 15–43)

PROGRESSION: Progress to lumbar flexion routine or deep water lower extremity exercises (Chapter 6).

REFERENCES

1. Rasch P, Burle R. Kinesiology and Applied Anatomy. Philadelphia: Lea & Febiger, 1972.
2. Cailliet R. Understand Your Backache. Philadelphia: F.A. Davis, 1984.
3. Thomson A, Skinner A, Piercy J. Tidy's Physiotherapy. 12th ed. Toronto: Butterworth-Heinemann, 1991.
4. Lind B, Sihlbom H, Nordwall A, Malchau H. Normal range of motion of the cervical spine. Arch Phys Med Rehabil 70:692–695, 1989.
5. Arnheim D. Modern Principles of Athletic Training. St. Louis: Times Mirror/Mosby College Publishing, 1993.
6. Magee D. Orthopedic Physical Assessment. Philadelphia: W.B. Saunders, 1987.
7. Pitman A. Awesome Aqua Abdominals. Canadian Aquatic Leaders Alliance Conference, Guelph, Ontario, 1994.

Fibromyalgia Syndrome and Aquatic Exercise

CHAPTER 16

WHAT IS FIBROMYALGIA SYNDROME?

Subjective Complaints in Fibromyalgia Syndrome

Fibromyalgia syndrome (FMS) is a nonarticular rheumatic disorder, one of a group of painful musculoskeletal conditions that emanate from periarticular structures outside the joint capsule and periosteum. FMS is referred to as a syndrome because it is identified by a number of symptoms rather than by one specific malfunction. It is characterized by diffuse musculoskeletal pain, aching, stiffness, fatigue, disturbed sleep, and tender points (Table 16–1). The pain is usually described as a burning sensation from "head to toe" or a pain that "hurts all over," similar to the aching and stiffness reported by patients with rheumatoid arthritis (RA). The pain may change locations, and it is most severe in the parts of the body used often. For some patients, the pain may be intense enough to interfere with daily tasks, but other patients feel only a mild discomfort.

The fatigue experienced may range from a feeling of tiredness to extreme exhaustion. The

TABLE 16–1. A Summary of the Subjective Complaints Reported in Primary Fibromyalgia

Generalized muscular aches and pains
Morning stiffness
Chronic fatigue and poor work tolerance
Sleep disturbance
Symptoms influenced by the weather—worse with cold or rain, temporary relief with heat

subjective symptoms associated with FMS can be further described in terms of a series of exacerbations and remissions. The symptoms are often made worse by cold and humid weather, tension, and inactivity and are eased by heat, moderate activity, or relaxation.

Historical Examination of Fibromyalgia Syndrome

The condition that is recognized as FMS today is not new. There have been countless historical references to "disturbed sleep, deep pain and exhaustion."[1, 2]

In 1904, Growers[3] introduced the term "fibrositis." His clinical observations identified various tender points, some of which are used today in the diagnosis of FMS. Growers was the first to describe asymmetric regional pain syndromes, as opposed to referred or diffuse body pain. He recognized that there was a difference between "spontaneous pain" and "sensitiveness." The sensitive sites, he observed, produced pain or discomfort only when pinched or when muscle action occurred; otherwise, they remained asymptomatic. Unfortunately, Growers regarded the hypersensitive sites he encountered as inflammatory, and he believed the condition to be a form of "muscular rheumatism."[1, 4]

In the 1930s, Kellgren and Livingston made a significant contribution to the understanding of pain mechanisms. They found that they could reproduce referred pain symptoms by injecting a hypertonic saline solution into the deep structures of the muscle. They recorded the "segmental reference of pain" and noted that it "related to deep structures within the segments rather than dermatomes."[1, 5, 6] By 1935 there was still no proof of local inflammation in FMS, and by 1950 the term "fibrositis" was abandoned completely. Researchers found it difficult to explain the symptoms these patients complained of, but they were reluctant to equate the symptoms with psychogenic factors.

After the American Rheumatism Association chose "morning stiffness" as the first criterion for RA, many patients with FMS were diagnosed as "probable RA" because they complained of that particular symptom.[7, 8] Over the next decade, much research was conducted into sleep deprivation, tender points, physical fitness, and many other pathophysiologic mechanisms.[9] However, it was not until the 1970s that two Canadian doctors, Hugh Smythe and Harvey Moldofsky, developed a method of diagnosing FMS. Soon afterward, FMS received recognition as a condition that is very real but often frustrating for both the physician and the patient. In 1990, an international medical symposium published requirements for the diagnosis of FMS that are now widely accepted.[10]

THE DIAGNOSIS AND ASSESSMENT OF FIBROMYALGIA SYNDROME

Primary versus Secondary Fibromyalgia

FMS is most commonly divided into two categories: primary and secondary. An individual who has primary FMS has no other concurrent condition. Those who have FMS in association with another disease (such as RA) are said to have secondary FMS; these patients have an "associated" or "concomitant" condition. These terms refer to any clinical disorder that may be contributing to the individual's musculoskeletal pains. A patient can have both arthritis (such as RA) and a form of nonarticular rheumatic disease (such as FMS) concurrently. The two conditions are no longer considered mutually exclusive and are treated and managed individually.[11]

Differential Diagnosis

In order for a true diagnosis of secondary fibromyalgia to exist, there must be (1) a diagnosis for FMS according to the American College of Rheumatology Criteria for diagnosis (Table 16–2) and (2) an associated condition that can be con-

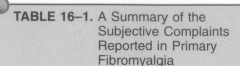

TABLE 16–2. The American College of Rheumatology 1990 Criteria for the Classification of Fibromyalgia

For classification purposes, patients will be said to have fibromyalgia if both criteria are satisfied. Widespread pain must have been present at least 3 months. The presence of a second clinical disorder does not exclude the diagnosis of fibromyalgia.

Criterion 1: History of Widespread Pain

Pain is considered widespread if all of the following are present: pain in the left side of the body, pain in the right side of the body, pain above the waist, and pain below the waist. In addition, axial skeletal pain (cervical spine, anterior chest, thoracic spine, or low back) must be present. In this definition, shoulder and buttock pain is considered as pain for each involved side. Low back pain is considered lower segment pain.

Criterion 2: Pain in 11 of 18 Tender Point Sites on Digital Palpation

Pain, on digital palpation, must be present in at least 11 of the following 18 tender point sites:
Occiput: bilateral, at the suboccipital muscle insertions.
Low cervical: bilateral, at the anterior aspects of the intertransverse spaces at C5-C7.
Trapezius muscle: bilateral, at the midpoint of the upper border.
Supraspinatus muscle: bilateral, at origins, above the spine of the scapula near the medial border.
Second rib: bilateral, at the second costochondral junctions, just lateral to the junctions on upper surfaces.
Lateral epicondyle: bilateral, 2 cm distal to the epicondyles.
Gluteal muscle: bilateral, in upper outer quadrants of buttocks in anterior fold of muscle.
Greater trochanter: bilateral, posterior to the trochanteric prominence.
Knee: bilateral, at the medial fat pad proximal to the joint line.
Digital palpation should be performed with an approximate force of 4 kg.
For a tender point to be considered positive, the subject must state that the palpation was painful. "Tender" is not to be considered "painful."*

*See Table 16–5.
From Wolfe F, Smythe HA, Yunus MB, et al. The American College of Rheumatology 1990 Criteria for the Classification of Fibromyalgia. Report of the multicenter criteria committee. Arthritis Rheum 33:160–172, 1990.

firmed or made evident from abnormal test profiles or that may be eased by successful treatment of the disease in question. The physician conducts a brief patient history, an examination, and laboratory tests to screen for concomitant conditions.

Although the exact cause of FMS is unknown, it often seems to be triggered by some sort of trauma, such as a fall, car accident, viral infection, childbirth, or surgical procedure. Or there may be no obvious trigger. Studies indicate that up to 10% of the general population has some form of nonarticular rheumatic disease, including 1% to 2% with FMS. FMS seems to occur most often in women (9 out of 10 cases). The age of onset tends to be from 12 to 45 years; onset after 60 years of age is uncommon.[12–15]

American College of Rheumatology Criteria for Diagnosis

Diagnosing FMS is difficult, because it shares many symptoms with other dysfunctional syndromes such as irritable bowel syndrome and tension headaches that do not show up on standard laboratory tests or X-rays.[16] There are many published diagnostic criteria for FMS. Although the diagnostic criteria put forth by the American College of Rheumatology have been criticized as being too simplistic, they have made a significant difference to the evaluation of patients with FMS, and they are the criteria discussed here.[10]

Diagnostic Criteria

In order for a diagnosis of FMS to be confirmed, the patient must complain of "widespread" musculoskeletal pain in four quadrants of the body—that is, above and below the waist and on both sides of the body—for more than 3 months.[10, 13, 17] In addition, the physician must rule out the possibility of traumatic injury, structural rheumatic disease, infectious arthropathy, endocrine-related arthropathy, or abnormal laboratory tests.[17]

Secondly, the points of acute tenderness or pain must occur in at least 11 of the 18 tender points that are characteristic of FMS (Fig. 16–1) when they are pressed with a 4-kg digital pressure, and

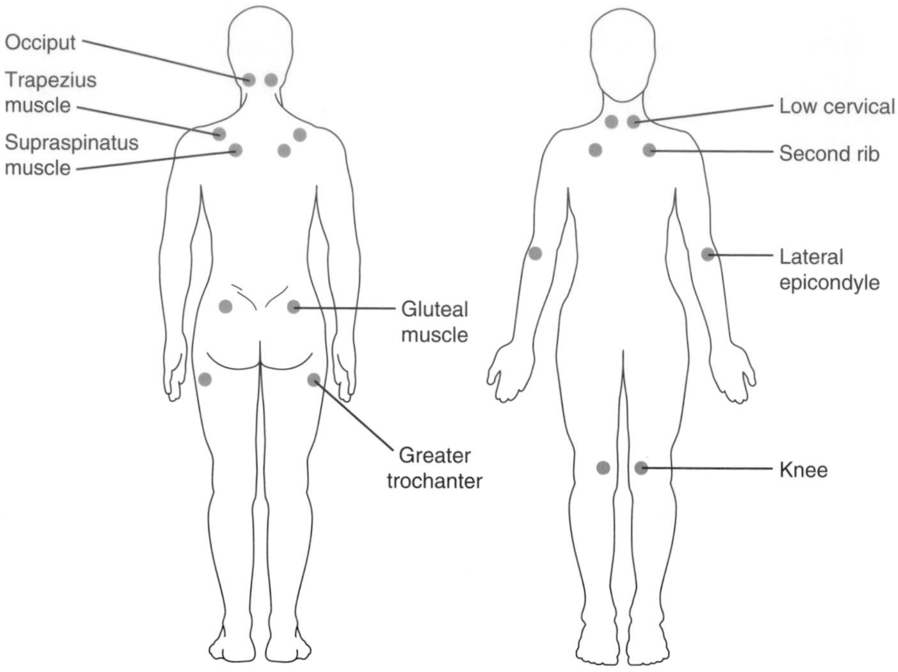

FIGURE 16–1. The tender points associated with fibromyalgia syndrome.

these responses must be reproducible on reexamination.[2, 10–12] (A 4-kg digital pressure is the amount of pressure necessary to cause the blood to blanch from the thumbnail for individuals with normal blood pressure.[12]) Patients with primary FMS have a generalized amplification of pain sensitivity.[18] At this level of pressure, the fibromyalgia patient reports feeling pain, whereas the normal individual reports feeling pressure.

In addition to the obligatory diagnostic criteria outlined, Yunus and coworkers[17] believe that 3 of 10 minor criteria should also be required in order to diagnose FMS:

- change in a symptom with activity
- change in a symptom with weather
- change in a symptom with anxiety or stress
- poor sleep
- general fatigue
- anxiety
- headache
- irritable bowel syndrome
- subjective swelling
- nonradicular, nondermatonic numbness.

Tender Points and Trigger Points

Patients with abnormalities of the periarticular soft tissue, such as bursitis, can have three types of painful sites. The pain may be *localized* and simply involve a tendon or bursa; it may be *regionalized,* as in myofascial pain syndrome and temporomandibular joint syndrome; or it may be *generalized* (involving multiple areas of the body), as in polymyalgia rheumatica, hypermobility syndrome, and fibromyalgia syndrome.[12] Although the sites of local tenderness are often referred to interchangeably as "tender points" or "trigger points," this usage in incorrect.[1] The two terms refer to different conditions, which respond to different treatments.

The tender points associated with FMS occur in specific locations.[11, 13] These locations of acute tenderness are widespread and are often unknown to the patient until they are touched. They vary in number and severity from patient to patient but are identical for everyone with FMS[13] (Table 16–3).

Trigger points, on the other hand, are "referred" points of pain on palpation. This is the type of pain characteristic of myofascial pain syndrome (some-

TABLE 16–3. Tender Point Sites Used in 1990 American College of Rheumatology Criteria for the Classification of Fibromyalgia Syndrome

Tender Points	
1, 2	*Occiput:* at the suboccipital muscle insertions
3, 4	*Low cervical:* at the anterior aspect of the intertransverse spaces at C5-C7
5, 6	*Trapezius muscle:* at the midpoint of the upper border
7, 8	*Supraspinatus muscle:* at origins, above the spine of the scapula near the medial border
9, 10	*Second rib:* at the second costochondral junctions, just lateral to the junctions on upper surfaces
11, 12	*Lateral epicondyle:* 2 cm distal to the epicondyles
13, 14	*Gluteal muscle:* in upper outer quadrants of the buttocks in anterior fold of muscle
15, 16	*Greater trochanter:* posterior to the trochanteric prominence
17, 18	*Knee:* at the medial fat pad proximal to the joint line
Control Points	
A, B	*Dorsal forearm:* mid-web space, midway between wrist and elbow
C, D	*Thumbnail:* middle of nail surface
E, F	*Metatarsal:* dorsal surface of third metatarsal at midshaft

Data from Ediger B. Coping with fibromyalgia (fibrositis). Toronto: LRH Publications, 1991; Wolfe F, Smythe HA, Yunus MB, et al. The American College of Rheumatology 1990 Criteria for the Classification of Fibromyalgia: Report of the multicenter criteria committee. Arthritis Rheum 33:160–172, 1990; Russell JI. Fibromyalgia syndrome: Recognition and management. Audioplus Teleconference, Annenberg Center at Eisenhower, Rancho Mirage, California, October 5, 1993.

times called "local fibrositis"), a tender point syndrome often confused with FMS.[11] The pain is regionalized and unilateral; for example, the pain may run through the hip and down the leg of the same side. Trigger points can be felt in the involved muscle and are tighter on palpation than the surrounding tissue ("taut bands"). Although the actual physiology of trigger points is unknown, there are many predisposing factors that are capable of causing such a reaction within a muscle (eg, a cold local draft, physical fatigue or muscle strain, muscle trauma, bad posture, stress, infection).[19]

Although the syndromes are different, patients with myofascial pain syndrome may have or may develop FMS syndrome as a result of their general poor conditioning[11] (Table 16–4).

It has been suggested that muscle microtrauma (tiny microscopic tears in the muscle) may be the underlying pathology of both myofascial pain syndrome and FMS and that myofascial pain syndrome may, in fact, represent the early stages of FMS.[11] Early diagnosis and treatment of myofascial pain may prevent the subsequent development of FMS. The most effective treatments for trigger point pain seem to be heat, massage,[19] direct pressure, acupuncture, injections of local anesthetic,[20] stretching, and the "spray and stretch" technique[21] (see description in the section on physical therapy).

Pain Severity

A tender point is defined as a site of severe pain with palpation.[21] When examining the patient with FMS, the clinician must determine the degree of palpation pressure and the number of total sites that elicit an acute pain response.[11, 17, 22] The "severity" of the response, which is usually 1+ or greater, is recorded, and the sum of severities at the 18 sites is called the tender point index (TPI) (Table 16–5). Assessing the total number of tender points goes beyond simple quantification, because pain is subjective and cannot be measured on an absolute basis.[15] The number of accepted sites depends on what the examiner considers to be a mild or moderate pain response to palpation.[15, 17]

Many studies have documented the acute tender point pain experienced by patients with FMS.[15, 23, 24] It is difficult to imagine that patients with FMS experience significantly more actual pain than those with RA who have damaged joints.[11, 12, 15, 17, 23, 24] However, when FMS and RA patients were compared with a normal control group in terms of functional ability (eg, lifting, taking items off shelves, squeezing things together), the control group had 100% functional ability but both the RA and FMS participants had 50%. Therefore, patients with FMS demonstrate either a lower pain tolerance or a higher pain amplification than patients with

TABLE 16–4. A Comparative Look at Fibromyalgia and Myofascial Pain Syndrome

	Fibromyalgia	Myofascial Pain
Diagnostic Criteria		
Characteristics of tender point pain	Multiple fibrositis "tender points" that occur at predictable sites on the body—local	The presence of one or more local "trigger" points—referred
Tender point distributions	Widespread aching of longer than 3 months duration—diffuse	Referred pain pattern specific to the "active" or "latent" trigger points—local
Tender point location	Muscle–tendon junctions	Muscle belly
Epidemiology		
Sex	Female predominance 10:1	Male predominance 2:1
Age	Median age 45	Median age 35
Subjective Complaints		
Stiffness	Widespread morning stiffness	Regional
Fatigue	A "nonrestorative" sleep pattern	Usually absent
Symptom Management		
Treatment	Tricyclics (antidepressants)	Local injections, "spray and stretch," heat and massage
Prognosis	Seldom cured—chronic	Usually good with treatment—possible recurrence

RA. They also have an impaired functional ability on objective assessment with a work simulator, although they do not have damaged bones or joints, as RA patients do.[11, 13, 25]

Pain sensitivity can also be used as an indicator of treatment effectiveness. For instance, patients with myofascial pain syndrome who receive successful treatment show an increase in their pain threshold levels toward normal values.[24]

PROPOSED PATHOGENIC MECHANISMS

Fibromyalgia is one of the most common diagnoses seen in rheumatology clinics. It is estimated that FMS constitutes 15% to 20% of outpatient rheumatology cases.[12, 23] In spite of the prevalence of primary FMS, the pathophysiology is not well understood. Clinical studies have identified a number of possible pathogenic mechanisms involved in

TABLE 16–5. The Severity Scale and Tender Point Index*

Severity	Patient Response to 4-kg Digital Pressure
0	No reported tenderness
1+	Tenderness reported verbally but indifferently, no physical response
2+	Tenderness reported plus an objective physical response (wince, withdrawal)
3+	Tenderness reported with emphasis, plus an exaggerated dramatic physical response (wince, jerk, withdrawal)
4+	Untouchable area; the anticipated pain is so severe that the patient avoids the expected palpation

*Tender Point Index = Sum of severities at 18 sites.

Data from Russell JI. Fibromyalgia syndrome: Recognition and management. Audioplus Teleconference, Annenberg Center at Eisenhower, Rancho Mirage, California, October 5, 1993; Russell JI, Vipraio G, Morgan WW, Bowden CL. Is there a metabolic basis for fibrositis syndrome? Am J Med 18(Suppl 3A):50–56, 1986.

FMS, some of which are reviewed here (Fig. 16–2).[26]

Psychologic Pathology

Patients with FMS have a lower than normal pain threshold.[24, 27] They often experience pain in response to a stimulus that does not normally cause pain; that is, they have "pain hypersensitivity."[27, 28] Usually no tissue damage or any likely pathophysiologic cause is detectable through routine laboratory tests. In the past, many physicians dismissed these patients as hypochondriacs and their symptoms as a "manifestation of hysteria," or they diagnosed them as suffering from "psychogenic rheumatism."[26–30] Patients who suffer from "psychogenic rheumatism," however, are influenced by changes to their internal environment (ie, the severity of their symptoms varies depending on their mood or emotional state).[27] However, patients with FMS report that their symptoms are influenced by factors in the external environment, such as the weather, heat, cold, and exercise.[16, 27] Today, physicians approach the psychiatric aspect of FMS by diagnosing patients as having a "somatoform pain disorder."[30, 31]

A number of psychologic tests and rating scales have been used in an attempt to establish a psychiatric pattern in patients with FMS.[28–31] As a result, some common psychologic characteristics of these patients have been found[30, 31] (Table 16–6). Many studies report a strong relation between FMS and a psychopathologic manifestation.

Individuals who suffer from a painful debilitating

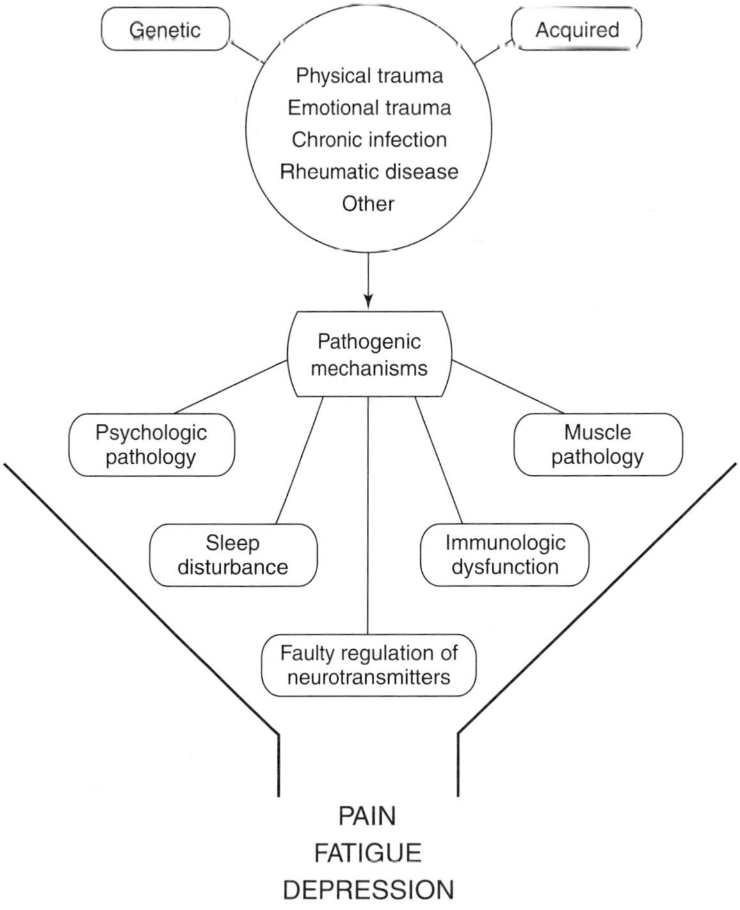

FIGURE 16–2. Possible pathogenic mechanisms of fibromyalgia syndrome.

TABLE 16–6. Common Psychologic Characteristics Found in Patients with Fibromyalgia Syndrome and Clinical Depression

Depression
Anxiety
Chronic pain
Insomnia
Irritability
Headache
Poor concentration
Loss of interest
Preoccupation with bodily functions

or limiting chronic medical condition often experience depression and anxiety and, consequently, more pain. Situational depression is observed in approximately 30% of FMS and RA patients, and it is not specific to any psychiatric disorder.[12, 28, 31] Furthermore, it is unclear whether pain is the cause or the consequence of the condition. Studies suggest that, while psychiatric factors might promote some cases of fibromyalgia, they are very unlikely to be a principal cause of the illness.[28] In fact, the psychologic characteristics associated with chronic pain tend to normalize after the pain subsides.[27]

Sleep Disturbance

Clinical studies show that persons with FMS have difficulty achieving refreshing, restorative sleep. This problem is associated with a physiologic electroencephalographic arousal disorder during sleep,[32, 33] a symptom that is prevalent in 80% to 100% of all FMS patients.[34] During the sleep-wake cycle, an individual experiences three different states: wakefulness, slow-wave sleep, and rapid eye movement (REM) sleep.[33, 34] These stages have distinct electronic frequencies, with defined patterns.[33] During wakefulness, the individual actively interacts with the surroundings; movements of the eyes, head, and body are characteristic of this state.

With the onset of sleep, movement stops. Slow-wave sleep is divided into four stages (1 through 4, or alpha through delta) and takes between 45 and 85 minutes to achieve.[33] Periods of slow-wave sleep then alternate with periods of REM sleep, which lasts between 5 and 45 minutes and during which dreaming occurs.

Each stage of slow-wave sleep represents a progressively deeper state of sleep, with 1 (alpha) being the lightest and stage 4 (delta) being the deepest; it is this stage that is lacking in patients with FMS. Stage 4 is restorative sleep; the hormones that are responsible for the body's growth and repair are most active during this period.

Although many features of FMS can be traced directly to sleep disturbance, it is unclear whether the symptoms are the cause or a result of sleep deprivation. Both conditions may be caused by a separate defective feedback system. Patients who suffer from other sleep disorders, such as sleep apnea (interrupted breathing) or nocturnal myoclonus (spasms in the arms or legs), not only complain of nonrestorative sleep (abnormal rhythm during stage 4 sleep) but also exhibit fibrositis tender points on examination. Fibrositis tender points can also be induced in normal healthy controls by selective stage 4 sleep deprivation.[35] Therefore, improving the quality of sleep might reduce the severity of the symptoms experienced by patients with FMS. However, some studies have indicated an inverse relation between pain severity and the ability to achieve restorative sleep that is related to the concentration of tryptophan. As tryptophan levels increased, so did the patients' ability to sleep; however, their pain became worse. (See next section.)

Faulty Regulation of Neurotransmitters

Changes in neurotransmitters such as serotonin, endorphins, and substance P influence the sleep-wake cycle and the perception and modulation of pain.[35–38] One theory suggests that the symptoms associated with FMS may be caused by a relative deficiency of serotonin.[35, 37, 38] Serotonin is a neurotransmitter that has a dramatic effect on blood vessels, the smooth muscle around blood vessels, and the blood flow through small vessels.[12] It also plays a role in the regulation of deep restorative sleep and in the perception of pain.

Patients with FMS may also have low levels of tryptophan, an essential amino acid and a metabolic precursor of serotonin synthesis that is obtained from the digestion of dietary proteins. Actively transferred across the blood-brain barrier, tryptophan in the form of serotonin is distributed to the areas around the brain where and when it is needed

(Fig. 16–3). Patients with FMS show lower levels of serum tryptophan and other amino acids than normal controls, and those with the lowest levels of free plasma tryptophan have the most severe pain.[38]

Peptides involved in the transmission and modulation of pain in the peripheral and central nervous systems have been identified. Vaeroy and colleagues[39] found that patients with FMS and Raynaud's phenomenon had three times the normal level of substance P in their cerebrospinal fluid. Substance P is a neurotransmitter and chemical mediator that initiates the pain process. Normal levels of substance P, together with serotonin, reduce or maintain normal pain perception, whereas substance P alone tends to amplify the pain signal so that what is perceived by the brain is not normal (minimal) pain but much pain. In other words, the perception of the severity of pain is chemically altered.[12]

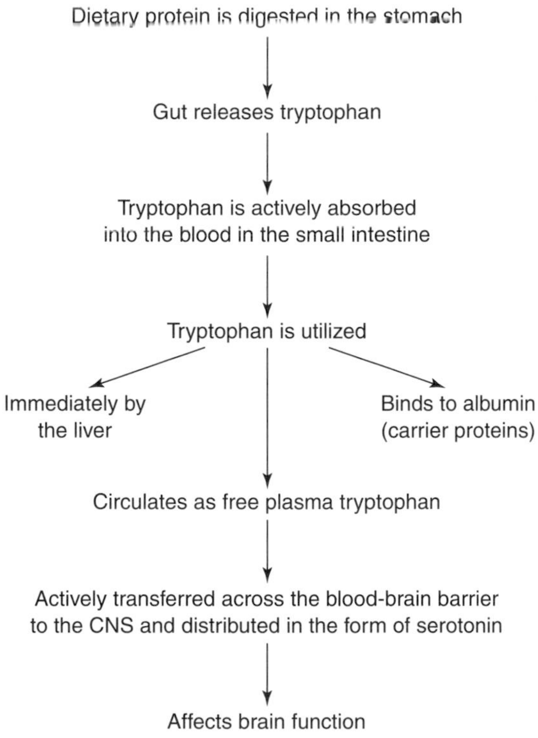
Dietary protein is digested in the stomach
Gut releases tryptophan
Tryptophan is actively absorbed into the blood in the small intestine
Tryptophan is utilized
Immediately by the liver
Binds to albumin (carrier proteins)
Circulates as free plasma tryptophan
Actively transferred across the blood-brain barrier to the CNS and distributed in the form of serotonin
Affects brain function

FIGURE 16–3. The metabolic pathway of tryptophan. (Modified from Russell IJ, Michalek JE, Vipraio FA, et al.: Serum amino acids in fibrositis/fibromyalgia syndrome. J Rheumatol 16(Suppl 19):158–163, 1989.)

Immunologic Dysfunction

Many patients with FMS report that their condition began suddenly after a flu-like viral illness.[26] The search for a specific viral cause has been disappointing. However, there is a link between sleep deprivation, infectious disease, and the direct involvement of bacterial products in sleep regulation. Important chemicals necessary for immunologic function are produced during stage 4 sleep. Muramyl peptides, for example, have the ability to alter cytokine production and are also involved in a variety of physiologic processes.[40] Cytokines such as interleukin-1 are known to enhance slow-wave sleep. A damaged immune response or damaged regulation of cytokines could explain the lack of restorative sleep and the flu-like symptoms reported by many patients with FMS.[26, 40] Furthermore, patients with FMS were found to have reduced levels[41] and reduced activity[42] of natural killer cells, compared with normal controls, which indicates that these patients may suffer from some type of immunologic dysfunction.

Muscle Pathology

Skeletal muscle represents an important end organ in FMS because many patients believe that the muscle is responsible for the pain and stiffness they experience. Abnormalities of muscle structure that have been identified histologically include atrophied fibers and reticular or elastic fibers not seen in normal muscle tissue. Functional abnormalities include a decrease in high-energy phosphate concentration, reduced tissue oxygenation, and impaired blood flow.[43]

The musculoskeletal pain, stiffness, and fatigue that are symptomatic of FMS may be the result of muscle microtrauma.[44] The muscle–tendon junctions have the highest concentrations of pain receptors and correspond to many of the tender points characteristic of FMS. The fibers involved in the transmission and sensation of pain in skeletal muscles have a relatively high threshold to normal stimuli. In the presence of neurotransmitters such as serotonin, these fibers become hypersensitive to repetitive or noxious stimuli and hence transmit pain at a low level of exertion.[43]

Muscle soreness appears to be related to the intensity of the exercise rather than to the duration.

Microtrauma to muscles also apparently results from unaccustomed exercise, particularly eccentric contractions.[44] A muscle produces the greatest amount of force when it is contracting eccentrically (lengthening) against resistance. Examples of exercises that have a high eccentric component are running (when the foot comes in contact with the ground), arm raises (when the arm is lowered), and situps (when the body returns to the starting position). Moderate swimming and cycling are good examples of low-intensity eccentric activities. For the fibromyalgia patient, pool exercises offer movement without eccentric forces.

One study found that there was "no difference in the degree of exercise-induced muscle soreness between subjects who perform concentric isokinetic contractions and those who perform eccentric isokinetic contractions" and that it is the workload that contributes to muscle soreness.[45] The amount of pain experienced because of microtrauma is directly related to fitness level, and patients with fibromyalgia are usually physically[43] and aerobically[44] unfit.

In addition, muscle blood flow studies have demonstrated that muscles and other tissues in patients with FMS suffer from hypoxia (lack of oxygen).[43] This condition is caused partly by faulty control of blood flow at the cellular level, which alters factors involved in the transport of oxygen to skeletal muscle and its subsequent use in the generation of high-energy phosphates. As a result, oxygen and nutrient supplies are restricted and waste materials are not properly flushed out.

Reduced levels of phosphoserine (important to efficient muscle contraction) have been found in patients with FMS.[46] The inability to effectively contract the muscle suggests the inability to effectively perform a given task.

Patients with FMS usually become unfit as a result of limiting their exercise because of pain or fatigue. Lack of stage 4 (delta) sleep increases fatigue, which in turn reduces the will to exercise; on the other hand, lack of exercise reduces the amount of restorative sleep. Both depletion of slow-wave sleep and inactivity influence the release of growth hormone. The suboptimal secretion of growth hormone not only inhibits slow-wave and REM sleep[37] but also influences protein synthesis.[38] Decreased amino acid levels in blood and the structural and functional abnormalities in skeletal muscle may be the result of an insufficient supply of substrate amino acids to meet the demands of normal muscle repair. An imbalance of this type may delay the healing of exercise-induced muscle microtrauma and so produce the painful muscular symptoms reported by fibromyalgia patients.[38, 44]

THE CONVENTIONAL APPROACH TO THE TREATMENT OF FIBROMYALGIA SYNDROME

Addressing the Emotional Factors

A chronic painful condition such as FMS lends itself well to a multidisciplinary rehabilitative team approach (Fig. 16–4). The treatment of FMS is aimed at reducing the symptoms rather than curing the condition itself. Reduced pain and improved sleep are accepted successful results of treatment because they help the individual cope and function more effectively.[12, 35, 41–45, 47–51]

Before physical therapy begins, the physician must make a confident diagnosis of FMS based on the accepted diagnostic criteria and evaluation process. The physician must also identify any associated medical illnesses, which often influence the severity of FMS symptoms. The fibromyalgia patient needs reassurance and an explanation of the nature of the illness and the steps that can be taken to alleviate the severity of the symptoms. General educational or counseling sessions can help teach the patient with FMS to manage both the emotional and physical aspects of the condition.

The therapist should perform a brief evaluation of social issues. The role of lifestyle and emotional factors (eg, marital discord, loss of work, litigation) must be examined, because these factors can affect the treatment outcome. Adequate support from family, friends, a support group, or other people with FMS is also important; if the patient is unable to cope with the added stress, depression, or anxiety, the appropriate psychiatric intervention may be necessary. The therapist should also evaluate patients' present mechanical stressors such as activities of daily living, family responsibilities, and working conditions, which may need to be altered depending on how well they are able to manage their symptoms.

Physical Therapy

Physical therapy techniques used in the treatment of FMS include the following:

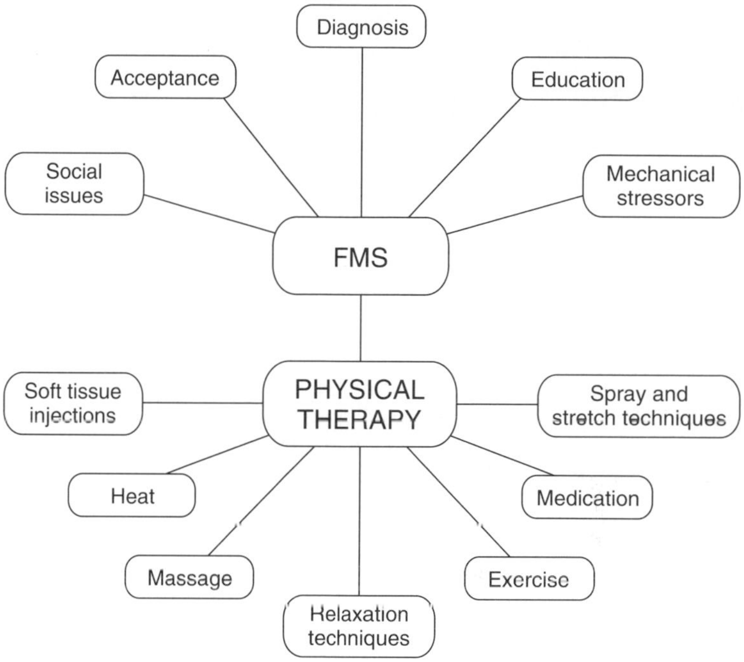

FIGURE 16–4. Factors involved in the treatment of fibromyalgia syndrome (FMS).

1. Local heat for 30 minutes to the neck, back, and shoulders
2. Deep tissue massage for 10 minutes to most symptomatic areas, as tolerated. This is very individualized because the patient may get worse before reporting any benefit
3. Instruction in relaxation techniques such as biofeedback, which helps the patient to recognize and control adverse muscular tension responses that are normally unconsciously performed, and relaxation training programs geared to relaxing the mind and body with the help of tapes, lectures, or books
4. A gradual progressive physical exercise program with aerobic and isotonic exercises such as walking and pool exercises
5. Some therapists use "spray and stretch" techniques, which involve spraying the skin at a tender site with a coolant such as Fluori-Methane that inhibits the pain sensation, then gently stretching the involved muscles.[21] Soft tissue injections are also used; a local anesthetic is injected into the tender sites to offer temporary relief from the pain.

Medication

Many fibromyalgia patients take painkillers such as acetaminophen (Tylenol) that help to reduce the pain to a tolerable level. Nonsteroidal anti-inflammatory drugs that have painkilling properties are used occasionally for arthritic conditions. However, because inflammation is not characteristic of FMS, these medications have limited benefit for fibromyalgia patients.

Some patients are also prescribed antidepressants, which help to treat the symptoms of musculoskeletal pain and sleep disturbance in FMS. The medications prescribed most often are amitriptyline (Elavil) and cyclobenzaprine (Flexeril). Patients who received low doses of amitriptyline showed a significant reduction in morning stiffness and self-reported pain, with improved sleep, global assessment scores, and tender point scores, and a greater sense of well-being.[24, 51, 52] Fibromyalgia patients have also reported improvements in localized pain, sleep disturbance, and trigger point scores after treatment with cyclobenzaprine.[38, 51–53] Both of these drugs are tricyclic medications (antidepressants), but cyclobenzaprine has the additional ability to reduce muscle tension by inhibiting the gamma efferent discharge to muscle spindles. As a result, the pain-spasm-pain cycle characteristic of FMS is broken, allowing the muscles to function more normally.

THE IMPORTANCE OF EXERCISE PROGRAMMING

Ability to Sustain Activity

Patients with FMS have a lower than average cardiovascular or aerobic fitness level, and their muscles do not utilize oxygen well.[49] As a result, these individuals tend to become unfit very easily, which further decreases their cardiovascular efficiency and peripheral circulation. In many instances, FMS leads to a reduction in habitual activity, which, if sustained, causes a cycle of deconditioning (Fig. 16–5).[44] Newham and Edwards[54] documented a number of symptoms that result from enforced inactivity in their analysis of "effort syndromes." Many of these symptoms are also reported by patients with FMS (Table 16–7).[43]

During endurance training, skeletal muscles undergo many physiologic adaptations (Table 16–8).[43] Unfit muscles, however, respond in the opposite direction, leaving the individual more susceptible to muscle microtrauma and pain. Patients with FMS are unable to perform high-intensity, long-duration activities.[49] Furthermore, these patients are usually so unfit that beneficial results can be achieved at a relatively low intensity of exercise.[49]

A graded exercise program to improve aerobic fitness is of therapeutic benefit to patients with FMS. Patients who participate in an aerobic program of low intensity for an extended period of time reduced some of the fibrositis-like symptoms caused by sleep deprivation[49]; specifically, they show improvement in tender points, global ratings, and cardiovascular fitness.[39, 55] Aerobic exercise not only increases cardiovascular conditioning but helps improve the transportation and utilization of oxygen by the tissues.

Patients with FMS also benefit from stretching and strengthening exercises. Stretching exercises help to maintain or increase flexibility and relax tight, stiff muscles. Strengthening exercises help

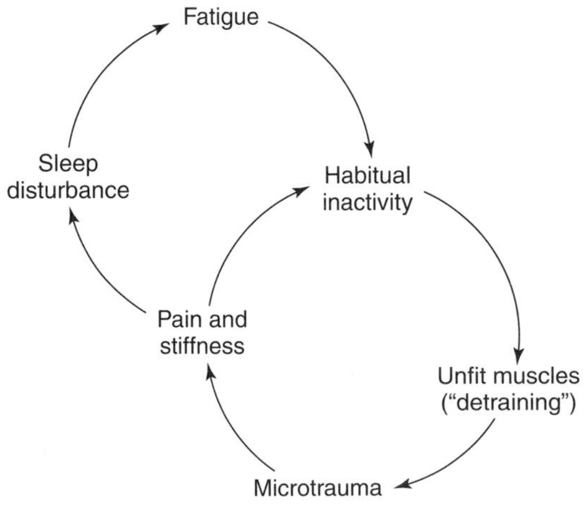

FIGURE 16–5. A feedback loop depicting the consequences of exercise-induced microtrauma: a self-sustaining cycle of muscular pain and fatigue.

TABLE 16–7. Common Symptoms Related to Habitual Inactivity

Cardiovascular system
Palpitations
Tachycardia
Neurological
Dizziness
Headache
Paraesthesia
Respiratory system
Breathlessness
Chest pain
Gastrointestinal system
Abdominal pain
Dysphagia
Musculoskeletal system
Muscle pain
Tremor
Autonomic nervous system
Excessive sweating
General symptoms
Fatigue
Weakness
Tension
Anxiety

TABLE 16–8. The Physiological Adaptations of Skeletal Muscle to Endurance Training

Increased muscle mass
Increased muscle strength
Increased oxidative enzymes
Increased adenosine triphosphate and phosphocreatine
Increased myoglobin
Increased capillary density
Increased arterial collateral circulation
Increased buffer capacity

to reduce the strain placed on the muscles. Most importantly, an effective program helps the patient with FMS to manage both the emotional and physical aspects of the illness.

Pain seems to be the central complaint in FMS. Whether it is primary or secondary to the symptoms of FMS, musculoskeletal pain is always present. Patients who persist in a regular routine of sustained physical activity despite the pain show improvement in their symptoms and can lead fairly normal lives.[43–45, 49–51]

Most patients respond best to a progressive aerobic exercise program that addresses stretching and strengthening, particularly of the neck, arms, legs, and spine. Pool exercises performed in a *heated* pool are perhaps the most beneficial activities for patients with FMS, because there is a lack of eccentric forces and the movements are slowed by the water, reducing the chance of microtrauma. Furthermore, the physiologic changes that occur in response to warm water immersion help to reduce perceived pain and increase ease of movement. About 50% of the people who begin any exercise program drop out during the first 6 months. Those who remain seldom adhere to the prescribed exercise routine. In order to ensure compliance, it is important not to base the program on guidelines formulated from data on healthy subjects, but to consider the ultimate goals of the exercising patient.

The goal of the fibromyalgia aquatic exercise therapy program is to help increase an individual's exercise tolerance and endurance level, thereby gaining a general increase in fitness level. As one's fitness level improves, the severity of symptoms such as postexertional pain, stiffness, and muscle weakness often decreases. Each exercise program should match the ability of the individual and should be flexible in response to the symptoms or pain experienced during each session. Regardless of fitness level, patients should start with only one-quarter of the amount of activity that they feel they can manage. It is important to progress slowly rather than start too aggressively and experience unnecessary setbacks. Fibromyalgia patients experience more pain after exercise to begin with than those who do not suffer from this condition. Postexertional pain is most prominent in the transitional phase between an unfit and a more fit state. Patients often need encouragement to persevere with their exercise routine through this phase, because there is a fine line between doing enough and doing too much.

Guidelines for Implementing a Progressive Aquatic Therapy Program

In the human body, the physiologic response to exercise directly depends on several factors: (1) the *frequency* of exercise performance (eg, sessions every week, every month), (2) the *intensity* of the exercise relative to individual's ability to perform the chosen task, (3) the *duration,* or the time it takes to perform the exercises in one session, and (4) the *type* of exercise performed. These factors influence the adaptations made by the physiologic systems,[49] and changing any one of these variables alters the physiologic response.

The more specific the goals of the exercise program, the greater the likelihood that the exercise will be appropriate for the purpose. Because there are no universal guidelines for exercise prescription, patients with FMS should be encouraged to exercise at their own rate or within their own capacity. It is important to consider carefully the type and severity of exercise, because activities with high intensity and high eccentric components are unsuitable for fibromyalgia patients.

The following exercise guidelines should be used in planning the exercise program:

1. The patient should try to exercise a minimum of two to three times per week.
2. Always start with three repetitions of each exercise when the patient begins each phase of the program.
3. Increase exercise intensity by adding two repetitions of each exercise every 2 to 3 weeks. Before each progression, the patient should be able to perform three consecutive sessions without a substantial increase in pain.
4. While exercising, use the Borg Scale of perceived exertion (see Fig. 17–9).
5. The patient should start gradually, exercising for 5 to 10 minutes, and increase by 2 to 3 minutes each week. The exercise program should last at least 30 minutes for maximum benefit.
6. Choose aquatic aerobic activities such as walking or deep water walking, deep water running, or cycling.

Patients with FMS benefit most from a low-resistance training program in which the intensity is increased at a slow rate, permitting gradual acclimation. It is difficult to evaluate the actual exercise tolerance (perceived pain threshold) of each patient because many feel they can do more than they actually can. Each exercise session results in post-exertional pain and stiffness, regardless of level. Progressively increasing the number of repetitions in each session increases the muscular endurance, but no change occurs in either actual pain threshold or perceived pain. As patients continue to exercise despite pain, however, they will eventually be able to do more exercise for the same amount of pain. Finally, with continuation of the endurance training program, the actual pain threshold begins to approach the perceived pain threshold, thereby reducing the severity of symptoms and resulting in a gradual acclimatization to exercise (Fig. 16–6).

Sample Fibromyalgia Pool Program

Warm-up

Stretch

- Calf Stretch (see Fig. 14–7)
- Hamstring Stretch (see Fig. 13–10)
- Quadriceps Stretch (see Fig. 13–5)
- Hip Flexor Stretch (see Fig. 12–5)
- Cross-Shoulder Stretch (see Fig. 8–11)
- Triceps Stretch (see Fig. 9–7)
- Forearm Stretch (see Fig. 9–9)
- Deep Water Shoulder Press (see Fig. 6–8)
- Back Stretch (see Fig. 15–18)
- Neck Range of Motion (see Figs. 15–28 to 15–32)

Strengthening

At the beginning, the strengthening program should alternate between the upper body one day and the lower body the next day. Begin slowly and apply all the guidelines, slowly integrating onto land.

Upper Body

- Resistive Shoulder Flexion (see Fig. 8–32)
- Resistive Shoulder Extension (see Fig. 8–33)
- Resistive Shoulder Adduction and Abduction (see Fig. 8–31)
- Resistive Horizontal Abduction and Adduction (see Fig. 8–34)

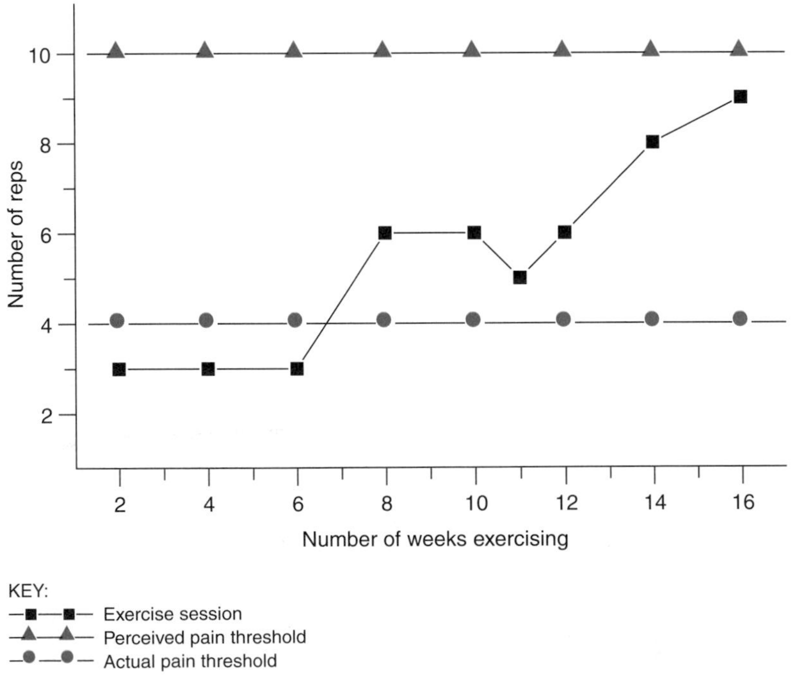

FIGURE 16–6. Response to a progressive aquatic exercise program.

- Rowing (see Fig. 8–36)
- Upright Rowing (see Fig. 8–38)
- Biceps Curl (see Fig. 9–11)
- Triceps Extension (see Fig. 9–14)
- Wrist Curl (see Fig. 10–17)

Lower Body

- Heel Raises (see Fig. 14–16)
- Toe Flexion and Extension (see Fig. 14–19)
- Thigh Extension (see Fig. 13–13)
- Hamstring Pull-back (see Fig. 13–14)
- Squats (see Fig. 13–16)
- Hip Flexion (see Fig. 12–11)
- Hip Extension (see Fig. 12–12)
- Hip Abduction and Adduction (see Fig. 12–13)

Abdominals

- Standing Crunches (see Fig. 15–35)
- Thigh Side Bends (see Fig. 15–50)
- Resistive Trunk Rotation (see Fig. 15–46)
- Pelvic Curl (see Fig. 15–34)

Aerobic Component

Stretches

REFERENCES

1. Smythe H. Fibrositis syndrome: A historical perspective. J Rheumatol 16:2–6, 1989.
2. Ediger B. Coping with Fibromyalgia (Fibrositis). Toronto: LRH Publications, 1991.
3. Mitchell SW, Moorehouse GR, Keen WW. Gunshot Wounds and Other Injuries of Nerves. Philadelphia: J.B. Lippincott, 1864.
4. Growers WR. A lecture on lumbago: Its lessons and analogues. BMJ 1:117–121, 1904.
5. Kellgren JH. Observations on referred pain arising from muscle. Clin Sci 3:174–190, 1938.
6. Livingston WK. Pain Mechanisms. New York: Macmillan, 1943, pp. 4–6.
7. Proposed diagnostic criteria for rheumatoid arthritis. Bull Rheum Dis 7:121–124, 1956.
8. Ropes MW, Bennett GA, Cobb S, et al. Proposed diagnostic criteria for rheumatoid arthritis. Ann Rheum Dis 16:118–125, 1957.
9. Smythe HA, Moldofsky H. Two contributions to the understanding of the "fibrositis" syndrome. Bull Rheum Dis 20:928–931, 1977.
10. Wolfe F, Smythe HA, Yunus MB, et al. The American College of Rheumatology 1990 Criteria for the Classification of Fibromyalgia: Report of the multicenter criteria committee. Arthritis Rheum 33:160–172, 1990.
11. Bennett R. Confounding features of the fibromyalgia syndrome: A current perspective of differential diagnosis. J Rheumatol 16(Suppl 19):58–61, 1989.
12. Russell JI. Fibromyalgia syndrome: Recognition and management. Audioplus Teleconference, Annenberg Center at Eisenhower, Rancho Mirage, California, October 5, 1993.
13. Turk D, Flor H. Primary fibromyalgia is greater than tender points: Toward a multiavial taxonomy. J Rheumatol 16(Suppl 19):80–86, 1989.
14. Felxon DT. Epidemiologic research in fibromyalgia. J Rheumatol 16(Suppl 19):7–11, 1989.
15. Rollman GB. Measurement of pain in fibromyalgia in the clinic and laboratory. J Rheumatol 16(Suppl 19):113–119, 1989.
16. Waylonis GW, Heck W. Fibromyalgia syndrome: New associations. Am J Phys Med Rehabil 71:343–348, 1992.
17. Yunus MB, Masi AT, Aldag JC. A controlled study of primary fibromyalgia syndrome: Clinical features and association with other functional syndromes. J Rheumatol 16(Suppl 19):62–71, 1989.
18. Mikkelsson M, Latikka P, Kautiainen H, et al. A comparison of muscle and bone pressure pain threshold and pain tolerance in fibromyalgia patients and controls. Arch Phys Med Rehabil 73:814–818, 1992.
19. Wale JO, ed. Tidy's Massage and Remedial Exercises. 11th ed. Bristol: John Wright & Sons, 1968.
20. Sola AE. Myofascial trigger point therapy. Res Staff Phys 49:38–45, 1980.
21. Travell J, Simmons DG. Myofascial Pain and Dysfunction: The Trigger Point Manual. Baltimore: Williams & Wilkins, 1983.
22. Russell JI, Vipraio G, Morgan WW, Bowden CL. Is there a metabolic basis for fibrositis syndrome? Am J Med 18(Suppl 3A):50–56, 1986.
23. Scudds RA, Trachsel LCE, Luckhurst BJ, Percy JS. A comparative study of pain, sleep quality and pain responsiveness in fibrositis and myofascial pain syndrome. J Rheumatol 16(Suppl 19):120–126, 1989.
24. Scudds RA, McCain GA, Rollman GB, Harth M. Improvements in pain responsiveness in patients with fibrositis after successful treatment with amitriptyline. J Rheumatol 16(Suppl 19):98–103, 1989.
25. Cathy MA, Wolf F, Kleinheksell SM. Functional ability and work status in patients with fibromyalgia. Arthritis Care Res 11:151–171, 1988.
26. Goldenberg DL. Fibromyalgia and its relation to chronic fatigue syndrome, viral illness and immune abnormalities. J Rheumatol 16(Suppl 19):91–93, 1989.
27. Sheon RP, Moskowitz RW, Goldberg VM. Soft Tissue Rheumatic Pain: Recognition, Management, Prevention. Philadelphia: Lea & Febiger, 1982.
28. Merskey H. Physical and psychological consideration in the classification of fibromyalgia. J Rheumatol 16(Suppl 19):72–79, 1989.
29. Goldenberg DL. An overview of psychologic studies in fibromyalgia. J Rheumatol 16(Suppl 19):12–14, 1989.
30. Goldenberg DL. Psychological symptoms and psychiatric diagnosis in patients with fibromyalgia. J Rheumatol 16(Suppl 19):107–130, 1989.
31. Hudson JI, Pope HG. Fibromyalgia and psychopathology:

Is fibromyalgia a form of "affective spectrum disorder?" J Rheumatol 16(Suppl 19):15–22, 1989.
32. Moldofsky H. Sleep–wake mechanisms in fibrositis. J Rheumatol 16(Suppl 19):47–48, 1989.
33. Jones BE. The sleep–wake cycle: Basic mechanisms. J Rheumatol 16(Suppl 19):49–51, 1989.
34. Moldofsky H. Nonrestorative sleep and symptoms after a febrile illness in patients with fibrositis and chronic fatigue syndromes. J Rheumatol 16(Suppl 19):150–153, 1989.
35. McCain GA, Tilbe KS. Diurnal hormone variation in fibromyalgia syndrome: A comparison with rheumatoid arthritis. J Rheumatol 16(Suppl 19):154–157, 1989.
36. Hamaty D, Valentine JL, Howard R, et al. The plasma endorphin, prostaglandin and catecholamine profile of patients with fibrositis treated with cyclobenzaprine and placebo: A 5-month study. J Rheumatol 16(Suppl 19):164–168, 1989.
37. Moldofsky H, Warsh JJ. Plasma tryptophan and musculoskektal pain in non-articular rheumatism ("fibrositis syndrome"). Pain 5:65–71, 1978.
38. Russell JI, Michalek JE, Vipraio FA, et al. Serum amino acids in fibrositis/fibromyalgia syndrome. J Rheumatol 16(Suppl 19):158–163, 1989.
39. Vaeroy H, Sakurada T, Forre O, et al. Modulation of pain in fibromyalgia (fibrositis syndrome): Cerebrospinal fluid investigation of pain related neuropeptides with special reference to calcitonin gene related peptide. J Rheumatol 16(Suppl 19):53–57, 1989
40. Krueger JM, Johannsen L. Baterial products: Cytokines and sleep. J Rheumatol 16(Suppl 19):52–57, 1989.
41. Caligiuri M, Murray C, Buchwald D, et al. Phenotypic and functional deficiency of natural killer cells in patients with chronic fatigue syndrome. J Immunol 139:3306–3313, 1987.
42. Russell JI, Vigraio GA, Tavar Z, et al. Abnormal natural killer cell activity in fibrositis syndrome is responsive to in vitro IL-2. Arthritis Rheum 81:824, 1988.
43. Bennett RM. Physical fitness and muscle metabolism in the fibromyalgia syndrome: An overview. J Rheumatol 16(Suppl 19):28–29, 1989.
44. Bennett RM. Bevond fibromyalgia: Ideas on etiology and treatment. J Rheumatol 16(Suppl 19):185–191, 1989.
45. Fitzgerald GK, Rothstein JM, Mayhew TP, Lamb RL. Exercise-induced muscle soreness after concentric and eccentric isokinetic contractions. Phys Ther 71:505–513, 1991.
46. Bengtsson A, Henriksson KG. The muscle in fibromyalgia: A review of Swedish studies. J Rheumatol 16(Suppl 19):144–149, 1989.
47. Rodnan GP, Schumacher HP, Zvaifler NJ, eds. Primer on the Rheumatic Diseases. 8th ed. Atlanta: Arthritis Foundation, 1983.
48. Henry JL. Concepts of pain sensation and its modulation. J Rheumatol 16(Suppl 19):104–112, 1989.
49. Klug GA, McAuley E, and Clark S. Factors influencing the development and maintenance of aerobic fitness: Lessons applicable to the fibrositis syndrome. J Rheumatol 16(Suppl 19):30–39, 1989.
50. Littlejohn G. Mediocolegal aspects of fibrositis syndrome. J Rheumatol 16(Suppl 19):169–173, 1989.
51. Buckelew SP. Fibromyalgia: A rehabilitation approach. Am J Phys Med Rehabil 68:37–41, 1989.
52. Goldenberg DL. A review of the role of tricyclic medications in the treatment of fibromyalgia syndrome. J Rheumatol 16(Suppl 19):137–139, 1989.
53. Quimby LG, Gratwick GM, Whitney CS, Block SR: A randomized trial of cyclobenzaprine for the treatment of fibromyalgia. J Rheumatol 16(Suppl 19):140–143, 1989.
54. Newham DQ, Edwards RHT. Effort syndromes. Physiotherapy 65:52–56, 1979.
55. Nichols DS, Glenn TM. Effects of aerobic exercise on pain perception, affect, and level of disability in individuals with fibromyalgia. Phys Ther 74:327–332, 1994.

Integrating Land-Based Exercises into Aquatic Rehabilitation Programs

Chapter 17

RECONDITIONING AFTER AN INJURY

Tissue Healing

Factors Affecting Healing

Regardless of the type of injury, all tissues (except cartilage, which does not regenerate) require a specific time for healing and remodeling to occur (Table 17–1). The most critical aspect of a rehabilitation program is increasing the intensity of the training stimuli. Structures that are involved too soon and have not had enough time to heal may experience tissue failure or breakdown. Damage usually occurs when the healing structure is subjected to repetitive loads without adequate rest or to a single maximal workload.[1] This is the type of injury observed in overuse syndromes and stress fractures.

After an injury, healing requires certain conditions. First, there must be an adequate blood supply. Structures with a good blood supply heal quickly. Circulating blood provides oxygen and nutrients to healing tissues while removing retained metabolites. An inadequate blood supply tends to slow the healing process. Lack of blood to the healing structures results in tissue death, which produces more scar tissue.[2]

Second, an adequate inflammatory reaction must occur for satisfactory healing of both soft tissues and bones. Inflammation usually lasts 3 to 4 days after the injury and is necessary for the clotting and subsequent growth of new tissue.

Third, the injured site or wound must be clean. Infection delays the healing process and causes damage to the tissue.

TABLE 17–1. Blood Supply and Healing Time of Various Body Tissues

Tissue Type	Blood Supply	Healing Time
Skin	Good	3–14 days
Muscle	Average	3 wk
Tendon/Ligaments	Poor	6 wk
Bone	Good	Upper limb (3–12 wk) Lower limb (12–18 wk) Femur (4–5 mo) (Young children, 4–6 wk)
Cartilage	None	No healing process

Fourth, irritation must be avoided during healing. Persistent irritation, such as the removal of a bandage, slows the healing process. Removing a dressing that is stuck to the wound breaks down newly formed granulation tissue by tearing the capillaries. Stress or strain can also cause this delicate tissue to break down and can slow repair.

Finally, adequate time is required for the healing process. As one ages, tissue collagen loses its elasticity and the capillary blood supply is decreased, which reduces the healing capability.[1] Therefore, in older persons, body tissues need more time to heal.

During the healing process, injured soft tissues and bones undergo three major phases: the inflammatory phase, the repair phase, and the remodeling phase.[3]

Healing of Soft Tissues

Injury to soft tissues can occur as a result of compression, tension, or shear forces. A compression force crushes the tissue. Tension forces pull and extend the tissue, as in strains and sprains. Shear forces are applied perpendicular to the collagen fibers. Tendons and ligaments are designed to tolerate tension force, but they cannot withstand shear or compression forces[3] (Fig. 17–1).

After an injury has been sustained, the inflammatory phase is initiated. The apparent signs of inflammation include redness, heat, swelling, pain, and loss of function.[3] Inflammation occurs during the first 24 hours as fluid accumulates in the injured area. This process is intended to protect, localize, and eliminate unwanted byproducts of the injury, in preparation for healing.

The repair or regeneration phase is associated with tissue death, which continues after the initial injury as a result of lack of oxygen. During this phase, healing occurs through increased cellular formation across the gap of the wound. Delicate granulation tissue is formed. After this new granulation tissue is formed, it is replaced by the type of tissue that was originally injured, then by fibrous or scar tissue.

During the remodeling phase, scar tissue is laid down quickly without much organization. The early introduction of exercise helps to provide some uniformity to this otherwise random process. As new tissue is laid down, more flexibility is achieved.

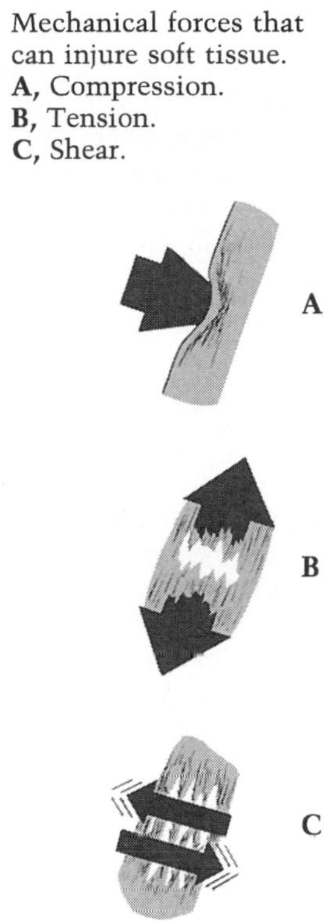

FIGURE 17–1. Mechanical forces that can injure soft tissues. *A*, Compression; *B*, tension; *C*, shear. (From Arnheim DD, Prentice WE. Principles of Athletic Training. 8th ed. St. Louis, Mosby–Year Book, 1993.)

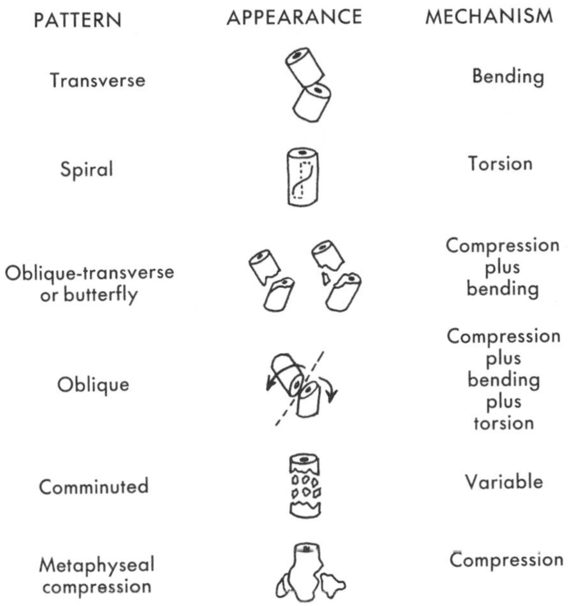

PATTERN
APPEARANCE
MECHANISM
Transverse
Bending
Spiral
Torsion
Oblique-transverse or butterfly
Compression plus bending
Oblique
Compression plus bending plus torsion
Comminuted
Variable
Metaphyseal compression
Compression

FIGURE 17–2. Mechanisms of bone fractures. (From Arnheim DD, Prentice WE. Principles of Athletic Training. 8th ed. St. Louis, Mosby Year Book, 1993.)

Healing of Fractures

Healing begins immediately after the injury. The inflammatory phase lasts approximately 4 days and is characterized by hemorrhage and bone death. When exercising in the acute stages, it is best to avoid movements that are similar to the mechanism of injury (Fig. 17–2).

During the repair phase, the cells adjacent to the fracture site proliferate. Granulation tissue begins to form a bridge between the ends of the broken bones. The cells mature as osteoblasts form immature bone, known as callus or woven bone. This process begins within 3 to 4 weeks of the injury and lasts approximately 3 or 4 months until the hard callus forms.[3]

Primary bone forms during the remodeling stage. The excess callus bone is reabsorbed, and trabecular bone is laid down along the lines of greatest stress. Remodeling continues until the fractured bone is restored to its original shape and structure.

Progressive Adaptation onto Land

After an injury there is pain, inflammation, swelling, loss of mobility, loss of function, and a rapid deterioration of fitness. The immediate concerns of the therapist should be to protect the involved area from further damage or strain; to reduce pain, inflammation, and swelling; to initiate an active rest program; to increase range of motion; and to educate and inform the patient about the nature of and restrictions imposed by the injury. The purpose of any rehabilitation program is to restore the damaged structures to a preinjury state through the use of therapeutic exercise. An integrative program employing aquatic and land-based exercises can achieve this goal much sooner than land-based exercises alone.

Rehabilitation programs that focus on increasing strength and endurance allow the patient to participate in continuous exercise while reducing the chance of reinjury. Patients who improve their strength and endurance from "sedentary" to "sedentary/light" or to "light" improve their chances for re-employment by 60%.[4] The reconditioning of a sedentary individual differs from that of an athlete only in the type and intensity of the exercises used in the program. Regardless of the condition, the therapist must determine which exercises will be most effective without endangering the injured structures or slowing the healing process. These exercises should be focused on increasing musculotendinous flexibility, increasing muscular strength and endurance, improving balance (proprioception), maintaining or restoring cardiorespiratory fitness, restoring biomechanical function, and progressively returning the patient to land activities as quickly as possible.

Rehabilitation should begin as soon as possible in order to prevent "disuse degeneration," which often results in atrophy, muscle contractures, loss of flexibility, and delayed healing because of circulatory impairment.[5] Integration of land-based exercises into the aquatic program should also begin as soon as possible. This process can be broken down into five levels of adaptation (Table 17–2).

Level One—Acute

In this stage, approximately 90% of the exercises are performed in the water and only 10% on land. Before proceeding to level two, the patient should be able to perform the exercises in Phase One of the prescribed aquatic exercise therapy program.

TABLE 17–2. Percentage of Water and Land Exercises Performed at Each Level of Adaptation

Level		% Water	% Land
1	Land (acute)	90	10
2	Introduce loading	80	20
3	Increase loading	60	40
4	Transfer adaptation	40	60
5	Maximize land integration	10	90

The land-based exercises at this stage should include only the uninvolved body parts and joints to help to maintain an acceptable level of strength, flexibility, and endurance. Exercise of the proximal and distal surrounding structures causes a "transfer effect" to the injured site, which in turn improves the patient's motor skills and function.[5] The patient should be able to perform a specific movement in the water with the correct "resistive pattern" before attempting it on land.

Level Two—Introduce Loading

In this stage, approximately 80% of the exercises are performed in the water and 20% on land. When introducing loading, it is important not to elicit pain in the injured part or exacerbate the symptoms.[5] The patient should be in Phase Two or Three of the aquatic exercise therapy program. The therapist should introduce minimal land-based exercises of the injured part. The exercises should be precisely regulated and performed in a controlled fashion with no abrupt movements. The environment should be controlled and predictable in order to eliminate risk of injury. Cyclic movements, such as bicycling, are best because they are composed of distinctive phases that are always identical and repetitive.[6] Isometric exercises can be introduced at this level. The patient should attempt to achieve full muscle contraction without pain. Avoid dynamic loading and power movements.

Level Three—Increase Loading

In this stage, approximately 60% of the exercises are performed in the water and 40% on land. The patient should be in Phase Four of the aquatic exercise therapy program. At this point the therapist should begin to specifically increase the load on the injured structures. The goal is to restore up to 50% of the original strength and range of motion. Before proceeding to the next level, the patient should be able to perform 50% of the exercise program on land and 50% in the water.

Level Four—Transfer Adaptation

At this level, only 40% of the exercises are performed in the water. The therapist should continue to increase loading and to reduce the aquatic emphasis wherever possible.

Level Five—Maximize Land Integration

At this level, the patient performs only 10% of the exercises in the water. The aquatic program may involve only stretching of tender structures after the land program has been completed. Before integrating onto land completely or returning to their prior activities, patients should have 95% of their full strength and flexibility in the injured structures.[6] The level of integration onto land and the phases of the aquatic exercise therapy program tend to overlap to achieve this goal (Table 17–3).

THE PRINCIPLES OF TRAINING

The Progressive Overload Principle

Most reconditioning programs are based on the progressive overload principle, which states that a body adapts when loaded beyond what it is normally required to accommodate. After the adaptation has occurred, the load must be further increased (progressed) to achieve adaptation at a higher level. In order to achieve a specific training result, each training stimulus should be specific with regard to speed, resistance, duration, muscle groups used, and joint actions required. All these factors influence the magnitude of the desired response.

The Intensity Principle

Intensity refers to the strength of the stimulus required to perform a movement or sequence of movements. This principle usually works in conjunction with the progressive overload principle. In order to develop strength or cardiovascular endurance, for example, a specific intensity (or force) must be exerted over a particular period of time. The physiologic adaptations produced by the stimulus depend on progressively increasing the workload or encountered resistance, the number of repetitions, and the rate (speed) and force of the repetitions performed.

The Frequency Principle

Each training session should be sufficiently spaced with rest periods to allow for responsive tissue growth, nutritional replenishment, and biochemical synthesis (the progressive overload principle). However, sessions must be frequent enough to provide a positive stress for physiologic development to occur. After a structure is overloaded, it exhibits some breakdown. The body then rebuilds that structure and adapts at a higher level. Depending on the intensity of the stimulus, the rebuilding process can take 12 to 48 hours. Constantly maintained stress does not provide favorable adaptations, whereas frequent intermittent stress is beneficial.

The Duration Principle

Any body structure, when exercised under a uniform load over an extended period of time, becomes accustomed to the work performed. Although there is a direct relation between the extent of a stimulus and its strength,[5] endurance exercises are usually performed at a low intensity (25% to 60% of maximum capacity). The ultimate goal of an endurance program, however, is to increase both the extent and the strength of the stimulus.

TABLE 17–3. Overlap Between Aquatic and Land Exercise Therapy Programs

Aquatic Exercise Therapy Phase	Level of Integration Onto Land
1—Postsurgical/acute	1—Land (acute)
2—Early exercise phase	2—Introduce loading
3—Intermediate exercise phase	3—Increase loading
4—Advanced exercise phase	4—Transfer adaptation
5—Integration onto land	5—Maximize land integration

TABLE 17–4. Physiologic Changes That Occur After Strength Training

Increased number myofibrils per muscle fiber
Increased capillary density per muscle fiber
Increased amount of protein
Increased number of muscle fibers
Increased muscle size (cross-sectional area)

The Specificity Principle

The specificity principle can be applied in a rehabilitation setting by relating the specific physical requirements necessary for activities of daily living to the movement patterns that elicit the biologic responses required to achieve the desired goals. Each program should be geared to the condition and desired movement patterns of the individual patient.

TRAINING FOR THE FUNCTIONAL COMPONENTS OF PERFORMANCE

The use of specific therapeutic exercises to improve performance requires an adaptation process. During adaptation, the organism is exposed to specific training stimuli in order to achieve the desired results. To optimize performance, one must understand how to train for the necessary motor functions.

Strength Training

Strength is the ability to apply force. Strength training is necessary to restore the patient to a preinjury state. The physiologic changes that occur after a strength training program are well documented (Table 17–4). The manifestations of strength gains from training include

- General strength—the strength of the whole muscular system as opposed to a specific muscle group
- Maximum strength—the greatest possible force produced in one attempt
- Power—the ability to overcome resistance in a short period of time (the product of strength and speed)
- Muscular endurance—the ability to perform work for an extended period of time (the ability to defeat fatigue when training for strength and endurance)

When developing a strength training program, the therapist must consider a number of factors. By adjusting these factors, the therapist and patient can effectively produce the desired training adaptations (Table 17–5).

Number of Exercises

The exercise program should include an adequate selection of exercises specific to achieve the desired treatment outcome without causing fatigue or damage to the healing structures. Strength assessments provided to the therapist are usually graded on the

TABLE 17–5. Summary of the Dominant Parameters in Strength Training and the Emphasis to be Placed on Each

	Exercise-Goals*		
	Maximum Strength	*Power*	*Muscular Endurance*
Load	H	M → L	M
No. repetitions	L	M	H
No. sets	H	M	L
Rhythm of performance	L	H	L → M
Rest interval	H	H → M	L

*H = high; M = medium; L = low.
From Bompa TO. Theory and Methodology of Training. Dubuque, Iowa: Kendall/Hunt, 1985.

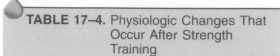

TABLE 17–6. Duffield's Scale of Muscle Power

The Oxford Scale of Muscle Power (On Land)	Modification of Scale in Water
0 = No contraction	1 = Contraction with buoyancy assisting
1 = A flicker of movement	2 = Contraction with buoyancy counterbalanced
2 = Movement with gravity counterbalanced; weak	2+ = Contraction against buoyancy
3 = Movement against gravity; fair	3 = Contraction against buoyancy at speed
4 = Movement against gravity and resistance; good	4 = Contraction against buoyancy and light float
5 = Normal	5 = Contraction against buoyancy and heavy float*

*Note that grade 5 cannot be accurately tested in water.
From Skinner AT, Thomson AM. Duffield's Exercise in Water. 3rd ed. East Sussex: Bailliere Tindall, 1983.

Oxford Scale from 0 to 5. Duffield has modified that scale for use with exercises performed in the water (Table 17–6).[7] The exercises chosen depend on the severity of the condition, the degree of immobilization, the flexibility, the patient's age, the patient's previous fitness level, and most importantly, the desired training effect.

Training Load

Various load magnitudes can be used in strength training. Each can be expressed in terms of one's maximum capacity: maximal (90%–100%), great (60%–90%), medium (30%–60%) and low (0%–30%).[6] The rehabilitation patient should begin at a low or medium capacity.

Number of Repetitions

The type of strength developed depends on the number of repetitions and the rhythm (or speed) of execution. Both factors are a function of load: the higher the load, the lower the number of repetitions and the slower their rhythm of execution[6] (Table 17–7).

TABLE 17–7. Number of Repetitions and Speed of Execution Used to Develop Maximum Strength, Power, and Muscular Endurance

Desired Strength Manifestation	Number of Repetitions	Speed of Execution
Maximum strength	Low (1–3)	Slow
Power	Moderate (5–10)	Dynamic
Muscular endurance	High (10–30)	Slow to medium

Number of Sets

A set consists of a specific number of repetitions of a particular exercise, followed by a period of rest. One to six sets are performed in each exercise session, depending on the number of prescribed exercises. The fewer the exercises, the greater the number of sets.

Rest Interval

As the patient acclimatizes to the training load, the rest interval decreases. The duration of the rest interval depends on the type of strength adaptation desired, the patient's level of conditioning, and the number of muscles involved in the exercise. For example, the rest interval for maximum strength is longer, between 2 and 10 minutes. Muscular endurance, on the other hand, requires a shorter rest interval, 1 to 2 minutes, to produce the desired adaptations.

Endurance Training

Endurance refers to the ability to perform repeated movements under load over a prolonged period of time. It is the ability to withstand fatigue, which is the limiting factor in repetitive work. In order to increase endurance, the muscle group must overcome fatigue by adapting to the training demands. Successful adaptation is reflected in improved endurance. Muscular endurance and cardiovascular endurance are two separate factors and are trained for independently.

Muscular Endurance

Strength is a significant component of muscular endurance. However, the limiting factor of performance is the energy production in the muscles. Aerobically, energy production depends on the amount of oxygen supplied to the working muscles and, ultimately, on the circulatory capacity of the body. On the other hand, the ability of the muscles to work anaerobically depends on the capacity of energy storage and the ability to compensate for lactic acid buildup during anaerobic energy production.[5]

Although developed to improve general fitness, a circuit training program can be designed to improve specific motor functions, including muscular endurance. The circuit may be short (6 exercises), normal (9 exercises), or long (12 exercises), with a duration of 10 to 30 minutes. The circuit may be repeated up to three times in a given exercise session. The duration, number of repetitions, and rest interval depend on the patient's condition, level of fitness, and level of integration. The program should be arranged to alternate muscle groups, and the intensity should be progressively increased. This progression can be achieved by increasing the load, increasing the number of repetitions, or reducing the time allowed to perform the circuit without changing the number of repetitions or the load.[6]

Aerobic Endurance

Aerobic endurance activities train the uptake and transport mechanisms of oxygen. These activities consist of low-intensity, long-duration, continuous work, and they should be performed in cooler water, from 82° to 86°F (28°–30°C).[8] In the water, it is best to determine intensity by the velocity, or the time required to perform a movement over a given distance. The training intensity should remain below 70% of the maximum velocity on land. The cadence can be controlled by a metronome and the heart rate recorded at various levels of cadence. The therapist can then choose a cadence level that elicits a heart rate within the target heart rate range.[9] The therapist can also use heart rate alone as an indicator; on land, it should be between 140 and 164 beats per minute (bpm), and in the water, 123 to 147 bpm (see the section on monitoring the intensity of aerobic exercise).

The rest interval should be between 45 and 90 seconds; it should not exceed 3 to 4 minutes. The heart rate should not drop below 120 bpm. In the water, there should be no rest interval, because heart rate tends to decrease when the body is submerged to shoulder level.[10] The exercise activity should consist of long repetitions, sometimes varying in magnitude. The water is an effective training medium because the metabolic requirement of exercise performed in water is greater than when the same exercise is done on land.[10] Research has found that there is a crossover effect from improvement in maximal oxygen uptake achieved in the water to that achieved in land-based exercises.[9] In aquatic conditioning, significantly different oxygen demands are placed on the body by various activities[11] (Fig. 17–3).

Training Methods to Increase Aerobic Endurance

Continuous Training

Continuous training methods may be long to intermediate in duration. The long slow distance training method involves uninterrupted work, usually 60 minutes or longer. The heart rate should remain between 150 and 170 bpm on land (133 to 163 bpm in the water). This type of training should be reserved for athletes and should not be performed in water temperatures greater than 86°F (30°C).

Intermediate slow distance training uses uninterrupted work of a shorter duration, usually between 20 and 60 minutes. This is perhaps the most popular form of continuous aerobic exercise for the general public because it improves cardiorespiratory fitness while decreasing body fat. Again, this type of high-intensity, long-duration training should not be performed in therapeutic waters because the temperature of the water is too high.

Interval Training

Interval training consists of repeated work cycles of high-intensity exercises interspersed with intervals of light exercises or recovery periods. This is an excellent method in the rehabilitation setting or for introducing aerobic exercise in the water or on land. The low-intensity intervals can be aerobic or anaerobic in design.

An aerobic interval arrangement is best for recovering patients or for individuals with poor cardiorespiratory fitness. Each exercise bout should last from 2 to 8 minutes (5–15 for more fit individuals). The intensity should be between 60% and 80% of the patient's functional capacity, according to the restrictions of the condition (70%–80% for more fit individuals). The combination of a high-intensity exercise (80%–85% of functional capacity) and a

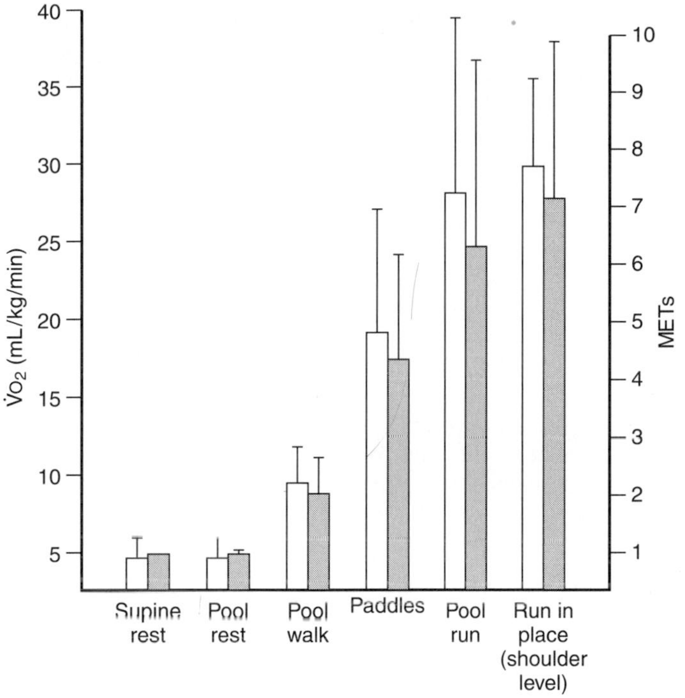

FIGURE 17–3. Oxygen consumption of various aquatic activities during exercise in a heated pool. (Modified from Kirby RL, Sacamano JT, Balch DE, Krielaars DJ, et al. Oxygen consumption during exercise in heated pool. Arch Phys Med Rehabil 65:21–23, 1984.)

low-intensity exercise (60%–70% of capacity) produces one work cycle. The heart rate fluctuations should remain within the aerobic heart rate training zone established for that patient. For interval programs performed in the water, the therapist must adjust the type of exercises performed or the duration of each exercise bout to offset the rapid slowing of the heart rate when the exercise intensity is reduced. The total duration of the program should be between 20 and 50 minutes (Table 17–8).

An anaerobic interval training program should be used only for healthy individuals with a high cardiorespiratory fitness level and completely healed injuries. The goal of this type of training is to increase speed and overall aerobic power. The training stimulus should be 30 seconds to 4 minutes long, and the intensity should be at 85% to more than 100% of functional capacity (maximal oxygen uptake). With this type of training, the speed and force of muscle contraction is greater, and so is the potential for musculoskeletal injury. It is imperative

TABLE 17–8. Sample Deep Water Interval Training Program

Exercise	Duration (Minutes)
Deep water running (see Fig. 6–12)	3
Deep water stride jump (see Fig. 6–18)	1
Deep water running	3
Deep water cross-country skiing (see Fig. 6–15)	1
Deep water running	3
Deep water seated leg extension (see Fig. 6–22)	1
Deep water running	3
Deep water double knee bend (see Fig. 6–21)	1
Deep water running	3
Deep water flutter kick (see Fig. 6–19)	1
Deep water running	3
Deep water double knee lift (see Fig. 6–18)	1
Deep water running	3
Deep water bum squeeze (see Fig. 6–25)	1

Total time = 28 min

that the referring physician or therapist approve the program before the patient is allowed to participate. At the beginning of the program, an aerobic warm-up should be performed, and the involved structures should be stretched.

Fartlek Training

Fartlek training is very similar to interval training but is far less structured. With this method, the high- and low-intensity exercise bouts are not systematically or accurately measured. The patient simply changes the intensity of performance over a predetermined distance or period of time. For example, over a 20-minute exercise bout, the pace or intensity can vary every 5 to 10 minutes for 2 to 10 minute intervals. In terms of rehabilitation, this method is still effective if the intensity is kept average to high within the restrictions of the condition.

Circuit Training

Circuit training uses a series of exercise stations that alternate between aerobic activities and strengthening or toning exercises. The number of exercise stations is usually between 4 and 12, with the workload at each station between 50% and 70% of functional capacity.[12] The combined duration of the aerobic exercises should be between 20 and 50 minutes. The strengthening or toning exercises should be arranged to work alternating body parts. The objective is continuous movement that keeps the heart rate within the target training zone (see next section).

Monitoring the Intensity of Aerobic Exercise

The simplest methods of monitoring intensity that can be used on land and in the water are the Rating of Perceived Exertion (RPE) scale and the talk test. Although these are not scientific methods, they do rely on the patient's reaction to exercise.

The RPE scale is a new, simplified version of the Borg Scale whereby the participant rates perceived effort of activity on a scale of 0 to 10 instead of 0 to 20 (Table 17–9). The Brennan Scale of perceived exertion used at the Houston International Running Center was developed for deep water running. The scale ranges from 1 to 5, with 2 being very light, 3 somewhat hard, and 5 very hard (eg, a 100- or 200-meter sprint).[9]

The talk test is used as an indicator of maximal intensity: if the patient is unable to talk during exercise it is probably because all the available oxygen is needed to supply the primary requirements of the body. Because talking is a secondary response of the respiratory system, the patient is unable to talk if the intensity is too high.

TABLE 17–9. Ratings of Perceived Exertion

RPE Scale	New Rating Scale (Borg Scale)
6 =	0 = Nothing at all
7 = Very, very light	0.5 = Very, very weak
8 =	1 = Very weak
9 = Very light	2 = Weak
10 =	3 = Moderate
11 = Fairly light	4 = Somewhat strong
12 =	5 = Strong
13 = Somewhat hard	6 =
14 =	7 = Very strong
15 = Hard	8 =
16 =	9 =
17 = Very hard	10 = Very, very strong
18 =	
19 = Very, very hard	Maximal
20 =	

From Borg GA. Psychophysical basis of perceived exertion. Med Sci Sports Exerc 14:377–381, 1982.

A commonly used method for determining target heart rate training zones is the maximal heart rate formula (Table 17–10). This method is similar to the Karvonen formula but does not require that the resting heart rate of the participant be known. The target zone is between 55% and 90% of the individual's maximum heart rate as recommended by the American College of Sports Medicine.[13] In order to maintain or improve general fitness, patients should exercise three to four times per week for a duration of 20 to 60 minutes, at an intensity of 55% to 90% of maximal heart rate.

Flexibility Training

There are various methods of developing flexibility: active (static or ballistic), passive, and combined (see Chapter 1). Flexibility exercises should be performed after the warm-up, or they may be incorporated into the warm-up. Stretches should be held for 30 or more seconds, and the amplitude of the stretch should be increased progressively within the precautions of the patient's condition.

TABLE 17–10. Using the Maximal Heart Rate Formula to Determine for Land-Based and Aquatic Exercise Target Heart Rate Training Zone

1. 220	−	Age	=	Maximal HR	
2. Maximal HR	×	0.60	=	Minimum Working HR (land-based exercise)	Lower limit
Maximal HR	×	0.90	=	Maximum Working HR (land-based exercise)	Upper limit
3. Minimum Working HR (land-based exercise)	−	17 bpm	=	Minimum Working HR (aquatic exercise)	
Maximum Working HR (land-based exercise)	−	17 bpm	=	Maximum Working HR (aquatic exercise)	

bpm = beats per minute; HR = heart rate.

Coordination Training

Coordination training is complex because it is interrelated with the other motor functions. Damage to the motor pathways, the cerebral cortex, the cerebellum, or the sensory nerves can result in jerky, arrhythmic, or inaccurate movement. The types of exercises used to restore harmonious movement vary according to the location of the lesion causing the condition. Conditions of incoordination that benefit from aquatic and land-based exercise therapy include those associated with weakness or flaccidity of a particular muscle group, those associated with spasticity of the muscles, those resulting from cerebellar lesions (ataxia), and those resulting from loss of kinesthetic sensation (sensory ataxia). The following principles of re-education should be applied for the indicated conditions.

Weakness or Flaccidity of a Particular Muscle Group

The body avoids uncoordinated movement whenever possible. As a result, the pattern of movement is altered in such a way that the function of the affected muscles is transferred to other groups. To correct the imbalances, the treatment program should include many repetitions of a skill and should integrate normal muscle action of all muscles into the performance of functional movement patterns.

Spasticity of Muscles

The water is perhaps the best medium for spasticity because it promotes relaxation. Warm-water immersion produces a sensory overflow that affects the skin's nerve endings significantly, including those sensitive to temperature, touch, and pressure.[14] Active exercises based on everyday movements are most beneficial. The more proximal joints should be exercised first, and all movement should be performed smoothly to reduce fatigue and assist relaxation.

Cerebellar Ataxia

The focus on treatment should be to restore stability to the trunk and proximal joints. In cases of severe weakness, a strengthening program, usually isometric, should be performed first. Resistive exercises should be limited to functional movement patterns.

Loss of Kinesthetic Awareness

The awareness of one's position in space is fundamental to neuromuscular coordination. During re-education, the patient's sense of sight can compensate for the loss of kinesthetic sense. Mimicking of normal body movements may recruit undamaged nervous pathways that are capable of conveying the impulses of kinesthetic sensation. Exercises that require concentration of attention, precision, and repetition are effective. The goal is to establish control of the movement. After this is achieved, progression can be made by altering the speed, range or difficulty of the exercises (eg, from lying to sitting to standing).

Summary

Early integration of land-based exercises into the aquatic program is intended to maximize development of each fitness component and prevent injury while increasing patient's compliance at each stage of rehabilitation. Many of these methods can be combined. Creativity in program development will help prevent boredom for all concerned.

REFERENCES

1. Kisner C, Colby L. Therapeutic Exercise: Foundations and Techniques. 2nd ed, Philadelphia: F.A. Davis, 1990.
2. Thomson A, Skinner A, and Piercy J. Tidy's Physiotherapy. 12th ed. Toronto: Butterworth-Heinemann, 1991.
3. Arnheim DD, Prentice WE. Principles of Athletic Training. 8th ed. St. Louis: Mosby–Year Book, 1993.
4. Davis VP, Fillingim RB, Doleys DM, Davis MP, et al. Assessment of aerobic power in chronic pain patients before and after a multi-disciplinary treatment program. Arch Phys Med Rehabil 73:726–729, 1992.
5. Krejci V, Koch P. Muscle and Tendon Injuries in Athletes. Chicago: Year Book Medical Publishers, 1976.
6. Bompa TO. Theory and Methodology of Training. Dubuque, Iowa: Kendall/Hunt, 1985.
7. Skinner AT, Thomson AM. Duffield's Exercise in Water. 3rd ed. East Sussex: Bailliere Tindall, 1983.
8. Kinder T, See J. Aqua Aerobics: A Scientific Approach. Dubuque, Iowa: Eddie Bowers 1992.
9. Wilder RP, Brennan DK. Fundamentals and techniques of aqua running for athletic rehabilitation. J Back Musculoskel Rehabil 4:287–296, 1994.
10. Johnson BL, Stromme SB, Adamczyk JW, et al. Comparison of oxygen uptake and heart rate during exercises on land and in water. Phys Ther 57:273–278, 1977.
11. Kirby RL, Sacamano JT, Balch DE, Kriellaars DJ. Oxygen consumption during exercise in heated pool. Arch Phys Med Rehabil 65:21–23, 1984.
12. Sudy M, ed. Personal Trainer Manual: The Resource for Fitness Instructors. San Diego: American Council on Exercise, 1993.
13. American College of Sports Medicine. Guidelines for Graded Exercise Testing and Prescription. 4th ed. Philadelphia: Lea & Febiger, 1991.
14. Becker BE. The biologic aspects of hydrotherapy. J Back Musculoskel Rehabil 4:255–264, 1994.

INDEX

Note: Page numbers in *italics* refer to illustrations; page numbers followed by t refer to tables.